dical Beauty

DEEPAK CHOPRA, M.D.,
AND KIMBERLY SNYDER, C.N.

Radical Beauty

HOW TO TRANSFORM YOURSELF
FROM THE INSIDE OUT

RIDER • SYDNEY • AUCKLAND • JOHANNESBURG

1 3 5 7 9 10 8 6 4 2

Rider, an imprint of Ebury Publishing,
20 Vauxhall Bridge Road,
London SW1V 2SA

Rider is part of the Penguin Random House group of companies
whose addresses can be found at global.penguinrandomhouse.com

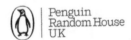

Penguin
Random House
UK

First published in Great Britain by Rider in 2016
This edition published in 2020
Published in the United States by Harmony Books, an imprint of Crown Publishing Group,
a division of Penguin Random House LLC, New York

Photographs by Kimberly Snyder and John Pisani except where noted in the photograph insert.

www.penguin.co.uk

A CIP catalogue record for this book is available from the British Library

ISBN 9781846046537

Printed and Bound in Great Britain by Clays Ltd, Elcograf S.p.A.

Penguin Random House is committed to a sustainable future for our business,
our readers and our planet. This book is made from Forest Stewardship Council®
certified paper.

This book is dedicated to you,
who is reading this right now.

May you fully accept and embrace
the unique Radical Beauty
that you already are.

CONTENTS

Radical Beauty: A Shift in Your Personal Reality

You are a wildflower, a beauty unsurpassed. In each soul is the unique imprint of the grace of God. Nowhere in the world is there another exactly like you. Of that you can justly be proud!

—Paramahansa Yogananda

Here's a scene being repeated thousands of times a day somewhere in America. You may even see yourself in the scene. Two women have stopped by the cosmetics counter of a large department store. They've been lured by a salesperson holding out the latest wonder foundation or skin cream. Or the two women caught a glimpse of themselves in the makeup mirror sitting on the counter.

One woman is twenty-three, in the prime of her youthful looks. But she frowns when she catches a glimpse of herself in the mirror. Her hair doesn't look quite right to her; maybe it's the fault of the new hairstylist she tried. Her skin looks dull, and ever since she started reading weekly tabloids, she's been critical of her thin lashes and a neck that isn't glamorously long and thin. With a sigh the young woman sits down and asks to try the new product. Anyway, the beauty game is still fun for her, and it takes only a few minutes before she's eagerly trying several other trendy products.

The other woman has perched on a stool close by. She's a few years over forty and, looking out of the corner of her eye, she's envious of the young woman. So fresh, so untouched by age. Catching sight of herself in the mirror, this older woman catches every flaw, every wrinkle that's beginning to show, either real or imagined. For her, it's work to keep herself looking acceptable, forget beautiful. She needs all kinds of products just to stop feeling insecure.

This is a scene we want to abolish from your life and from the life of any woman, of any age, who devotes time, energy, and emotion in search of beauty. We want you never again to feel insecure about your looks. For most women, feeling beautiful is connected to feeling lovable and desirable. We want you to stop being insecure about those two things, too. Beauty, love, and desirability are yours to possess naturally—this we promise. There's a great journey awaiting you that will restore you to your natural beauty, rekindling the inner light that shines from every child but somehow got dimmed over the years. What has faded isn't your beauty, because that will always be your birthright. What has faded is your optimism, confidence, and sense of control. This book will show you how to restore them, and then the light of beauty will rekindle itself, naturally and for the rest of your life.

What Is Beauty?

The journey to Radical Beauty begins with the most basic question: what is beauty? We feel that a new definition is sorely needed, and society is ready for one. Beauty is no stranger. In many ways we're obsessed by it.

As you move through your daily life, you inevitably encounter the word *beauty*. If you glance up while shopping at your local pharmacy, you'll find numerous aisles stocked with products claiming to make you more beautiful. There are countless magazines and websites dedicated to beauty, teaching us different ways to lose weight, choose the perfect lipstick, create smoky celebrity eyes, and copy the latest hairstyle trends. If you stop and look around at our culture, the concept of beauty seems very important. But what exactly is beauty, and when you think of the word, what does it mean to you?

The mainstream media provides an onslaught of images and messages about beauty that are meant to sell products. If you believe these messages, you might be inclined to think that beauty is defined by the external—having "perfectly" formed facial features, an on-trend hairstyle, and a physical shape that matches up with the current idealized expression of beauty (such as being pencil thin but having a perfectly rounded bottom). If you don't naturally possess these "beautiful" qualities, you've been led to believe that the primary way to bolster your own beauty is to fill your drawers with makeup and skin-care products while preening your hair with highlights, blowouts, and chemical straightening treatments. It may also seem mandatory to spend a sizable portion of your waking hours at the gym, experimenting with the newest workout class to sculpt the perfect figure. We've been taught to believe that when it comes to products, treatments, and workouts, more equals better results and therefore more beauty.

Unfortunately, this definition of beauty is all about image. There's nothing new about defining beauty externally. It's the equivalent of empty calories: they seem appealing at first, and then you end up with an unsatisfied feeling. The specifics of what is considered beautiful may shift as one fad fades in favor of another, but one thing remains constant: our fascination with beauty. People have appreciated beauty and grasped for it for centuries, beginning with the earliest human civilizations. Ancient Egyptians and Babylonians used primitive forms of kohl eyeliners to dramatize their eyes. In ancient Greece women applied rouge made from crushed mulberries to brighten their cheeks. Images of porcelain-skinned, sleek-haired women have been discovered painted onto centuries-old Asian rice-paper scrolls.

While the shape and size of idealized features vary between cultures, there tend to be a few commonly held beliefs about beauty. First, there is the idea that beauty is a limited and fleeting commodity, as if being beautiful is reserved only for the young and a small, genetically gifted portion of the population. Another widely held conviction in many cultures is that beauty is a relative phenomenon, meaning that it is measured by comparison against others. One woman's hair or eyes are beautiful only if they are more beautiful than another woman's. This idea perpetuates the unfortunate and unnecessary rivalry that is still far too common among women.

A New Approach: Radical Beauty

In the twenty-first century we all need a new concept of what real beauty is. For both authors, it's something we like to call Radical Beauty. What does that mean? Radical Beauty has nothing to do with trendy makeup, fleeting fads, or insecure comparisons with other women. Radical Beauty extends beyond the physical, encompassing all parts of your inner and outer being. It is something that exists universally, and, at the same time, it is completely unique to you. It nurtures and highlights your magnetism and confidence, vitality, and overall health, from your bodily tissues to the outer, visible parts of yourself. You achieve Radical Beauty when you reach the highest and most authentic potential of your natural true beauty. This means that Radical Beauty is a birthright for each and every one of us.

Certain makeup and hair and skin products are fantastic for temporarily defining your eyes or smoothing out your skin, but there is so much more you can do to augment your inherent natural beauty. That is what Radical Beauty is all about. Instead of being shallow or limited to external body parts, Radical Beauty goes deep below the surface.

For some women, it will be a brand-new concept to think of beauty as more than the shape of their face, the size of their body, and the color of their hair and skin, but look around in nature. What do you see? Beauty and harmony are universal forces that manifest everywhere. A graceful willow tree and a mighty oak are both beautiful in their own way. Nature is infinitely generous with the variety of beauty that exists, and this holds true for human beings, too. In the natural scheme, every creature has its own pure and unique beauty. Hold a single rose petal in your hand and you will realize that beauty isn't relegated to spectacular waterfalls and dramatic sunsets. You can discover a marvelous harmony in the most common things: cutting open a grapefruit, looking at the mottled pattern on a rock, or examining the interconnected, vein-like inner structure of a houseplant's leaves. Beauty truly exists in every single expression of nature once we allow ourselves to see it.

You are part of nature, so you have the right to claim your natural beauty's highest potential—your Radical Beauty.

You were born to claim your share of universal beauty. Unlocking your highest potential of beauty, including your greatest possible levels of energy, vitality, and health, will help put you at one with the universe. The very nature of the universe is to express profound beauty. The ocean waves ebb and flow effortlessly. The rain simply falls, and the shells along the beach just lie in the sand, embodying their lovely colors and shapes. As your Radical Beauty unfolds, you, too, will become an increasingly more authentic expression of your own beauty.

Your uniqueness makes it totally unnecessary to compare yourself with anyone else. For too many people, beauty involves feeling inferior by comparison. This always creates a gap, a duality between what is now and what is the ideal. When it comes to Radical Beauty, there is absolutely no space for comparison or competition. Each of us is here to express our highest beauty, which no one else's beauty can diminish. But you can add to another person's beauty—your mother's, your daughter's, your friend's—by making this an aspect of your own beauty. You are free to fully celebrate others' beauty while feeling confident in your own. What a change that would be!

"You are the mirror of divine beauty. Nothing is more beautiful than naturalness. Not trying to be something you are not, but being the most authentic, uncovered expression of yourself. We all look to images of actors and models who are supposed to be the ideal in society. In reality, many of these people are likely to be extremely insecure about their desirability, since their value is subject to the constant fluctuations of a public that they have not met, that is a moving target. Aspiring to be exactly like these images of those in the media is aspiring to be something you are not. When you are trying to be something other than yourself, you cannot be beautiful, which by nature is the truest aspect of you and you alone."

—*The Path to Love,* by Deepak Chopra

The Six Pillars of Radical Beauty

We've begun with an inspiring vision. Next come the practicalities, the how-to that makes any vision come to life. You can achieve Radical Beauty by following the six Radical Beauty Pillars, which make up the firm foundation of powerful lifestyle teachings that support your highest expression of beauty. A series of practical guidelines, rhythms, and routines not only will benefit you but also will promote beauty and health for the whole planet.

In Ayurveda, the traditional medical system of India, there's a saying about how everything in nature works together in harmony: "As is the macrocosm, so is the microcosm. As is the great, so is the small." A healthy body is meant to be part of a healthy planet. What's truly good for one is naturally good for the other. Our pillars restore this natural harmony. Just as pollution, chemical tampering, and toxic dumping disrupt harmonies in nature, your beauty becomes diminished from congestion and toxicity buildup in your digestive system when you eat the wrong foods, use toxic beauty products, and inhabit improper sleep and lifestyle routines.

As you read through each of the six pillars, start applying the specific tools and lifestyle changes that make the most sense to you. You can dip your toe in slowly or dive in as completely as you want. Whatever pace you choose will be the right one, because it is your own. More and more, you will be able to unlock your highest beauty potential to serve you wherever you are. Here is a quick overview of the Radical Beauty Pillars and the benefits you can expect to receive from each one.

PILLAR 1: INTERNAL NOURISHMENT

Beauty has to emerge from the inside out, so your dietary choices and digestion are a primary influence. The way that you eat is a critical factor in determining the vitality of your beauty. Everything you put into your body is used to create the foundation upon which your body, hair, and skin are built.

In this pillar you'll learn dietary shifts that will optimize your digestion, create nutritional balance, and bolster your nutrient absorption. This will result in a clearer, smoother, and more radiant complexion, a flatter midsection, more natural muscle tone throughout your body, higher sustained energy, and—over time—healthier and more lustrous hair.

PILLAR 2: EXTERNAL NOURISHMENT

This pillar will identify the most effective ingredients to apply directly to your skin, as well as the most beneficial Radical Beauty skin-care routines. These will ensure that you nourish your skin in the best way possible, while avoiding toxins that can tax your skin and migrate to your inner body, polluting your bloodstream and liver and contributing to toxic congestion.

When done properly, simple daily routines, such as *abhyanga* oil massage (which you will find out how to do in Pillar 2, page 121), can soothe your nervous system and create powerfully rejuvenating effects, including a reduction in the pent-up stress that contributes to wrinkles. Such routines can help your organs actually grow younger and help restore the vitality and glow to your skin. The powerful shifts in this pillar also promote detoxification by manually supporting your lymphatic system from the outside in.

PILLAR 3: PEAK BEAUTY SLEEP

Your sleep rhythms are an essential component of Radical Beauty, and this pillar will outline numerous tips and tools to enhance this important part of your life.

Proper sleep enables your blood to flow more efficiently to your skin, which is important for supporting your skin to heal itself daily. It also helps reduce dark under-eye circles and stress. Reduced stress can help improve eating habits and digestion, which in turn can lead to even clearer skin with fewer breakouts. You will also learn optimal sleep methods to enhance your body's creation of growth hormone, which boosts your collagen production and is critical for keeping your skin firm and resilient.

PILLAR 4: PRIMAL BEAUTY

This pillar focuses on how to live closer and more in tune with nature, which is a powerful way to bring out your natural beauty. You will learn how to align your energy with the larger natural rhythms of nature by shifting your daily patterns in accordance with the solar and lunar cycles and the seasons. This alignment with the macrocosm will help you harness the force to support your overall energy and vitality.

You will also learn how to reduce the toxic chemicals, electromagnetic radiation, and pollution in your personal space, which will reduce their negative impacts on your hormones and biorhythms. This pillar also teaches the benefits of simple practices like "earthing," or physically touching the earth's surface, which have been shown to help balance your body with negative ions and help neutralize aging free radicals.

PILLAR 5: BEAUTIFUL MOVEMENT

This pillar will delve into the best ways to move your body to promote natural grace, tone, and beauty, as well as which forms of movement are aging and should be avoided. You can actually overdo certain types of workouts—excessive levels of physical exertion can create oxidative stress in your body. When it comes to movement, balance—not total hours spent at the gym—is the key to getting the most tangible, visible results for a toned, fit body.

You'll learn powerful breathing techniques that can make a tremendous difference to your beauty, as well as specific yoga poses, appropriate for all levels, to promote vitality and detoxification. Such movements can promote inner healing and rejuvenate everything from your digestion and circulation to your skin and hair health.

PILLAR 6: SPIRITUAL BEAUTY

This pillar is all about how self-love, heart-based living, and a peaceful mind foster natural beauty from the inside out and increase your natural glow and magnetic presence. Chronic anger, worry, and fear are as acidic and inflammatory to your body as refined junk food. To avoid toxicity from negative emotions, the practice of meditation is perhaps the most powerful step you can take. When you meditate, you reach the prime source of beauty. We can call it spirit, the soul, or the true self; the exact word isn't important.

What's important is to have the inner experience of being connected to your source, and then integrating meditation into your life. Spiritual beauty brings another dimension to who you are and what your purpose is. Nothing is more beautiful than being able to live as a whole person, someone who shines with an inner light. Then the true union of body, mind, and soul is complete.

All of the pillars work together to round out the Radical Beauty lifestyle that will allow you to express your highest and most authentic beauty. We are thrilled for you to embark on your own personal journey, and to see the many transformations marking your onward path.

You can get excited about the many improvements that are on their way to you: higher energy, a sense of calm, and a vital connection to yourself, not to mention more beautifully smooth and radiant skin, healthy hair, bright eyes, and—perhaps best of all—more confidence and the ability to tap into and be in touch with the true beauty that is already within you. The experience of feeling and seeing results will inspire you to keep going. And the further along you journey to discover your own natural beauty, the more you will convey your own expression of Radical Beauty, which is reflected uniquely by you.

With great love.
Deepak and Kimberly

Internal Nourishment

Knowledge is power, and in this pillar you'll gain the power to choose the best foods to fuel your Radical Beauty. As you learn an entirely new way of looking at food, the choices you begin to make will result in radiant skin, high energy, and healthy hair. The Radical Beauty approach stops looking at food in terms of vigilantly watched calories or thinking about eating as an anxious, tightly controlled activity. Beauty and enjoyment are connected, and the greatest enjoyment comes from fulfillment, which begins within. The Radical Beauty approach is something we call Internal Nourishment, a program of strategies to incorporate into your daily dietary rhythm, along with natural, powerful beauty secrets based on enhancing your natural beauty.

You won't achieve Radical Beauty with one particular measurement like tallying up daily grams of carbs and fats. There is not one set of definitive guidelines that work for everyone. Instead of dictating that we all must eat an exact percentage of carbohydrates, fats, and proteins, the latest wisdom is that each body processes these basic food components individually. Your unique response determines the benefits and drawbacks of consuming certain foods. Individual balance is the key, looking at your total diet and how each part works together. This is known as synergy, a dynamic process that takes place in every cell.

We want everyone to wean themselves off fad diets and nutritional trends that are overly simplistic. So many of them falsely demonize one ingredient or even a single macronutrient, whether it is sugar, salt, fat, carbs, or some other culprit. On the other side of the coin are the false promises made on behalf of a "miracle" food that supposedly makes you thin and beautiful, healthy and totally immune to disease and aging. Demonized foods and miracle foods are both fantasies—not to mention that they constantly keep changing.

In contrast, we are going to dive much deeper into creating long-term shifts in your personal attitudes, coupled with practical tips to support your highest level of authentic, natural beauty. Nourishing yourself with food should be a source of joy, not a source of anxiety.

Shifts, even seemingly slight ones, can powerfully help to raise your consciousness and expand the reality of what's possible. If the *Titanic* had only shifted its course by a few degrees, a great disaster would have been avoided. A few degrees turn into a huge change over the course of a hundred or thousand miles.

In your life, a small shift can bring huge benefits over the course of months and years, so the time to start is now. Why deprive yourself of Radical Beauty when your entire well-being can improve so easily? As you start to take baby steps, you will feel empowered to go forward as it feels right for you, so it won't feel jarring or like a big struggle. You can do it! You can create the life and beauty you want, starting with smaller shifts and building up naturally.

Let Go of Your Preconceived Notions About Food

The Four Common Reasons We Choose Foods

If you're like most people, you choose what to eat for one of four primary reasons, or a combination of them. Everyone has their own individual priorities based on their background, how they perceive foods, and their personal goals.

REASON #1: TASTE

The number one reason we eat the way we do is because of how food tastes. This one is obvious. After years of dietary habits, we are all naturally wired to reach for whatever we find tasty. The alarming trend toward obesity in America is blamed on consuming too much fat, sugar, and too many overall calories. One could just as easily blame our addiction on the taste of salt and sugar, which permeate fast food and junk food. Advertising has programmed us to salivate at the mere thought of more and more saltiness, sugariness, and other tastes that zing the tongue, like the spicy, sour tang found in everything from buffalo wings to the "special sauce" on a Big Mac. Of course, personal tastes vary according to factors such as how we were raised. Many of us continue to choose the same foods we ate as children because we find their tastes familiar and comforting.

Unfortunately, many of the most obvious "bad for you" foods, such as the hamburgers and milk shakes peddled by chain restaurants, taste delicious to a large percentage of Americans, who persist in leading with a few strong, habit-forming tastes in their default food choices. For them, taste rules despite ever-mounting evidence against eating salty, sugary, fatty foods in large amounts. The fact that you are reading this book right now says that you're interested in looking deeper into the nourishment food can provide.

It may be hard right now to imagine your life without eating your favorite treat every day, but rest assured that you won't feel this way forever. First of all, you don't have to be "perfect" all the time. Don't be afraid that you can't ever have your treats again. Also remember that your tastes can (and will) change over time. You may gravitate toward processed, sugary foods now, but after making several small dietary shifts, biochemistry changes will cause you to crave different foods. Your body will be able to more thoroughly cleanse itself, and you'll experience more vitality that will make you look more alive and energetic. These shifts will cause the intense cravings you may have had in the past to diminish naturally.

REASON #2: WEIGHT

The second thing most people think about when choosing what to eat is how it will impact their weight. After a quick mental rundown based on the nutritional philosophy you currently subscribe to, you may reduce any and all foods down to one overarching characteristic: "fattening" or "not fattening." Depending on how diet focused you have been over the years, you might also do a quick scan of the nutritional information on the food's label, assessing the number of calories, grams of carbs, amounts of sugar and protein, and so on. Some of us perform these mental calculations continuously, day in and day out. It's exhausting.

The idea that the key to weight loss lies in a simple formula—"calories in minus calories out"—is so pervasive that it is considered a fact in the mainstream belief system. The truth is that this formula is far too one-dimensional. Our bodies digest different foods in different ways, and everything we eat affects our cellular structure. The Radical Beauty shifts will allow you to effectively lose or maintain weight with a much simpler formula that will make calorie counting obsolete.

CHEMICALS IN PROCESSED FOOD CAN MAKE YOU FAT

New research is highlighting the fact that tracking calories or other numbers isn't the best way to control your weight. A study from the journal *Nature* found that chemicals added to processed and junk foods can alter gut bacteria, which can cause intestinal inflammation. This may in turn lead to various bowel issues and weight gain.[1] Instead of becoming a label-reading junkie, use nature as your truest beauty food guide. The closer a food is to its natural state the better, and the more processed a food is, the more you should avoid it.

REASON #3: HEALTHINESS

The third major reason people eat what they do is how "healthful" they consider a food to be. Here the choices are not necessarily related to weight loss but are based on the belief that a certain food will promote good health. A good example of this is when someone chooses to drink a glass of milk because he or she thinks it's a great source of calcium. (This is actually not a good idea for everyone, by the way, but more on that later.) Your health is certainly a major reason to choose a particular food over another, but unfortunately there is a lot of confusion and misinformation circulating about what's truly healthful and what isn't. We will clarify this confusion throughout this pillar.

But the bottom line is that natural, organically raised food *is* healthful. Over millions of years, the human digestive system has been interacting with the environment. Our hunter-gatherer ancestors left us an incredible legacy—the ability to digest and gain nourishment from the widest possible range of foods. We are the planet's most successful omnivores. The key to this ability is twofold: our genes and the thousands of kinds of bacteria that reside in our digestive tract. No other creature, so far as science knows, has diversified its diet the way *Homo sapiens* has.

The upside is that you are equipped to choose almost any dietary plan, with a balance of food groups and nutrients, that suits your climate, body type, and personal preferences. The downside is that there is wide latitude for abusing the body. Pandas cannot survive if their single food source, bamboo leaves, isn't available, and koalas can't survive without eucalyptus leaves. Humans, on the other hand, can adapt to unhealthy diets and survive for decades on them—but not without a cost. Healthful eating comes down to using our ancestral gift as wisely as possible while avoiding the abuses we're tempted into by the forces behind junk food, fast food, and all the processing and artificial ingredients that go into so much packaged food on grocery shelves.

REASON #4: CONVENIENCE

The fourth reason we choose what to eat is convenience. Life is busy, and food seems like an easy place to cut corners and save time. Whether it's fast food, takeout, grabbing something premade from the local deli or the prepared section at the grocery store, or stocking the freezer with a variety of microwavable meals like family-sized pizzas and burritos, convenience looms as a very big reason that many people and families choose what to eat.

Even though awareness of natural, organically raised food is growing—for instance, the largest retailer of organic food in America is Walmart—for countless Americans convenience is paramount. Around one out of every ten meals in this country is eaten at a single fast-food chain: McDonald's. We can't expect to turn back the clock. Unlike a traditional village in India, Tuscany, or South America, our lifestyle doesn't include extended families in which typically a woman, either the wife, mother, or grandmother, is expected to make a daily round of the baker, vegetable monger, fruit seller, and possibly butcher, bringing home the ingredients and cooking every meal of the day. Social roles have changed too much for this way of life to be more than a romantic fantasy (or a daily grind, if you are the designated cook for everyone). The real question is how to balance convenience with freshly cooked meals in such a way that everyone is satisfied, no one is overly stressed, and the resulting meals are truly nourishing and delicious.

A New Reason to Choose Food

So much for the reasons that shape our eating right now. There needs to be a better way. With this book, we hope you will consider an entirely new reason to choose certain foods, and that is to build your dynamic, authentic beauty. The foods you choose to eat have a profound effect not only on your level of health but also on your tissue quality and therefore your outer expression of beauty. Achieving Radical Beauty also means you will achieve superior health.

Waking up to this awareness is, in itself, liberating and very empowering. You have a choice. Each day with every meal you eat, you can choose to apply this knowledge and eat in a specific way that enhances and supports your natural beauty. What's on your fork, the foods you reach for at the grocery store, and even the way you prepare and eat those foods are all vehicles for great change. You can employ any and all of these strategies to claim your Radical Beauty.

There is so much confusion about the connection between food and beauty. Despite all of the information circulating out there (including Kimberly's Beauty Detox books), many people struggle to apply these concepts. They use artificial sweeteners to quell cravings and try to avoid white sugar despite the fact that artificial sweeteners are even more detrimental to their beauty. People are scared to eat bananas because of their natural carbs and sugar, yet they nosh on packaged bars filled with fragmented, processed ingredients such as soya or whey protein isolates, fractionated palm kernel oil, and invert evaporated cane syrup.

You are not what you eat but what you assimilate and digest.

Perhaps you, too, are confused. We don't blame you! When bombarded by snippets of information from casual conversations, a fitness app on your phone, or the latest diet circulated in the media that guarantees fast results, many people react by growing afraid of real food. They choose "safer" items that have their nutritional information neatly printed out on the label. Over time, they ignore their constant bloat, the din of a rumbling belly, or the increasing rate of acid reflux, and are too embarrassed to bring up the fact that they don't go to the bathroom every day. Then they wonder why they have deepening bags under their eyes, breakouts and patchiness, and increasingly brittle and lackluster hair.

Here's the truth: it's all connected. What we eat and the whole basis of integrating these foods and our bodies—*digestion*—must be approached properly to support our inner glow and our outer beauty. Digestion is truly a key to unleashing your Radical Beauty. Referred to as *agni* in Ayurveda (the oldest known medical system, founded in India about 5,000 years ago), digestion is at the center of our health and our beauty. You are not what you eat, but what you assimilate, or absorb and utilize as nourishment in your body, and digest. Numbers alone will never give you an accurate sense of that picture.

Chronic Diseases and Premature Aging: Not Natural or Necessary

Numbers-based dietary assessments have no place in traditional wellness systems such as Ayurveda and Traditional Chinese Medicine. Both have become popular in the West over the past few decades, as people have become heavier and more prone to illness and aging because of damaging lifestyle choices, especially in the typical American diet. Some negative trends, given our aging population, are advancing upon us faster than ever before. Until around World War II, the leading causes of death were infectious diseases such as tuberculosis, influenza, and pneumonia, which are airborne, along with waterborne diseases like cholera.[2] Degenerative diseases, which involve the deterioration of the structure or function of tissue, such as type 2 diabetes, were actually quite rare. At the turn of the twentieth century, it was considered highly unusual for a physician in a general practice to see a patient complaining of angina, the typical chest pain due to heart disease. With improvements in sanitation and medical care since then, we've fortunately seen an immense reduction in infectious diseases.

People are still dying from diseases, but today it's the *type* of diseases that has dramatically shifted. In modern America noncommunicable, chronic, or degenerative disorders are the leading cause of death. Some rates are falling dramatically, such as deaths from stroke, while others, like most forms of cancer, budge very slowly. But even more important is the discovery that if we look at the most common lifestyle disorders, such as heart disease, obesity, type 2 diabetes, and various forms of preventable cancers, their outset can be traced back years before the first symptoms appear.

It's been known for a long time that skin cancer, for example, is related to how much sun exposure without sunblock occurred early in life, even though the cancer doesn't appear until adulthood in most cases. Similarly, diet and exercise at an early age make a major difference in someone's risk of osteoporosis later in life. Now it seems more than probable that most chronic disorders follow this pattern, and in some cases, such as autism, schizophrenia, and Alzheimer's disease, the time for prevention and early treatment may actually be in the first few years or even months of life.

Today, we are becoming more and more aware that lifestyle affects our overall health. According to the World Health Organization, in 2012 noncommunicable diseases, namely cardiovascular diseases, cancers, diabetes, and chronic lung disease, were responsible for 68 percent of all deaths globally.[3] As Dr. James Pacala from the University of Minnesota states, "Some people can have a family history of heart diseases, but it's actually a history of smoking, overeating, and [an inactive] lifestyle. And if you adopt that lifestyle, you're going to run into the same problems your parents did."[4]

Most degenerative diseases and lifestyle disorders can't be cast off as "natural." If that were the case, they would have occurred in similar percentages throughout history. But they haven't, because when underlying factors change, such as sanitation, clean air and water, and diet, disease changes with them. Over the last fifty years in particular, there has been an explosion of "unnatural" diseases as various populations ignore best advice about the basics of well-being: healthy diet, physical activity, and reduced stress. On average we live longer today than we did in the past, but the quality of life for many is greatly diminished, and damaging lifestyle choices are sustained through a multitude of medications and treatments that have a host of side effects.

Just as chronic diseases aren't natural, neither is premature, accelerated aging in the many forms it takes, such as dull skin, cloudy eyes, or chronic fatigue. Though these symptoms of aging are pervasive, they aren't inevitable. Of course, skin may naturally wrinkle or fold over decades, but this does not have to happen prematurely. There are women in their twenties with chronic dark circles under their eyes, crow's feet, and thinning hair, while some women well into their fifties and beyond maintain vital energy, shining eyes, and healthy, more elastic skin and muscle tone. While genes can play a factor, to a great extent the rate at which you age can be determined by your lifestyle. Following dietary fads, eating processed foods, and consuming chemicals, additives, and preservatives leads to compromised digestion and skin that can repair itself less and less.

Premature aging, including hair and skin issues, can be seen as the weakening and suppression of your body's natural healing response. By approaching your diet strategically, you have more control over your immunity, natural healing response, and therefore beauty. It's as simple as that. Your food choices can help you retain the glow of health and authentic beauty at any stage.

Each of the shifts in this pillar represents broader and simpler ways to modify your eating habits. Incorporating these shifts is far easier to understand and follow than obsessing over the minutiae of complicated programs, trying to source the exact food listed out in a meal plan, or trying to calculate the exact numbers of calories or carbs in any given meal. Embracing these overarching shifts in your daily rhythms will help you to achieve the Radical Beauty that is your birthright.

Regain Control over Your Body's Natural Processes

The next shift is about accepting your body's natural ability to renew itself. Life *is* renewal, and therefore so is beauty. Although you can't see it, a renewal process is constantly taking place inside your body. Some cells, such as the villus cells in your intestinal tract (which help you absorb nutrients) and the taste buds in your mouth, might be replaced in a few days, while other body parts, such as bones, take much longer to renew. Yet even the most solid-looking parts of your body are exchanging molecules that move in and out of each cell. Some experts believe that the average age of all the cells in an adult's body is seven to ten years.[1] This doesn't mean that you have to wait that long to see results. Rather, everything in your body is relatively new, even the bones that seem so permanent and fixed. You are actually renewing all the time. This is exciting news, for it means that you can start fostering exceptionally healthy new cells today.

Your red blood cells, which carry oxygen to your skin and provide a glow, course through almost 1,000 miles of arteries, veins, and capillaries; red blood corpuscles have a life span of only about 120 days before being deposited into your spleen.[2] According to which researchers you consult, the cells that make up your liver—the all-important filter of toxins, pesticides, and drugs—can be turned over in as little as 150[3] to 500 days.[4]

The State of Your Skin

Fresh, glowing skin is very important to any woman who is beauty conscious, but your skin is also an extension of your overall health. When you shift your attitude in this direction, you can use this very visible aspect of your outer appearance as a message from every cell in your body about your well-being. Before we delve

SKIN VERSUS HAIR RENEWAL

The state of your hair and skin is an extension of your overall health, and many people experience major transformations from lifeless and brittle hair to thicker, fuller hair after implementing the lifestyle shifts recommended in Radical Beauty. But you have to be patient, as hair, in particular, doesn't transform overnight. The surface layer of your skin, however, is renewed approximately every four weeks. So you can expect to see clearer and more vibrant skin after about a month of making a conscious shift to living more healthily and beautifully. It's also possible to see more of a "glow" to your skin in as little as a few days, as wastes clear from your system and circulation and nutrient flow to your skin improves.

No doubt about it, it does take longer for your hair to regain its natural health and beauty. Depending on your hair's length, it can be anywhere from three to six years old. On average, it grows about one centimeter, or just under half an inch, every month. You can start nourishing healthier hair follicles to produce healthier hair, but it will take additional time to see more dramatic improvements since it needs to grow. By making the proper shifts starting today, you can rest assured that beautiful hair is on the way.

into this shift, please do a quick examination on the current state of your skin. Go to the closest mirror and check out your face, neck, and hands. What is really going on?

IS YOUR SKIN DRY?

Dry skin can indicate a deep level of dehydration, which needs to be addressed from within by hydrating with the right-temperature liquids and foods (more on this on page 91) as well as with proper skin-care products. You also might not be getting enough of the proper kinds and amounts of nourishing beauty fat. Some undernourishment or malabsorptive digestive issues may also be at play.

IS YOUR SKIN OILY?

Excessive oil buildup in your complexion might indicate that your liver is overloaded and needs extra care or that you are not adequately metabolizing and assimilating your foods. Are you constipated? Perhaps you are overeating fats, especially the worst kinds (cooked, fried fats and heated vegetable oils). You also may be eating foods that are congestive or allergenic, or that you aren't digesting completely.

IS YOUR SKIN BREAKING OUT?

Breakouts can indicate a toxic buildup in your system. Your elimination organs may be overwhelmed, which can encourage impurities to push out through your skin. There may be excessive phlegm buildup from overeating congestive, difficult-to-digest foods (such as dairy), or your digestive system may be compromised.

IS YOUR SKIN RED OR RASHY?

Inflamed, red, or rashy skin might indicate that you are consistently eating something that is triggering an inflammatory or allergic response. Alternatively, you might be eating foods that are too "hot" for your system. In Ayurveda, internal overheating, known as excessive *Pitta,* is considered a major cause of aging.

If you are experiencing any of these skin conditions, don't worry! We bring these up so you have an honest base of assessment as we start to delve into dietary remedies. These skin issues can be balanced, starting with establishing powerful new nutritional rhythms for your long-term lifestyle. Let's dive in.

Boost Your Circulation

Optimal circulation is extremely important. Consider a huge, majestic apple tree. The roots of the tree, buried deep in the soil, have to absorb minerals and water from the earth and then pull them upward into the trunk and outward branches of the tree to nourish each tiny burgeoning twig and, ultimately, the fruit—in this case, the apples. Without proper circulation throughout the tree, the apples would not get the nourishment they need, and they certainly would not be as juicy, delicious, or beautiful.

It's the same with your body. Circulation ensures that nutrients flow efficiently throughout your entire body, including up into your hair follicles to nourish every hair on your head. It also allows oxygen to reach all of your cells so they can turn over and the new cells grow healthily. Tissue healing is an intricate process that is also regulated by circulation.[5] Fat stored in your fat cells needs to be accessible so it can be flushed out to help you maintain your ideal weight. This process also removes aging toxins, pollutants, chemicals, and additives from your body.

Think back to the tree analogy. In your case, the "fruits" of your beauty include the outer, visible parts. But your body cannot possibly be expected to build healthy hair or glowing skin without excellent circulation supplying all its needs and efficiently removing the waste that constantly builds up in your system.

QUICK BEAUTY CIRCULATION TEST

Take a look down and examine your fingernails. Do you see a white half-moon shape at the base of each fingernail? This can indicate that you have good circulation and vitality flowing through your body. If all or part of the half-moon is missing, it can mean that your circulation needs a boost. Either way, there is much you can do to improve your circulation further and allow your beauty to shine through. Check back in the future to see if the half-moon shapes eventually emerge or grow more prominent as you take steps to improve your beauty circulation.

Excessive toxins, mucus, arterial plaque, and waste buildup can congest your system and reduce your circulation. Capillaries, which are very tiny and narrow, carry nutrients and oxygen-rich blood through their thin walls to surrounding tissues. They also allow for cellular waste to return to the blood so it can be excreted from the body. If there are buildups or obstructions in your circulatory system, beauty-building nutrition and oxygen become blocked, and your hair, skin, and nails all suffer. A buildup of toxicity in your system also taxes your whole body and contributes to accelerated aging. For instance, research shows that heavy metals, one of the many types of toxins we are exposed to from the food and water supply, as well as the environment, contribute to aging.[6]

Your outer beauty isn't the only element of Radical Beauty that requires excellent circulation. Magnetic energy is also captivatingly beautiful and dependent on this process. Have you ever met someone who was so full of passion and life that you couldn't help but feel drawn to her? A certain light pours out of her eyes and her authentically joyful smile. Her gestures and movements and even the way she walks all seem fluid and full of liveliness. We're all attracted to that kind of energy. Energy comes from the combustion of fuel, which requires oxygen. *Prana,* or your life-force energy, is circulated through the blood, or *rakta.* The better your circulation, the more oxygen is available to all of your body's cells, and the more naturally energized you will feel. This will make you all the more positively energetic and, in turn, all the more beautiful.

There are actually two different circulatory systems that work together to keep your body healthy: the *cardiovascular circulatory system* and the *lymphatic circulatory system.* The lymphatic system is discussed in detail later (see page 120); here we focus on using foods to boost your cardiovascular circulation. But both systems have to be supported in order to maximize your beauty results.

Supporting Your Cardiovascular System for More Beautifying Oxygen and Nutrient Flow

Perhaps you've only thought of your cardiovascular system in terms of how it impacts your heart health, but it also has a big effect on your beauty. The cardiovascular system pumps nutrients throughout the body to nourish the glowing skin and the strong hair and nails you desire. With each heartbeat, oxygen- and nutrient-rich blood is distributed to every cell. To boost your beauty, you need this pumping action to efficiently reach all your cells and carry the maximum amount of oxygen and nutrition.

FOODS TO INCORPORATE FOR
OPTIMAL CIRCULATION

Listed below are some of the most effective foods for boosting your cardiovascular system. Eating these foods is not a quick fix; you can't munch on a handful of blueberries and expect dramatically thicker hair the next day. But these are excellent foods to incorporate in order to see gradual but long-term shifts in your hair, skin, and energy. Going at your own pace, start incorporating them into your regular routine.

BLUEBERRIES, STRAWBERRIES, GRAPES, AND CHERRIES: All delicious bounty from nature, these tasty fruits contain flavonoids that protect your blood vessels and heart from cell-damaging free radicals.

CITRUS FRUITS: Citrus fruits are high in vitamin C, which helps to prevent plaque buildup in your arteries, are alkalizing upon metabolism (see page 54 for more discussion on this), and have cleansing properties to help flush out your system. Lemons are forever and always a top Radical Beauty fruit with many versatile uses. Just squeeze them into water or use them as a base for salad dressings. Other great citrus fruits include grapefruit, limes, oranges, and pomelos. (Be sure to seek these out when traveling in Asia and India, where they are natively grown and extra delicious.)

BEE POLLEN: Besides being rich in protein, antioxidants, and minerals, bee pollen contains a compound called rutin, which is an antioxidant bioflavonoid that has been found to strengthen capillaries and blood vessels and improve circulation. It has a faint honey taste, but it's not sweet per se. The best place to source it is from a local beekeeper. (Check out your local farmer's market.) Store extra amounts in your freezer. Bee pollen is a great addition to smoothies, and you can also take just a little spoonful of it plain and chew well. Note: As with any new food, be sure to start with a tiny amount first to see how your body reacts. If you have a honey or pollen allergy, bee pollen may not be suitable for you.

AVOCADOS: Avocados supply skin-softening, beautifying, and circulation-supporting monounsaturated fats, as well as lots of folic acid, B vitamins, and fiber. All of this will help support healthy blood flow.

THE GLOWING GREEN SMOOTHIE (GGS)

Drinking the Glowing Green Smoothie in the morning is part of the foundation of Kimberly's Beauty Detox philosophy. Yes, it's green . . . but it is delicious! Its taste is balanced between greens, lemon, and fruit, and it is packed with fiber, antioxidants, minerals, vitamins, and countless other nutrients to give you sustained high energy. The GGS is also the ultimate health and beauty fuel for glowing skin, immunity, strong hair, bright eyes, and overall vitality. By blending, you are in essence "predigesting" the foods, and your body does not have to work to break down the foods and waste unnecessary energy in digestion.

The Glowing Green Smoothie uses entire vegetables and fruits, including the juice and fiber, so you are truly eating whole foods. The fiber doesn't have extra calories but is a beauty and detox friend because it naturally controls appetite, sweeps out wastes, and balances blood sugar levels. If you don't have time to make it daily, you can whip up multiple batches and store them in your fridge for two or three days, or even freeze portion sizes to have later in the week. The most important thing is that you make the GGS a part of your daily life!

GLOWING GREEN SMOOTHIE

YIELD: about 3 pints (1.7 litres) (3 to 4 servings)

NOTE: Mix and match your greens and fruits for nutritional variety, depending on what looks fresh and is seasonal. It's best to avoid melons, which digest better on their own. Be sure to always include the lemon. Use organic produce as much as possible.

16 fl oz (500 ml) cool filtered water
3 lbs (1.5 kg) chopped spinach
14 1/2 oz (450 g) chopped cos lettuce
5 oz (150 g) cups chopped celery (about 2 stalks)
1 pear, cored and chopped
1 apple, cored and chopped

1 ripe banana, peeled
2 tablespoons fresh lemon juice
1 oz (25 g) chopped coriander (optional)
1/2 oz (15 g) chopped parsley (optional)

Add water, spinach, and chopped lettuce to the blender. Start the blender on a low speed and mix until smooth. Next add the celery, pear, apple, banana, and lemon juice, plus the coriander and parsley, if desired. Blend on high until smooth.

CHIA SEEDS: These are a great source of omega-3 fatty acids, which help contribute to healthy and increased blood circulation. It is very important to consume chia seeds after they are fully hydrated (soak chia seeds in about a one part seed, nine parts liquid medium of water, almond milk, or coconut milk, for at least half an hour) in order to get their full beauty benefits. They also include both soluble and insoluble fiber. Chia pudding is always a great bet, not only because it's delicious but also because it has a perfect gelatinous form that is as cleansing as it is filling.

DARK CHOCOLATE: Dark chocolate contains flavonols that can improve your blood circulation. Pick up some organic, raw cacao powder and add it to your afternoon smoothie. When choosing chocolate bars, go for a high percentage of cacao and a low percentage of sugar. Also be sure to avoid milk chocolate and white chocolate, which do not contain flavonols. Dark chocolate is a great source of beauty minerals, and a moderate amount will help nip your sweet tooth in the bud.

DOCOSAHEXAENOIC ACID (DHA) SUPPLEMENTS: This algae-based healthy fat helps lower triglycerides, reduce blood pressure, thin the blood, and ensure optimal circulation. Your body can make DHA from omega-3 fats, but you can also supplement for extra insurance. Fish obtain their DHA from algae, so rather than take a fish oil pill, which may be rancid, you can go right to the primary source and take an algae-based supplement. (For more about DHA, see page 53.)

WARMING SPICES: Ginger and cayenne pepper are great for helping clear congestion and increase your blood circulation. They also boost your metabolism and help strengthen your arteries and blood vessels. Be sure to keep cayenne handy to sprinkle onto wraps or sandwiches. Keep fresh ginger in the fridge, perhaps in a small bowl near eye level so you remember to use it often. Grate it into stir-fries or slice it and add it into soups and teas.

GARLIC: Garlic contains a compound known as allicin that helps open up your circulation and loosen congestion throughout your body. Garlic is a natural blood thinner that can improve blood flow to your limbs.[7] It's especially potent in its raw form, so try adding garlic to raw dips and salad dressings. Garlic still has benefits when heated, so you can add it when cooking, too. Radishes, onions, and leeks are also helpful in a similar fashion.

PUMPKIN SEEDS AND ALMONDS: These both have high levels of vitamin E, which is great for keeping blood flowing freely throughout your body. They're both also great sources of beauty minerals such as calcium and zinc.

WHOLE GRAINS: High in fiber, gluten-free whole grains such as brown rice help lower cholesterol by binding to bile acids and escorting them out of the body. (Bile acids, manufactured by the liver using cholesterol, are used to digest fat.) Because the fiber helps remove bile acids from circulation, the liver has to manufacture new acids and then uses up more cholesterol. This process lowers the amount of cholesterol circulating in the body. Soak all of your grains (and nuts) overnight to make them easier to digest for nutrient absorption.

Foods to Avoid for Optimal Circulation

While the foods above will help boost your circulation, there are some foods that will have the opposite effect, slowing down your circulation and promoting aging throughout the body. For the best beauty-boosting results, try limiting or omitting the following foods from your diet.

VEGETABLE OILS

When heated, vegetable oils produce large amounts of beauty-destroying free radicals.[8] Free radicals are basically "damaged" atoms or molecules with unpaired electrons that are believed to cause and accelerate aging and tissue damage. Stick to cooking and baking with coconut oil, which is made up largely of medium-chain fatty acids that can withstand high heat without becoming rancid and digests well, supplying energy and even boosting metabolism.

DAIRY

In vegan diets as well as in some Asian societies, dairy products are absent. In veganism the contention is that dairy is mucus forming, contains no fiber, and is very hard for many people to digest. The National Institute of Diabetes and Digestive and Kidney Diseases estimates that 30 to 50 million Americans are lactose intolerant.[9] Many people experience digestive relief after eliminating dairy from their diets for various reasons. As the Harvard School of Public

Health states, "Clearly, although more research is needed, we cannot be confident that high milk . . . intake is safe."[10]

Of the two authors of this book, Kimberly feels strongly that cow's milk is not in tune with the human body and its nutrition requirements. It's debatable that people have been conditioned to believe that dairy is automatically healthy to consume, but that does not make it biologically right for everyone. Many people worry that without drinking cow's milk, they won't get enough calcium and will therefore have bone density issues, but this is not true. Clinical research shows that dairy products actually have little or no benefit for bones. There are numerous studies to back this up, including a 2005 review published in the journal *Pediatrics*, which concluded that milk consumption does not improve bone integrity in children.[11] As for women, the Harvard Nurses' Health Study followed more than 72,000 women for eighteen years, and its results showed that there was no protective effect of increased milk consumption on fracture risk.[12] The consumption of dairy products has also been linked to higher risk for various cancers. The Iowa Women's Health Study found that women who consumed more than one glass of milk daily had a 73 percent greater chance of developing ovarian cancer than women who drank less than one glass per day.[13]

Besides, there are plenty of great plant sources of calcium to work into your diet, including Brussels sprouts, spring greens, mustard greens, cabbage, celery, oranges, sesame seeds/tahini, spinach, Swiss chard, and turnip greens. These have beneficial calcium but none of the risks associated with drinking cow's milk.

Deepak respects the research but feels that milk has been a part of traditional diets in India as well as Western societies for centuries. In keeping with our policy in this book that no food should be demonized, our position is that personal experience can be the best guide if you stay receptive and intuitive to how you react to certain foods after you eat them. Certainly there is no medical harm to giving up dairy as long as you have adequate vitamin D both in your diet and through some exposure to sunlight. Try giving up dairy for two weeks and see if you personally experience any improvements in your digestion and energy.

PROCESSED SOYA

In the United States, soya is now largely genetically modified. It is also a top food allergen that many people don't digest well. Though your first reaction is probably to think of soya in the form of tofu, derivatives and highly processed forms of soya are actually in all kinds of packaged foods. For instance, if you look on the label of most packaged energy or protein bars you'll see "soya protein isolates" listed as an ingredient. This is a fragmented and highly processed soya derivative. If you can't get organic soya, which by definition means it is not GMO, or derived from a genetically modified organism, then you should avoid it completely, but organic miso, tempeh, and natto are all great choices you can rotate into your diet. These forms are fermented, and the long process of fermentation makes the soya easier to digest and assimilate properly.

GLUTEN

Gluten is the dominant protein in wheat, barley, and rye. Like soya, gluten is a top food allergen. Those with celiac disease cannot tolerate gluten, but many others are sensitive to gluten despite not having celiac disease. Gluten sensitivities can lead to bloating and inflammation in the intestinal tract, and gluten may also exacerbate or possibly contribute to autoimmune disorders.[14] Wheat is a top pesticide-sprayed crop that often is grown in largely mineral-depleted soil. Try eliminating gluten for two weeks and see if you notice a difference in any existing bloating or digestive issues, or if your overall energy improves. But be sure to avoid processed, low-quality gluten-free products and switch to more whole-foods-based choices instead.

CIGARETTES, CAFFEINE, AND ALCOHOL

No, cigarettes aren't a food, but they're worth mentioning here because of the disastrous effects they have on your beauty and your health. Along with caffeine and alcohol, they constrict your circulation flow and greatly contribute to accelerated aging.

ANIMAL FATS

Work to reduce your intake of red meat, dairy, and, especially, artificial trans fats such as margarine. While there is some debate today about whether or not cholesterol is as bad for you as we've been led to believe over the past few decades, it's still a good idea to be conservative with your consumption of animal fats. Plus, toxins and impurities like arsenic-based drugs,[15] *E. coli* bacteria,[16] and hormones[17] can get stored in the fat of animal foods. Choose lean cuts and avoid oily skins.

LIQUID GOLD CIRCULATION ELIXIR

This is a delicious way to incorporate beauty-building bee pollen into your routine. Remember to introduce bee pollen slowly, only a few granules at a time, to ensure your body tolerates it. (If you have a pollen allergy, you should avoid it.) Sip this midmorning or midafternoon as an energizing beverage.

12 fl oz (350 ml) coconut water
1 ripe banana, peeled
1 tablespoon bee pollen (more or less, adjust to your personal taste)

1 tablespoon chia gel (chia seeds soaked in water for at least 30 minutes)

Blend all the ingredients together.

Digestion and Aging

In addition to efficient circulation, optimal digestion is key for the proper nourishment of cells and tissues, leading to exceptional health, vitality, and beauty. The body expels solid wastes through the digestive tract, but if there is a blockage or an inefficient flow of elimination, then toxic overload may ensue. This can even lead to the reabsorption of toxins into the bloodstream, filtering through the wall of the colon (a problem commonly known as *leaky gut*).

Your kidneys, lungs, liver, and skin are other eliminative, cleansing organs able to complete their functions more efficiently if there is no backup in the colon. The gut-liver axis refers to the close anatomical and functional relationship between the gastrointestinal tract and the liver. There is an interaction and exchange between the two organs.[18] A study out of the *World Journal of Gastroenterology* found that taking probiotics to nourish the gut can help support the liver as well.[19] Many have reported that the alleviation of constipation has helped clear up the stubborn acne and oily skin that can be a function of an overloaded liver.

There is a strong connection between your gut health and the quality of your skin. One study found that small intestine bacterial overgrowth (SIBO), a condition involving inappropriate growth of bacteria in the small intestine, is ten times more prevalent in people with acne rosacea, and that correction of SIBO in these individuals led to marked clinical improvement in their skin.[20] We can also see evidence of the gut/digestion/skin connection as probiotics can help improve skin conditions. The first case that studied this was back in 1961, when physician Robert Siver tracked three hundred patients who were given a commercially available probiotic and found that 80 percent of those with acne showed some clinical improvement.[21] More recent studies, including one from Italy, demonstrated that probiotics taken by acne patients in addition to standard care led to better clinical outcomes than standard care alone.[22]

Even if you take isolated vitamin supplements such as biotin (B_7), vitamin C, or zinc (which is commonly recommended for acne) to improve your complexion or your hair, nothing will really work if you have compromised digestion. Digestion is the integrative process of absorbing and assimilating vitamins and other nutrients and expelling everything the body does not need. It makes sense that optimal digestion helps nourish and create beautiful, healthy skin.

More efficient digestion can also allow you to clean out toxins more productively and make it easier to restore and maintain your natural weight. It is well documented that those who struggle with obesity have significantly impaired gut function compared with the general population.[23] Obese individuals are shown to have problems with effective digestion and absorption of food, gastrointestinal illness, unstable or pathological intestinal microbiota, poor immune status, and overall lower well-being. This all strongly suggests a lack of gut health.[24] Diets high in vegetables or fiber lead to healthier functioning colons with a reduced risk of disease.[25]

If you are constipated, it is essential that you do something about it immediately for your beauty and health's sake. Another symptom of sluggish digestion is everyone's least favorite feeling: bloating. There's nothing beautiful about trying to peel out of your seat at dinner feeling like your belly is going to split your dress down the middle, or trying to focus on your staff meeting or be present to go over your kids' homework when your widening midsection

YOU MAY BE CHRONICALLY DEHYDRATED (EVEN IF YOU DON'T THINK YOU ARE)

Many of us don't realize when we are chronically dehydrated. This is a big problem because many chronic beauty issues, such as weakened hair and dry skin, are caused or exacerbated by chronic dehydration. Dehydration can cause your kidneys and the rest of your body to hold water. This can lead to metabolic waste not being properly flushed out of your body, which causes congestion and contributes to accelerated aging.

You may need to consume more water than you think to ensure that your system is properly hydrated. This is especially true if you live in a dry climate, sweat a lot in your workouts, consume alcohol, drink excessive amounts of caffeine, or are following a high protein diet..(The body has to use up more water to flush out the nitrogen in protein.)

So how much water do you really need? It depends on your size, physical activity, health status, and where you live. If you are looking for a goal number to try to plan around, a very general recommendation is to take your weight in pounds and divide that in two, and that's around how many ounces of water you need per day. For instance, if you weigh 140 pounds, then you need around 70 ounces of water per day. Monitor your urine and make sure it stays clear or pale yellow, and always avoid getting to the point of extreme thirst before having more water.

Be sure to also keep some room temperature water on your desk, in your purse, or in your car. If you drink smoothies or green juice, you are getting some hydration through those sources. Juicy fruits and veggies like cucumbers and celery are also good sources of hydration. If you drink alcohol, which is dehydrating, increase your water intake the next day and make sure to drink plenty of water while actually imbibing (as well as before and afterward!).

pushes past your pants seam, internally screaming at you to pay attention to it and it alone.

Bloating is more than unpleasant; it's a sign that your digestion has been compromised in some way. Luckily, there are many Radical Beauty recommendations to help you reduce bloat once and for all. The tips below will help increase your digestive power; alleviate constipation and irregular, uncomfortable, or incomplete elimination; banish bloat once and for all; and amplify your energy. All of this can contribute to the unfolding of your own natural beauty's expression.

Radical Action Steps to Improve Your Digestion and Banish Bloat

Now that you know how important good digestion is to your beauty, here are the most effective steps you can take to improve it.

PROBIOTICS

A high-quality probiotic supplement will help balance the bacteria in your gut and promote better digestion. When choosing a supplement, remember that it's not all about numbers; don't look just for the highest culture counts on the label. Instead, look for a product with the widest array of soil-based organisms (SBOs), which are the types of bacteria that can fully survive your stomach acid and take up long-term residence in your gut. This paves the way for continuing gut health and beauty. A formula containing both prebiotics and probiotics is also great, as the prebiotics serve as the "food" to help nourish the probiotics in your gut.

FIBER

To increase your fiber, eat more veggies in general and include them at all meals, as *only* plant foods contain fiber (while meat and dairy do not). It's also important to diversify. The bacteria that digest your food, known as intestinal flora, consume the fiber that we cannot digest. There are between 500 and 2,000 species of these microorganisms in the digestive tract, and they feed on all manner of fiber. Variety is therefore essential, covering the entire plant kingdom in your diet, which means fiber from whole grains, fruits, and vegetables. To maximize the effect of any fiber, use the whole food; choose whole fruits over straight fruit juice, for instance. Buy brown rice in place of white, and choose steel-cut porridge oats over sugary, processed cereals. This natural diversity is much healthier for you than commercial fiber supplements. Care should be taken with the rough bran in bran-rich cereals, however, since it can scrape against the intestinal wall and even injure it. See page 39 for tips to increase your fiber intake while avoiding excessive gassiness.

HOT WATER

Drinking hot water in the morning (with some lemon squeezed in) can encourage your bowels to let go and allow for more efficient elimination. This morning practice contributes to good hydration, which, as noted earlier, is really important. It's also a good idea to get up earlier. Your gut does not respond well to being rushed, so allow for ample bathroom time after drinking your hot water to let your body relax and do its thing!

AVOID HARD-TO-DIGEST FOODS

Processed foods, fried foods, and dairy are particularly hard on your digestive system.

The more detoxified your body is, the more beautiful you become.

TIME YOUR MEALS WISELY

Try waiting at least 3 hours between meals instead of constantly grazing during the day. This allows the foods in your system to digest more fully. Bloat (see page 35) may be compounded if your digestive system is constantly full of food, and you pile more and more food that doesn't have enough time to digest on top. Also try simplifying your meals by using fewer components.

USE SPICES STRATEGICALLY

Boost sluggish digestion, or *agni* in Ayerveda, with spices like turmeric, cumin, black pepper, and ginger. You can sprinkle these spices into stir-fries, soups, and salad dressings, or try adding them to hot water and make your own spice tea.

TRY A MAGNESIUM-OXYGEN SUPPLEMENT

This nonlaxative, non-habit-forming aid helps clear out accumulated waste in your system. Constipation and waste buildup may also contribute to bloating.

TAKE DIGESTIVE ENZYMES BEFORE MEALS

These are capsules you can take to help your food break down more efficiently and support better digestion and assimilation. There are various kinds of enzymes included in various formulations, but in a nutshell, proteases break down proteins, lipases break down fats and carbohydrates, and amylases break down carbohydrates.

AVOID FIZZY BEVERAGES

The carbon dioxide that makes soda and even plain seltzer bubbly can cause or exacerbate bloating.

STEAM YOUR VEGGIES

If your system is rebuilding, try steaming your veggies instead of eating them raw. This can help break down the fiber and make them easier to digest.

EAT MORE SLOWLY AND DON'T OVEREAT

The latter probably seems quite obvious, but if you scarf down your lunch while hunched over your computer or lap up a huge plate of food in record time as soon as you get home after a long workday (maybe because you skipped lunch), you may find that eating quickly has a sneaky way of contributing to overeating.

Slow down your consumption and you'll leave the space in your stomach needed to break down foods, which can help abate bloating.

LIMIT THE AMOUNT OF DENSE FAT IN EACH MEAL

Fat takes longer to digest than protein or carbohydrates and can make you feel uncomfortably heavy if you consume too much of it at once. Avoid bloating by limiting fats in your everyday diet. (You do need the right amount and type of fat, but you don't need to overdo it. See page 51 for more info.) A little bit of oil goes a long way when cooking. Try getting a ceramic (non-Teflon) nonstick pan that allows for easier cooking and cleanup while letting you use less oil overall.

SOAK BEANS, LEGUMES, AND GRAINS OVERNIGHT

These foods contain sugars called oligosaccharides, enzyme inhibitors, and phytic acid, which bind to essential minerals and inhibit their absorption. Soaking can help deactivate these substances, which in turn assists in preventing bloating while improving nutrient absorption.

CHOOSE YOUR VEGETABLES WISELY

Brassica or cruciferous vegetables like broccoli, cauliflower, Brussels sprouts, and leafy greens are fantastically high in nutrients but can be particularly gas inducing due to the sugars and starches they contain. If you are having major bloating problems or especially if you are transitioning your diet, try temporarily cutting back on broccoli, cauliflower, and Brussels sprouts and having leafy green salads instead of kale salads, as kale (a popular new "superfood" rich in minerals, vitamins, and amino acids) also happens to be in this vegetable family.

EAT PINEAPPLE

Pineapple contains the enzyme bromelain, which helps break down proteins in your body and aids digestion. Try using pineapple as the fruit component of your

HOW TO INCORPORATE MORE FIBER
(WHILE PREVENTING GASSINESS!)

Internal Nourishment is all about consuming plenty of veggies and natural foods, so by eating more veggies, plant-based meals, and health drinks such as Glowing Green Smoothie (page 27), you are going to naturally increase your fiber intake. This is a great thing, which is a bit of an understatement. Fiber is important for cleansing and helps move toxins out of your body so that your true beauty can shine through. *But* if you abruptly increase your fiber intake from a little to a lot, you may feel more gassy and bloated as your body adjusts.

The key is to drink more water to prevent gassiness. Fiber happens to be an indigestible carbohydrate. That's why it's great for bulking up meals without adding extra calories and helping you feel full when you eat lots of super-beautifying plant foods. But fiber also absorbs a great deal of water. If there is not enough water in your system, too much fiber can cause slower movement through the digestive system, which in turn leads to bloating and gassiness. Be sure to drink lots of room temperature water in between (rather than during) meals so it's there to be used by your digestive system when you need it to process all that fiber. Drinking too much water at meals can dilute digestive enzymes and slow down digestion, also contributing to bloating.

Steaming veggies rather than eating them raw can also make it easier to break down fiber, especially when transitioning your diet. Chew a little bit when drinking your Glowing Green Smoothie, rather than chugging it, as it is made up of whole foods. Soon enough, you'll get used to eating more fiber. You'll be more cleansed, and your belly will be more taut and tight to boot!

Glowing Green Smoothie (page 27) or having a bowl of cut-up pineapple mid-morning.

AVOID SPICY AND PUNGENT FOODS

Especially if your system is sensitive, hot sauces and spices like chili powder, garlic, onions, and vinegar can cause irritation in your stomach that can lead to bloating. Try using flavorful fresh herbs such as basil, oregano, and parsley instead.

AVOID STRAWS

Drinking through a straw makes it easier to swallow excess air, which can contribute to bloat. Along those same lines, give up chewing gum, which traps air and gas in your system, contributing to bloating. Chewing is a signal for your body to start breaking down food and begin digestion. Gum chewing is therefore useless and confusing to your body as it is not accompanied by anything nutritive to digest!

Daily Detoxification

Most of us do our best to focus on what we put into our bodies, but the truth is that what you clean out is just as important. To be your most beautiful, you have to constantly support the removal of toxins from your cells.

There are two kinds of toxins: *exogenous* toxins come from pollutants and chemicals in the environment, while *endogenous* toxins are the normal by-products of metabolism that are created within your body. Your cells are being renovated daily by two opposite processes, either building up (*anabolism*) or breaking down (*catabolism*). As a result, your body has to clear out an enormous amount of cellular debris each and every day. If this is done inefficiently, it can weigh down your body and contribute to toxicity buildup.

Detoxification happens naturally, but you can take steps to raise the level of efficiency. Supporting your daily detoxification processes is vital to maintain clear, glowing skin and a youthful appearance.

ARE YOU OVERLY TOXIC?

Which of the following apply to you?

_____ Unclear head, mental dullness

_____ Frequent upset stomach or bloating

_____ Chronic aches and pains

_____ Constipation and digestive distress

_____ Offensive body odors

_____ Bad breath

_____ Continual fatigue

_____ Sallow, aging skin

_____ Strong addiction to sweets

_____ Waking with a stuffy nose

_____ Coated tongue

If three or more of these pertain to you, your ongoing detoxification could probably use some extra support. Be sure to pay attention and apply the advice in this pillar to help enhance the ongoing cleansing mechanisms of your body.

Your Beautiful, Beauty-Building Liver

Your liver is a critical beauty organ. Weighing around 3 power-packed pounds, the liver is your primary organ for detoxification. It works tirelessly to cleanse your blood of toxins and bacteria and neutralize pollutants. In fact, it filters around one hefty quart of blood per minute, dealing with all the agrochemicals, toxins, pollutants, food additives, preservatives, residues, pesticides, and countless other unnamed residues and chemicals that you put into your body unknowingly (or knowingly, in the case of those margaritas you had at happy hour last Friday!). After processing all these toxins, your liver secretes them into the digestive tract to exit the body or into a water-soluble form to be filtered through the kidneys and excreted as urine.

It's extremely important to support your liver if you want beautiful skin, eyes, and hair. In addition to its role in detoxification, this organ is the keeper of some sacred beauty goods. It stores vitamins A, B_{12}, and D, as well as iron, copper, and glucose, releasing these nutrients into the bloodstream as needed.[26]

Your liver is also a major fat burner, since it produces bile and bile acids, which emulsify fats. One issue that brings home the importance of the liver is cholesterol. For decades the link between cholesterol and heart attacks, now the leading cause of death among women as well as men, has been controversial.

Does this surprise you? We've all taken for granted that cholesterol is bad for you. In fact, the majority of cholesterol is manufactured by the body itself and is a necessary part of building cells. There is no controversy over this fact, or the risk posed by "bad" cholesterol, or low-density lipoprotein (LDL). The thorny issue that arises is over the cholesterol you eat versus the cholesterol your body makes. There is ample proof that high cholesterol in the blood puts someone at risk for heart disease. But the same has not been proved for cholesterol in the diet. This is because of the liver, which stands midway as a kind of processing plant to turn all the fat you eat into fat for your body to use.

How your liver processes fat is genetically determined. Some people can eat a high-cholesterol diet and still have low cholesterol in the blood; they are lucky when it comes to their liver. Other people are unlucky, and they exhibit high levels of cholesterol in the blood even on a low-fat diet. But most people fall somewhere in between. Their liver will process the cholesterol in their diet into a moderate level of cholesterol in the blood. This natural ratio is considered healthy, but it must be noted that aging causes cholesterol levels to rise. This may be genetically programmed, but it is just as likely that eating a typical high-fat diet for decades causes the liver to decline in function. For the moment, it's probably best to be prudent, regularly eating the foods rich in the omega-3 fatty acids that we recommend on page 54, such as chia seeds, which have a beneficial effect on fats in the blood, and cutting out or greatly reducing the "hard fats" found in red meat.

After being produced by the liver, bile is stored in the gallbladder and secreted into the small intestine to break down those beauty fats and put them to good use. In Traditional Chinese Medicine (TCM), the liver is considered a primary organ responsible for circulating blood and qi throughout the body. According to TCM, a healthy, well-functioning liver is important for healthy menstruation and fertility.[27]

When the liver is overloaded by toxicity or mistreated, it becomes dysfunctional and cannot complete its important tasks—from detoxifying to fat burning and blood cleaning—as efficiently as it should. This can lead to premature aging and diminished energy and beauty. When your liver can efficiently process toxicity, your skin becomes brighter and more beautiful, more nutrition is able to reach your hair follicles, and you have more beautiful energy overall. The great news is that this is a resilient organ with super-regenerative powers. Unless you have an extremely damaged liver or a condition like cirrhosis, there is much you can do to help it rebuild and regenerate even if you've abused your liver in the past. Taking care of your liver is an essential beauty task. In addition to all of the tips for boosting digestion, following are some of the best techniques and foods to nourish your liver and increase detoxification within your body on a daily basis.

STAY AWAY FROM HIGH PROTEIN DIETS

High protein diets have become popular ways to lose weight, but they may also contribute to accelerated aging and disease.[28] Nowadays, most people consume far more protein than their bodies really need. Valter Longo, director of the Longevity Institute at the University of Southern California, states, "The majority of Americans are eating about twice as much proteins as they should."[29] Research has shown that long-term high protein intake results in increased cancer risk, precipitated progression of coronary artery disease, disorders of bone and renal function, and disorders of liver function.[30] Clearly, when it comes to protein, too much can have negative effects on your system (see page 72). Lesson: You can clearly overdo it, so be mindful of how much you are consuming.

Your liver plays a role in protein metabolism, including processing amino acids,[31] converting them into glucose for energy, and removing ammonia, a natural waste product of protein metabolism, from the bloodstream.[32] The liver also synthesizes nonessential amino acids. An overabundance of protein places a burden on the liver. Try cutting back on animal protein in particular and eating more nutrient-dense plant-based meals to help your liver stay on top of its vital health- and beauty-boosting functions.

LIMIT MEDICATIONS

Only use over-the-counter drugs when absolutely needed. This includes paracetamol, which research has shown has a particularly strong effect on the liver.[33] While drugs can be critical in emergencies and accidents, as well as very helpful in treating various medical conditions, your liver does have to detoxify them. Keep this in mind when choosing which medications to take. If you have a headache, resting and rehydrating instead of immediately popping a pill is better for your liver. Very often, drinking water, restoring B vitamins by eating a banana, or getting a massage to help alleviate stress will relieve a headache without taking any type of drug. Speak to your doctor about which prescription medications are absolutely necessary.

LIMIT PROCESSED FOOD AND GO ORGANIC AS MUCH AS POSSIBLE

All the preservatives, pesticides, artificial dyes, and chemicals that go into packaged foods can distort metabolic processes in the liver. Eat clean and have clean, beautiful skin.

EAT MORE PLANTS

Increase your intake of fruits and especially vegetables, which are very nourishing to your liver. This is easy to accomplish by drinking the Glowing Green Smoothie (page 27), eating bigger salads at meals, and keeping fresh, cut-up veggies around to munch on.

START YOUR DAY DRINKING HOT WATER WITH LEMON

Water helps flush out wastes and supports your liver, as well as the functioning of your entire body. Hot lemon water helps purify and stimulate the liver and liquefies bile while inhibiting excess bile flow. It supports your digestion and even has a similar atomic composition to saliva and hydrochloric acid, which are used in digestion.[34]

DRINK LIVER-SUPPORTING TEA WITH MILK THISTLE

Several studies suggest that substances in the milk thistle plant (especially a flavonoid called silymarin) protect the liver from toxins, although research has been limited, mixed, and preliminary.[35] If you are new to this herb, be sure to consult your health-care professional first.

AVOID FRIED FOODS

This particularly includes foods made from heated vegetable oils (such as potato chips). Cooked, reused, and rancid oils can put an especially big burden on your liver and on digestion in general.[36] In lab research, even olive oil cooked at high temperatures has been shown to induce oxidative stress on the liver.[37] It's best to cook with coconut oil, which can withstand high temperatures.

TAKE A TRADITIONAL CHINESE MEDICINE APPROACH

In Traditional Chinese Medicine, if someone has "liver yin deficiency," the liver has been compromised. This results in hair loss and sallow skin. To strengthen your liver, this ancient Asian medical system recommends eating courgettes, squash, potatoes, sweet potatoes, string beans, beetroot, mushrooms, tomatoes, spinach, carrots, parsley, apples, banana, mulberries, mango, coconut, peaches, lychees, melons, oats, tempeh, and black sesame seeds.[38]

AVOID FOIE GRAS

Radical Beauty is more about creating a balanced lifestyle than adhering to absolutes, but one hard-and-fast rule is to steer clear of beauty-diminishing foie gras. Foie gras sounds fancy, and some people claim it's delicious, but it's quite literally the toxic liver of geese and ducks that likely have been fed an unnatural diet of GMO corn. Such a diet creates fatty liver disease in these animals, and the excessive fat makes their liver taste rich and buttery, but it's a lot less tempting when you realize that it's disease making it taste this way, isn't it? Although consuming offal (the internal organs and entrails of butchered animals) has become an en vogue gourmet phenomenon, it's best to avoid consuming animal liver from any four-, two-, or no-legged creature (i.e., fish). Now that you understand the liver is the detoxifying center for the body, you probably want to avoid eating an organ full of toxins without any extra encouragement.

EAT MORE GRAPEFRUIT

Grapefruit is high in vitamin C and antioxidants and can help your liver flush out carcinogens and toxins. It also gives your liver a boost in dealing with various medications. In a lab study, grapefruit juice was shown to prevent damage to DNA molecules that were exposed to conventional anticancer drugs.[39]

TRY BEETROOT

Beetroot is high in plant flavonoids and cleansing fiber and can improve the overall functioning of your liver.

UP YOUR LEAFY GREEN INTAKE

Leafy greens like spinach and cos lettuce contain chlorophyll and thousands of phytonutrients that can help neutralize the metals, chemicals, and pesticides that may be in your food, thereby helping to protect the liver.

DRINK GREEN TEA

Green tea is full of plant antioxidants known as catechins, which improve the liver's functioning.

EAT MORE AVOCADOS

Avocados are a great source of an antioxidant called glutathione, which your liver uses to filter out toxins and harmful waste.

SLOWLY INCREASE CRUCIFEROUS VEGETABLES

Cruciferous veggies like broccoli and Brussels sprouts increase the amount of glucosinolate (organic compounds) in our bodies, thereby increasing the digestive enzymes that flush toxins and taxing pollutants from the body. (Temporarily delay or start slowly when introducing these veggies if you currently are prone to bloating or transitioning your diet.)

TRY TURMERIC

The spice turmeric is not only a fantastic anti-inflammatory aid, but it can also help detoxify your liver by stimulating the production of bile to help your body digest fats better. Start incorporating it into your cooking regimen—check out the Radical Beauty Liver Tonic recipe (below) and the Creamy Masala Vegetable Stew (page 298).

RADICAL BEAUTY LIVER TONIC

This toning, cleansing, and anti-inflammatory drink can be made at any time to help nourish and give your liver a boost.

1-inch (2.5 cm) piece of ginger, sliced thinly
Filtered water (enough to fill your tea mug)
Juice of 1/2 lemon

2 teaspoons raw honey (or coconut sugar or nectar)
1/4 teaspoon powdered turmeric
Pinch of cayenne pepper
Pinch of black pepper

Place the ginger slices in a tea mug. Heat the water in a kettle or small pot and then pour the hot water over the ginger slices, allowing them to steep for about 3 minutes. Add the remaining ingredients and mix well. Enjoy immediately.

GO FOR WALNUTS

Like avocados, walnuts are also high in glutathione and omega-3 fatty acids, which can support your liver's cleansing functions.

Detoxing Alcohol

It's probably obvious by now that if you want to be as toxin-free as possible, you should avoid alcohol. No one would suggest that alcohol is a beauty booster. But the divide between theory and reality can be wide! It's perhaps unrealistic to think you'll never drink an alcoholic beverage again. This may be the case for some of you, but for others, it's a distinct possibility that you may have a drink (or a few) here and there, as well as some big nights out. (Though if you are serious about preserving your beauty, these would be increasingly less frequent.)

Alcohol is a hepatotoxin, meaning it specifically damages your liver and impairs your body's ability to detoxify itself. Alcohol is also dehydrating and causes your skin to look less fresh and smooth, especially the day after imbibing. There is no doubt that alcohol is depleting. If and when do you decide to indulge, there's some important information to keep in mind when picking your poison.

LIMIT CONGENERS

Chances are you've never heard of congeners. But if you drink alcohol, you have unknowingly consumed them. Congeners are substances produced during fermentation that can include small amounts of chemicals such as esters, tannins, acetone, methanol, and aldehydes. Congeners are responsible for most of the taste and aroma of distilled alcoholic beverages and may contribute to the symptoms of a hangover.[40] Darker liquors such as whiskey or scotch contain more congeners than clear liquors. Research has suggested that whiskey and dark liquors can produce stronger hangovers due to their high levels of congeners.[41] This means that because of their extra impurities, darker liquors hit your body in a stronger and perhaps more damaging and aging way. If you are going to drink hard liquor, stick to clear varieties such as vodka or gin.

KEEP IT SIMPLE

The simplest drinks are, of course, shots, but these are definitely not the best idea as they go down way too fast and may lead you to consume far more than you realize. A better option is to nurse a simple drink of vodka, soda water, and lime. Avoid sugary mixers, which add inflammation on top of the toxic effects of the alcohol and further age your skin, adding a sallow appearance, dark under-eye circles, and puffiness. Skip the mojitos and other mixed drinks that call for pure cane sugar. Also avoid sugary mixers such as orange juice, sodas, energy drinks, margarita mixes, and the like. It's simply too much for your poor body to take all at once. If you really want a sweet drink, try adding some stevia, xylitol, or a little coconut sugar or raw honey to unsweetened and diluted cranberry juice and vodka. Of course, it would be hard to find this at a bar, but you could make it for yourself and your friends during a festive home hangout.

CHOOSE RED OVER WHITE

Red wine contains more antioxidants than white, so it is generally the better choice. However, red wine can also inflame the skin and trigger a histamine release in some people (especially those of Asian descent). This can cause redness and preexisting rosacea to flare up. Unfortunately, wine often comes with added sulfites, and the sugars in wine can contribute to candida and sugar-imbalance issues. Still, if you have none of these aforementioned issues, red wine (in moderation) is not a bad choice.

SKIP THE BEER

Beer shouldn't be your go-to alcohol of choice (minus those occasional tailgating parties, perhaps). Because of the hops that are used to brew it, beer has some estrogenic effects, meaning it can disrupt your hormones.[42] It can also be very bloating and often contains gluten.

Toxic Overload: How to Deal with a Hangover

Alright, so it happened. You woke up feeling completely lousy from one (or a few) drinks too many. It's too late now to try to alternate drinks with water or to pass on that last cocktail. (Who knew it would come back to bite you *this* badly!) What should you do?

Drinking lots and lots of room temperature water to rehydrate your entire system is a good place to start. You can also sip on hot water with lemon to help flush out your liver. Add some ginger, which will stimulate digestion and help you process the excess alcohol lingering in your system. Coconut water will also help, as it contains potassium, electrolytes, and some B vitamins that will combat dehydration and replenish your body.

For breakfast, eating fiber-filled foods will make you feel more balanced. A simple gluten-free avocado sandwich will stabilize you, and the carbohydrates in the bread will absorb the excess alcohol in your system while helping your achy head. Also try eating a banana, which contains potassium and B vitamins, to help replenish what your body lost from your little alcohol binge; some porridge oats with a banana would actually be a fantastic choice.

At lunchtime, a hummus and veggie wrap or sandwich (preferably with gluten-free bread) can also be comforting and digests well during this "delicate" time. A nice big lentil or veggie soup with some brown rice, or vegetarian sushi rolls, are also good choices. Try some chopped cabbage either in a salad or in a healthy slaw with a little tahini as the base. The cabbage will help stabilize your blood glucose levels. Stay away from greasy foods (as tempting as they may be) or the misguided "hair of the dog" approach (which refers to drinking more alcohol the next morning to ease a painful hangover), which will just add to the digestive burden and make it harder for you to get back to normal. Don't worry; this, too, will pass.

Radical Beauty Ratios and Macronutrient Balance

Whether they came from Ireland, Japan, or Namibia, our ancestors didn't approach health and beauty by hunching over calculators and calorie-tracking apps. They certainly had no intention of figuring out to the last milligram how much was needed of every nutrient and micronutrient. Analyzing numbers, which often leads quickly to obsessing over them, is not natural, and your goal is to move closer to your body's natural intelligence so you can express more of your own natural beauty.

Knowing what's in each food requires too much time and effort that is much better spent reaching a single goal: knowing just a few essential ratios. These ratios will be enough to allow your body to optimize its own ability to maintain health and beauty. Thankfully it's much simpler to stay on track this way. Starting today, look at your food from a big-picture perspective that will allow you to adhere to general guidelines instead of becoming a slave to numbers. Here are some of the top Radical Beauty ratios to know to help you bring forth your maximum beauty.

Radical Beauty Ratio #1: Essential Fatty Acids

Many people who are trying to lose or maintain their weight focus on steering clear of fat, but the correct kind and amount of fat is essential for optimal and sustained beauty. We all need fat to nourish our skin properly, sustain proper energy levels, regulate our hormones, and build shiny hair and strong nails.

Essential fatty acids (EFAs) perform many different functions in the body that are vital for health and beauty. In particular, they help build beautiful, radiant skin. These fats help maintain the integrity of cellular walls, which helps to maintain water and vital nutrients while allowing for the release of wastes. This is critical to skin health. When your skin is fully hydrated and able to retain water within its cells, it appears youthfully supple. This is where these EFAs are key, because they are the components that help keep your skin cells healthy and your skin's membrane functioning optimally. A more supple and flexible cellular structure may also reduce the appearance of cellulite.

A lack of these important fats can lead to dry skin that doesn't maintain its plump, healthy-looking structure and ends up sagging like a slowly deflating helium balloon (obviously the look you do *not* want). Healthy cellular walls, reinforced by essential fatty acids, help to continually remove wastes. This can also be very helpful for eradicating acne. When you consider acne you might naturally think it's better to avoid all oils, but getting in some essential fats is actually helpful. EFAs maintain an ideal level of fats so that your skin doesn't overproduce sebum. The wrong balance of fats and a deficiency of the right fats produce imbalances in sebum and leads to breakouts.[1]

In this section we will focus on the two main families: omega-6 fatty acids and omega-3 fatty acids. Excessive omega-6 fatty acids ingested through vegetable oils are thought to induce inflammation in the body (acting as "pro-inflammatory mediators") and have been associated with specific conditions like the development of inflammatory acne.[2] In the right balance, EFAs help ensure that wastes leave the skin in a healthy way, which prevents clogged pores. Essential fats also nourish skin that has already been damaged by blemishes (and from picking at your skin!).

The I-word—*inflammation*—should be everyone's concern. In 2015 the National Institutes of Health made this a major medical priority, assigning hundreds of millions of dollars to discover what the hidden damage of chronic inflammation actually is and how to prevent it. For most people, inflammation is a new issue, because they don't realize that low-level chronic inflammation is pervasive in society. When you burn or cut yourself, the inflammation response is a natural part of healing. There is warmth, redness, and swelling at the affected area. But inflammation can exist, not as a healing mechanism but due to the constant irritant of things like stress, leaky gut, and residual toxins in the tissues.

You will be hearing much more about chronic inflammation in years to come. Even without signs like warmth, redness, and swelling—in fact, without symptoms at all—inflammation contributes to serious health issues like cardiovascular disease and autoimmune diseases,[3] but it can also lead to free radicals[4] that exacerbate wrinkles and contribute to new ones,[5] aging your skin and body in general.

Fatty acids play a key role in inflammation on both the good and bad side. Omega-3 fats help oxygen circulate throughout the body, ensuring that cell activity is healthy and that your organs and red blood cells are functioning properly. This is essential for maximum energy. These fats are also important to help abate inflammation[6] and nourish the skin. Not having enough omega-3 fats can lead to a variety of issues, such as eczema, allergies, and depression.[7]

The major omega-3 acid is converted into two others—eicosapentaenoic acid (EPA) and docosahexaenoic acid (DHA)—which are also important for a healthy heart and brain (your brain is actually made up of 60 percent fat),[8] as well as helping to balance a person's moods.[9] Sometimes the conversion of fatty acids isn't optimal. If you are concerned, try algae-based supplements. Fish obtain most of their omega-3 fats from algae, and these supplements don't pose the possible contamination or rancidity risks of fish oil pills.

The other type of EFA, omega-6 fatty acids, is also important. As with omega-3s, it also converts into two other acids—linoleic acid (LA) and gamma-linolenic acid (GLA). Omega-6 fatty acids are a precursor for a hormone-like substance called prostaglandins, which have an impact on many functions of the body, including calcium movement, cell growth, the kidneys' filtration rate, and the constriction and dilation of the smooth muscle cells in your veins.

Whether your diet is well rounded or full of junk food, you're probably getting enough (or even more than enough) omega-6 fatty acids. That's because omega-6s are found in vegetable oils like corn, rapeseed, and soyabean, which are used in nearly every packaged chip, cookie, cracker, and treat on grocery shelves. Omega-6s are also plentiful in seeds, nuts, vegetables, grains, eggs, and poultry. You really don't have to boost this nutrient in your diet; it's already there. Omega-3s, on the other hand, are much less common in the standard Western diet. This is a problem because the ratio between these two types of EFAs can have a dramatic impact on your health and beauty.

The ideal ratio of omega-6 to omega-3 fats is anywhere between 1:1 and 4:1, but due to the large amount of animal products, fast food, processed foods, vegetable oils, and fried foods they eat, Americans tend to have anywhere from seventeen[10] to thirty or even fifty times more omega-6s than omega-3s.[11] The result of this out-of-whack ratio is a contribution to that silent beauty killer called inflammation that you can't feel sneaking up on you but that damages your skin by causing wrinkles and premature aging.

But don't worry; you can start balancing your EFA ratio today! To keep your ratio in check, try to consume *more* omega-3 fatty acids in whole-food forms from the following sources:

- Chia seeds
- Flaxseeds
- Walnuts
- Chlorella
- Hemp seeds
- Sesame seeds and tahini (made from ground sesame seeds)
- Cauliflower
- Purslane (as well as other weeds and greens)
- Brussels sprouts
- Algae-based omega-3 fatty acid supplement
- Dark, leafy greens such as spinach

And cut out or at least consume less of these top omega-6 sources:

- Sunflower, rapeseed, soya, cottonseed, and generic vegetable oils
- Margarine
- Junk foods such as chips, crackers, and popcorn that contain the above oils (Blends of these oils are often labeled "vegetable oils" in the ingredient list.)
- Fried foods, such as fried chicken, french fries, tempura, and so on.

Radical Beauty Ratio #2:
The Acid/Alkaline Ratio

If you were a chemist and looked at the body as a sea of chemicals, one of the first tests you'd perform would be to see how acid or alkaline someone's body is.

This test looks for the pH value, a simple scale that goes from very acid to very alkaline:

0 to 7 pH = acid

7 pH = neutral

7 to 14 pH = alkaline

This is the same measurement that can be done with litmus paper, which turns pink when dipped into an acidic solution and blue when dipped into an alkaline solution; purple is neutral. Your body has zones that need to be acid or alkaline—there's no single pH for everywhere. Blood must be maintained slightly alkaline, while the stomach needs to be highly acidic to digest food. In other areas, like your mouth, too much acidity leads to being vulnerable to cavities (candy and other sweets convert into acids due to the digestive activity of saliva).

Your body is incredibly precise about maintaining the right pH levels, and when they are off, it compensates by drawing upon specific micronutrients, particularly minerals. Calcium, magnesium, and potassium are chief among the minerals that are alkaline, and the good news is that restoring these trace minerals, particularly through a diet rich in fresh fruits and vegetables, can be a very quick, effective treatment for restoring bodily balance, as well as a preventive for many health and beauty conditions.

Every food you eat has either an acidic or alkalizing effect on the body, and even though these two authors don't adopt a so-called alkaline-ash diet, the ratio between acidic and alkalizing foods is another essential one for achieving true beauty. Alkalizing foods can help neutralize harmful acids,[12] and your body's pH has a big impact on your beauty and the rate at which you age.

A fascinating study from the *Journal of Environmental and Public Health*, outlined in an article entitled "The Alkaline Diet: Is There Evidence That an Alkaline pH Diet Benefits Health?" found that an alkaline diet, made up of an abundance of fruits and vegetables, has many health and beauty benefits, including helping to prevent muscle wasting (keeping your body beautifully toned), increasing growth hormone (which can help your skin smooth and youthful), improving lower back pain, and increasing available magnesium that is needed to activate vitamin D,[13] which aids in keeping your bones and teeth beautifully strong. A chronically acid-forming diet can lead to a loss of calcium through the urine, weaker bones, and the loss of other alkaline minerals, such as potassium and magnesium. The loss and imbalance of key minerals can lead to dry skin that cracks, is itchy, and ages prematurely.[14]

Acid diminishes the supply of oxygen available to all your body's tissues and cells. The lack of oxygen interferes with mitochondrial function, and the cell's ability to repair and replenish itself becomes impaired. The result is increased general aging of all your cells and increased fatigue, which can lead you to reach for external energy aids such as coffee and energy drinks, which are often acidic and make this imbalance even worse.

Increased acidity also can make you age more in other ways. An acidic environment can throw off your bacterial balance, imbalancing the proliferation of "bad" bacteria over the "good," and leading to more harmful microorganisms that can contribute to inflammation. Because acids are corrosive, additional tissue damage and inflammation can ensue. Free radicals can abound in your body, unleashing their beauty-squashing potential on your precious cells.

How pH Affects Your Beauty

Much of your beauty potential is determined at this cellular level. When your body is more alkaline, there is an increased flow of oxygen and nutrients into your cell walls, and cellular waste is disposed of more easily.[15] If you are chronically acidic, however, less oxygen and fewer nutrients are delivered to your cells. This can lead to a buildup of waste inside your cells, which contributes to a vast array of health and beauty issues, such as diminished energy, sallow skin, and wrinkles. Your body can fully absorb and utilize key beauty nutrients only within certain pH levels, so less nutrient absorption is the precursor to dull or dry skin and lifeless hair.

Our ancestors naturally ate an abundance of fruits, vegetables, nuts, and seeds. Their diets were also high in organic mineral compounds, especially magnesium, calcium, and potassium. These are all alkalizing foods. But because of the widespread availability of many less healthy foods today, both the types and portion sizes of what we consume have become dangerously imbalanced.

Just by shifting your overall diet to consist of 80 percent alkalizing foods, you might be able to correct energy and beauty issues that have plagued you for years. This shift in your overall way of eating can provide these benefits:

- Circulate more healing oxygen in your body
- Increase nutrient absorption
- Shift from sallow to radiant skin
- Transition from limp to thick hair
- Create boundless energy

Some foods, such as quinoa and almonds, are slightly alkalizing or acid forming (depending on various factors such as whether or not they've been soaked), but they are not highly acid forming like other foods, so even in their most acidic form it's okay to include them in the 80 percent. It's important that the bulk of your diet be made of the most alkalizing foods, namely fruits and veggies. The other 20 percent of your diet can be made up of acid-forming foods. Unfortunately, the typical Western diet is largely *acidogenic,* meaning it has an overall acidifying effect on the body that promotes chronic acidosis and results in the loss of minerals in the body, which are used to buffer against metabolic acids.

Remember that your body has complex mechanisms for maintaining the correct acid/alkaline balance. We are talking about potential imbalances that diet may be able to correct—you alone are the judge of the benefits you see when moving toward a more alkaline diet. If you stick to about 20 percent (or less) acid-forming foods, the acids will be balanced by the alkaline foods in your diet. So the great news is that you don't have to feel pressured to eat "perfectly"; you can still allow for some of these foods in your diet. The problems occur when the ratio creeps out of balance, and more than 20 percent of your food is highly acid forming. This is unfortunately the case for most Westerners or anyone consuming a modern Western diet. Just look around. Chronic fatigue, a "tired" face, poor skin quality, and cloudy eyes all indicate that a person's body is overly acidic.

Once you know which foods are alkaline and which are acidic, it's easier than you may think to implement this ratio (see some sample meal plans in Pillar 5, page 237). Remember, this doesn't mean that you can never eat any acidic foods again or that you have to become a vegan if you don't want to at this time. However, animal protein is by nature highly acidic, so if and when you choose to eat it, make sure it's a smaller portion size compared with the alkaline fruits and veggies on your plate.

Strive to apply this important Radical Beauty ratio in a broad sense to each plate of food you eat, and to your overall daily and weekly food consumption. Also try to avoid eating any meals or snacks that are composed of 100 percent acid-forming foods; seek balance every time you eat. It's not quite as effective for balancing your pH if some of your meals are very alkaline and others are completely acidic. For instance, a few eggs on their own are a very acid-forming meal that has a very different impact on your entire system than one egg on top of a big green salad. If there are at least some alkaline-forming foods present each time you eat, your body will be able to more efficiently buffer the acids that are produced as your meals are digested and metabolized. This can prevent further acidity and help your body expel any acidic toxins that have already accumulated.

Eighty percent of the foods you consume should be of varying levels of alkalinity, emphasizing foods from this list:

- Green vegetables
- Root vegetables (acorn, butternut or coquina squash, yams, turnips, sweet potatoes, etc.)
- All other veggies
- Fruit
- Gluten-free grains (quinoa, brown rice, and steel-cut oats from a gluten-free facility are great options), soaked overnight (These options are slightly more acidic than others on this list, but compared with the very acidic foods listed below, they are great grounding, filling options.)
- Herbs (parsley, coriander, basil, etc.)
- Sprouts
- Raw apple-cider vinegar
- Seeds (especially chia)
- Nuts, especially almonds and walnuts (ideally soaked overnight)
- Ginger, turmeric, and other roots that can act as spices in food
- Legumes, such as lentils (in moderation and ideally soaked overnight)
- Spices (paprika, cumin, etc.)

Twenty percent (or less) of the foods you consume should come from these highly acid-forming sources:

- Red meat
- Poultry
- Fish
- Dairy (in all forms, including yogurt)
- Eggs
- Coffee
- Alcohol (minimize as much as possible)
- Processed foods (minimize as much as possible); this includes anything packaged, from protein bars to chips. You can occasionally enjoy such foods, but remember that they do fall in the 20 percent group. Of course, junk foods like candy bars and Twinkies should be avoided altogether (see our no-no list below).

An easy way to work toward this balance is to ensure that most of your grocery cart is filled with whole foods, mostly from the outer edges of the grocery store, or the bulk bins, or whole plant foods from the farmer's market. Whole foods are largely more alkaline by definition than ones that have been processed and made into commercialized products.

Radical Beauty No-Nos

The following items are too acid forming and damaging to your beauty to ever consume. If you currently eat any of these items, try to wean yourself off them, go cold turkey, or do whatever you have to do to get these items completely out of your diet for the sake of your beauty and health!

ARTIFICIAL SWEETENERS

Man-made, synthetic, toxic, and acid forming, these can lead to neurotoxic effects in your brain and cause headaches, dizziness, and more problems. The term *excitotoxicity* means that such products have the ability to literally excite cells to death[16] and even encourage the production of free radicals that create tissue and organ damage—including skin that ages faster.

All artificial sweeteners should be avoided, as well as any products that contain them. This includes aspartame (found in Canderel), sucralose (found in Splenda), and saccharin (in Hermesetas). If you want a low glycemic sweetener with no calories, try stevia or erythritol. Though they undergo processing, for sure, they are at least derived from plants and are not associated with the toxic side effects associated with the aforementioned artificial sweeteners.

SODAS AND SOFT DRINKS

Sodas of any kind should be avoided, including diet varieties that include toxic artificial sweeteners.

REFINED SUGAR AND WHITE FLOUR

These probably should be eliminated from your diet, at first on an experimental basis if you have symptoms that could be traced to acid/alkaline imbalance. Americans consume vast quantities of refined sugar and grains, so making a reasonable restriction is sensible for everyone. Kimberly feels strongly that a broad range of common conditions—inflammation, weight gain, and low energy—is the curse of these beauty-busting white powders.

JUNK FOODS AND PROCESSED SNACKS

Reduce these as much as possible, relegating them to isolated treats from time to time. Hey, nobody's perfect, but junky items shouldn't be staples in your cupboard.

CANNED PRODUCTS

Canned goods often contain artificial preservatives and high levels of salt and sodium. In addition, the canning process destroys valuable nutrients found in fresh produce. It's best to go fresh. Some health advocates are wary of chemicals in the metal lining of cans that can leach into food. Get precooked beans in cartons instead of cans, or cook larger portions of fresh and freeze extras. Canned vegetables should be strictly avoided! If you are in a real pinch and can't source fresh vegetables, frozen vegetables would be the next best option.

COMMERCIAL SPORTS DRINKS

These contain beauty-depleting ingredients such as artificial food coloring, high fructose corn syrup, brominated vegetable oil, and artificial sweeteners.

See, the list isn't so long, is it? Most foods, even those that are less than ideal, can be absorbed into the 20 percent part of the overall ratio. Even alcohol, if you enjoy drinks from time to time, can be part of that 20 percent (of course, a *small* part!). It's not the best thing to put into your body, clearly, but Radical Beauty embodies a realistic plan that can be incorporated into to your lifestyle.

Radical Beauty Ratio #3: Macronutrient Balance

There are three macronutrients, the main elements that make up any given food: fat, carbohydrates, and protein. Historically, we've seen dietary philosophies cast one of these macronutrients as the evil root of weight gain, only to have it rage and then fade away. But it doesn't really make sense that one of the main components in food is inherently flawed and worthy of complete rejection. Eliminating any of these macronutrients from your diet and overemphasizing the other two creates an inevitable imbalance in your body, and natural balance is our primary goal here.

Balance is a key facet in nature creating optimal beauty. Imbalance in any form is a surefire way to diminish beauty.

If you track diet fads back to the 1980s, you will find a period when fat was aggressively pinned as the singular cause of weight gain. The widespread mentality at the time emphasized shunning all forms of fat as a way to lose weight and support health. Unfortunately, this campaign led to the overconsumption of carbohydrates, including refined carbohydrates like sliced bread, packaged crackers and snacks, and nasty, fat-free super-processed cheese varieties. A label of "fat-free" or "low-fat" was pretty much the gold standard for weight loss back then. Unfortunately, people's weights continued to rise, the aging phenomenon of inflammation grew overall, and sicknesses like heart disease and diabetes continued to soar rather than diminish.

A few decades later, we now look back in hindsight and see how demonizing the entire macronutrient of fat has led to disastrous health and beauty consequences. It's clear that a greater understanding of good fats versus bad fats is necessary to determine how to incorporate the appropriate amount of the right fats into your diet to create beauty balance.

What we are seeing today is the same staunch shunning of another macronutrient, except now the "bad one" is carbohydrates. Carbs are now often regarded as a weight loss foe as many people choose a high protein / low carb diet without fully understanding the ramifications. But avoiding carbohydrates in all its forms can also tip you out of balance and push you to eat too much protein and fat. This makes your body more acidic, which can accelerate aging and deplete your beauty. The answer is to balance all three macronutrients within your diet instead of eliminating any one of them, and to adhere to proper ratios between each macronutrient and the specific forms of each one.

FAT

As discussed on page 51, eating some fat is essential for beauty and health, but you don't need too much of it. Although fat should not be demonized as it was in the 1980s, the typical American diet still includes far too much fat—and the wrong kinds. If you look at some of the people around the world with the best health and longest lives, you'll see that many of them favor plant foods with lower fat and protein consumption. This is true of most traditional diets in Asia as well as the diets of the Hunzas from Pakistan, the Okinawans from Japan,[17] and the Vilcabamba peoples from Ecuador.

The source of fat in your diet is extremely important. You should get most of your beauty fat from whole plant forms, such as nutrient-dense seeds, nuts, and avocados. Coconut oil is great to cook with in small amounts, and natural oils like olive oil can be used in small quantities on already prepared foods or raw foods like salads (if you do want to cook with a little olive oil, stick to lower temperatures). Avoid congestive fats, such as trans fats in margarine and other prepared products, vegetable oils (especially in a cooked form as already noted), and excessive animal fats. Even lean cuts of animal protein can have upward of 50 percent of their calories coming from fat. Consider that the US Department of Agriculture defines lean minced beef, for instance, as containing no more than 10 percent fat, but this refers to product weight, *not* the percentage of calories from fat.

To get out of a strict numbers-based mentality, think visually: a whole avocado, a tablespoon or two of chia or flaxseeds, and a bit of coconut oil used when cooking your dinner are great ways you can get your daily fat in. As a guideline, 15 to 30 percent of your diet should come from healthy fats. This might sound broad, but this is where some individual customization based on your constitution comes into play.

In Ayurveda, different body types are categorized into what your main *dosha* type is: *Kapha, Vata,* or *Pitta.* If you are *Vata,* for instance, and tend to be more thin and willowy, you might do better with a higher ratio of fats in your diet. If you have a stocky *Kapha*-based frame and tend to put on weight more easily, you might feel more balanced and be better able to manage your weight at the lower end of this ratio. *Pitta* types, which have a medium, well-built, and strong frame, are advised to avoid oily and fried foods, as oil is believed to contribute to the naturally fiery nature of *Pittas,* and to consume moderate levels of fat overall.

Whether you subscribe to the *dosha* theory or not, you can still intuit your body type and what works best for you. Listen to your body, notice how you feel, experiment with different levels of healthy fat (primarily from all whole-food, plant-based sources), and determine the best specific ratio for you.

CARBOHYDRATES

Carbohydrates provide energy for your muscles, brain, and central nervous system. In fact, the human brain depends exclusively on carbohydrates for its

HIGH FRUCTOSE VS. CRYSTALLINE FRUCTOSE

Thankfully, the media has caught on to the fact that high fructose corn syrup, the main ingredient in most soft drinks around the world, is a big health and beauty no-no (not that its consumption has been curtailed much by the bad press). This is a highly processed liquid that puts a big burden on your liver[18] and metabolizes to fat very quickly. The fact that it is liquid and absorbed virtually instantly into your body only magnifies its harmful qualities. Sure, a small amount of fructose occurs naturally in fruits and vegetables, but these whole foods are vital sources of beauty fiber and nutrients, and they don't provide enough fructose to cause concern, as noted by *Diabetes Care*.[19]

But what about crystalline fructose? It has a sort of mysterious name that hasn't been demonized in the public—at least not yet. But if you start to poke around, you will see it listed as an ingredient in popular "health drinks," such as various flavored waters and certain sports drinks. What's scary is that crystalline fructose contains an even higher percentage of fructose than high fructose corn syrup. That's right, higher. High fructose corn syrup (HFCS) is made from cornstarch (read: cheap to manufacture), which consists entirely of glucose. After the starch is extracted, it goes through processing with enzymes that convert some of the glucose into fructose. Depending on the exact processing mechanisms, HFCS can contain 42, 55, or up to 90 percent fructose. Additional processing crystallizes the syrup, and upon drying you have—voilà!—crystalline fructose at a shocking 99 to 100 percent pure fructose.

Of course this is great for food manufacturers, as a nearly pure-fructose sweetener is up to 20 percent sweeter than sucrose,[20] meaning they can save money on sweeteners. If you happen to pick up a packaged food or beverage that includes crystalline fructose on its ingredient list, put it right back down.

energy. If you feel you are in a brain fog or easily become irritated or testy (let's be honest!), it might be because you aren't eating enough of the right form of carbohydrates. Read on.

Research has found that eating carbohydrates increases serotonin release.[21] As you probably know, serotonin elevates your mood, helps you feel balanced, and regulates your appetite, especially in terms of helping you feel satiated. Normal serotonin levels are also important for regular, healthy sleep patterns.[22] This may explain why someone who drastically cuts carbs from their diet gets really grumpy or moody. Emotional imbalance can often be a serious hint of a dietary imbalance.

Let's go back to ancient teachings for a moment: Traditional Chinese Medicine and Ayurveda both recommend carbohydrate consumption for nourishment by way of grains, root vegetables, and seasonal fruit, which are all prized in both systems for their healing, balancing, and health-elevating properties. According to Ayurveda, a high protein diet without grains will create a "doshic" imbalance and increase *Pitta*. A *Pitta* imbalance can manifest in "excess fire," which can exhibit personality-wise as irritability, grumpiness, impatience, and anger—qualities not conducive to beauty and peace. If you try to eat super-low-carb, you may find your sweet cravings getting out of control as your body naturally seeks the carbohydrates we were designed to consume.

When people try to restrict carbohydrates to lose weight, they break down fat incompletely, producing a by-product called ketones. The buildup of ketones can cause an imbalance that leads to excessive acid production,[23] which can lead to acidosis in your body. Diets that are excessively low in carbohydrates can help you lose weight, at least temporarily, but can also lead to fatigue, dehydration, constipation, and bad breath.

There are basically three types of carbohydrates, and they are certainly not equal when it comes to their impact on your beauty.

1. Simple and Refined Carbohydrates

These carbohydrates are broken down very quickly in your system and can create a surge in blood sugar levels and insulin release. A major intake of refined carbohydrates, which is epidemic in modern America, can lead to chronic inflammation,[24] and such inflammation produces enzymes that break down collagen and elastin, which can create or exacerbate wrinkles, contribute to sagging skin, and severely age your skin.[25] Excessive sugar can also lead to the overgrowth of "bad" bacteria in your mouth and intestinal tract, providing a potential breeding ground for a candida imbalance, for example, that contributes to acne, bloating, and constipation.

The sugar you add to your coffee or bake into brownies with your kids isn't the only simple carbohydrate you may be overeating. That breakfast bagel you grabbed during a conference room meeting, the English muffin you toasted up for breakfast, and those saltine crackers lurking in your cupboard are all plentiful sources of simple carbs, too. Maybe you've heard this before, but white flour converts pretty much directly into blood sugar, so try to think of the two as one and the same. Imagine a sugar cube dissolving into a cup of coffee. It almost immediately melts and becomes invisible. It's the same way with white flour. It looks like a different form, but upon consumption it melts right down into blood sugar.

These are the type of carbs you want to avoid, or at the very least minimize in your diet:

- White sugar
- Refined white flour and related products, including cereals, cakes, bagels, cookies, crackers, and so on (There are countless products that could fit into this one category, if you tally up all the products in the middle of the average grocery store. Just avoid those snack- and processed-food aisles and you can largely avoid most of these.)
- Jam and jellies
- Sodas and soft drinks
- Straight fruit juice (especially if pasteurized, which damages some nutrients)

2. Complex Carbohydrates (aka Starches)

These carbohydrates are more structurally complex and take longer to get broken down and digested by your body. As they enter the bloodstream more slowly and do not trigger a dramatic spike in insulin levels, they have a stabilizing effect on your body and provide sustained energy. Many of the benefits found in vegetarianism and whole food diets come from eating complex carbohydrates, because nature has "packaged" them in balance with fiber, vitamins, and minerals in a way that's the most healthful for digestion and assimilation.

Below are some good sources of complex carbs to incorporate into your diet.

WHAT ABOUT FRUIT?

Whole fruits contain a mixture of complex and simple carbohydrates. Fruit is one of the most beautifying foods of all, a crowning glory of nature. Clearly not refined or processed but grown on trees, fruit comes to us in a complete nutritional package of vitamins, antioxidants, minerals, fiber, and so much more. If you eat fruit in its whole form, the natural fiber in the fruit helps to slow down the digestion of the sugar.

It would be a huge beauty mistake to completely avoid fruit for fear of its sugar. It's grown in nature, and a fundamental Radical Beauty belief is that if you align yourself with and eat closer to nature, you will experience more of your natural beauty. Information on the Harvard Health Publications site references the work by Robert H. Lustig, an obesity specialist at the University of California, San Francisco. Lustig asserts that the fructose that occurs in smaller quantities naturally in fruits is not harmful, because one also gets the fiber from the fruit, which "affects the biochemical outcome."[26]

As you work on balancing your diet, you will find that you crave fewer junky and refined sugars and foods. The fruit you eat will largely replace those foods and satisfy your natural cravings for sweets. The high amounts of vitamin C, antioxidants, and countless other phytonutrients in the fruit (many of which haven't even been identified yet) outweigh its sugar.

Some say that all sugar is the same in the body, but that is not true if you look at it from the holistic perspective of the overall impact of a given food you eat. Fruit has so many fantastic beauty benefits; you can't just take the reductionist approach and compare it to table sugar. It's best to eat fruit alone and on an empty stomach to help it digest completely and easily. This also tends to reduce bloating.

If you have blood sugar issues (such as diabetes) or a candida imbalance issue, then you need to lay off fruit, with the possible exception (if permitted by your doctor) of non-sweet fruits, such as lemons and cucumbers, and sour fruits, such as cranberries and green apples (which are low in sugar), until you work toward a healthier balance. But a healthy body will be better able to handle natural foods, which very much include the peak of nature's beauty, the fruit.

Do not be scared to eat from this group of foods! They will help you feel good and digest your food well, and they are energizing and filling. They also contain a lot of minerals and other beauty nutrients. You can balance complex carb portion sizes by loading up on salads and nonstarch veggies alongside them, but the following are important energy and beauty foods with many different beautifying and health benefits:

- Starchy vegetables: tubers such as sweet potatoes, yams, pumpkins and squash of all kinds including acorn, butternut and coquina.
- Beans and legumes (soaked overnight)
- Whole, unrefined, and gluten-free grains such as brown rice, millet, buckwheat (handled in a gluten-free facility), oats and quinoa (As discussed previously, gluten can be difficult to digest for many.)

3. Fiber

These indigestible carbohydrates are not broken down finely enough for your body to absorb them, and therefore are not a source of energy or calories. But fiber, as we discussed on pages 35–36, is still important to your daily diet, as it lets you feel full and satisfied, helps you to sustain energy, and has stabilizing effects. Besides, fiber from veggies and fruit, green smoothies and porridge oats, for example, is extremely important for beauty because of its ability to help sweep out toxins. It's an amazing natural cleanser that forces wastes and toxins to keep moving along so that your true beauty can shine through.

Finding the Balance

So how many carbohydrates should you eat? Balance it out. As a general ratio, 50 to 70 percent of your diet can be made up from beauty carbohydrates, which include complex carbohydrates, vegetables, legumes (including beans, chickpeas, and lentils), and fruits. As with fat, customize this percentage to the right amount for *your* body. Refined carbs don't have a place in this ratio. As with fat, experiment and see what works best for you and your body type and constitution. Eat unlimited veggies, especially green veggies, throughout the day. You can have them in salads, green smoothies, steamed, or lightly sautéed. Starchy root vegetables also digest well and can be paired with greens and other nonstarchy veggies. Beans and grains don't have to be everyday foods (although some cultures and people do great consuming them on a daily basis), but they can be worked into your weekly rotation a few times a week at around one cup (cooked) or more, depending on your constitution, activity levels, and how you deal with digesting certain foods. Pay attention to your own body's needs and how you feel. Your body is unique to you.

PROTEIN

Protein is made of amino acids, the building blocks of every cell. Amino acids are found in all natural foods in varying amounts, from cos lettuce to kale to almonds. Amino acids are like alphabet blocks; they can be combined from smaller units into whole proteins, like letters being combined to form whole words. Therefore, a totally vegetarian or vegan diet, by combining amino acid groups, can achieve the full complement of proteins needed for health and beauty.

Because protein isn't used for energy by the body, we need much less of it than people believe when they consume steaks and burgers. Only a few ounces are really needed; there isn't much protein deficiency today in developed societies except among the very poor and malnourished. If your diet contains enough calories, it will be virtually impossible not to get enough protein, even without trying. The old belief that vegetarianism was dangerous because of protein deficiency was never true. There are no innate drawbacks to a plant-based diet.

The most complete protein source in the vegetable kingdom is soya, and for decades soya burgers, tofu, and soya-based supplements and bars were a mainstay of vegetarian diets, not to mention traditional regular diets in China and Japan. But current research casts doubt on consuming excessive amounts of soya as a major part of our diet, with the risk of genetically modified soya and inflammation being the most recent concerns (but as mentioned on page 31, organic forms of fermented soya, such as tempeh, natto, and miso, are easier-to-digest options that can be worked into your diet in moderation if you don't have a soya allergy). But virtually all foods contain varying levels of protein, and you can get a hefty amount on a plant-based diet. For instance, a cup of cooked lentils has around 18 grams of protein, and a cup of cooked spinach has around 5 grams of plant protein. Brussels sprouts, mushrooms—you name it—all whole foods contain protein-building amino acids that are easily assimilated into your body. (Long before amino acid combining became scientific, traditional diets delivered com-

WHAT ABOUT THE PALEOLITHIC (CAVE MAN) DIET?

One of the newer iterations of the high protein / low carb diet is the so-called Paleo diet, which was first outlined by Loren Cordain, an exercise physiology professor at Colorado State University. The views of this plan are founded on the extremely hypothetical habits of the Paleolithic (Stone Age) people and modern-day hunter-gatherers, which he suggested could be studied to make assumptions about the dietary habits of those in Paleo times.[27] But as pointed out by T. Colin Campbell, PhD, in his book *The Low-Carb Fraud*, Cordain "confesses in several places in his research papers[28] that estimates of dietary intakes in both of these groups are 'subjective in nature'" and furthermore "acknowledges that 'scores' attempting to rate these presumed intakes from a very large compendium of 862 of the world's societies are 'not precise.'"[29] Cordain notes that the true "hunter-gatherer way of life," devoid of Western influence, is "now probably extinct."[30]

Historically, anthropologists reached a consensus that only about 33 percent of the foods consumed by hunter-gatherer societies were animal based.[31] But in 2000, Cordain added a larger number of societies and changed some of the definitions, leading to a much higher estimate that about 66 to 75 percent of these "Paleo" diets were made up of animal foods.[32] Scientific literature and anthropologists have challenged Cordain's conjectures, including anthropologist Katharine Milton, who asserts that Cordain's assumption that modern hunter-gatherers are representative of Paleolithic hunter-gatherers is a stretch.[33]

Plant foods leave little or no traces in archaeological remains, making it hard to accurately assess ancient dietary habits, if we did want to use that as a guide for our modern-day diet. But we can see with certainty that we share a very similar gut anatomy (simple acid stomach, a small cecum, a small intestine, and a distinctly sacculated colon), as well as a lack of anatomical tools (sharp fangs, claws) to kill and eat larger animals, with our nearest genetic relatives, chimpanzees. Looking at their natural diet reveals that chimpanzees are largely plant eaters, and may only get upward of 4 to 6 percent of their diet from animal-based foods in the form of ants and termites.[34]

Assumptions and highly conjectural "evidence" from ancient history should not be used to assert the guidelines of eating such a high protein and high fat diet today (30 to 50 percent of each). Superior research directly refutes the high levels of protein and fat pushed by high protein diets such as the Paleo. For instance, it has been widely established that when diet and disease correlations for different populations are compared, diets like Paleo that are rich in fat and animal protein correlate strongly with higher rates of heart disease and breast, colon, and prostate cancer,[35] to name only a few major health conditions. Eating a largely (or all) plant-based diet that is lower in animal protein has been shown to prevent and even reverse such serious illnesses as certain cancers,[36,37] heart disease,[38] and diabetes.[39] And that is truly a beautiful thing.

plete proteins by serving grains and legumes together, the classic combination of rice and beans or rice and lentils that is still the staple for billions of people around the world.)

So far, protein is the one macronutrient that has never been demonized in mainstream diets, though you will find evidence against overconsumption of protein in movements instigated by the China Study and other research. The China Study was headed by Dr. T. Colin Campbell, professor emeritus in the Division of Nutritional Sciences at Cornell University, and was funded by such prestigious organizations as the National Institutes of Health, the American Cancer Society, and the American Institute for Cancer Research. It found strong evidence of the diet's role in cancer growth and a correlation between high protein intake and cancer growth.[40]

Unfortunately, what we see today, especially in modern Westernized societies and in big cities in many parts of the world, is a huge overconsumption of protein. This is the result of both larger portion sizes and more frequent consumption of animal proteins, which is a dangerous shift. Studies in Tunisia,[41] Beijing,[42] and Sweden[43] have shown that as traditional diets rich in plant foods started shifting to incorporate more animal foods, there has been a rise in heart attacks and cardiovascular-related deaths. Remember that our cardiovascular system is one of our circulatory systems, and optimal circulation is a key contributor to health as well as your highest beauty. A recent study found that those who ate high protein diets were 75 percent more likely to die from *any* cause,[44] and the recommendations arising from the study, namely to reduce animal proteins and consume more plant foods, were in keeping with the protein consumption recommendations from the World Health Organization and the Institute of Medicine.

Excessive protein puts a heavy burden on digestion, as digesting protein is energy exhaustive and requires a great deal of enzymes. It is especially taxing on your liver and kidneys, which have a limited capacity to expel uric acid. This leads to an increased possibility of an accumulation of uric acid in the body. High protein foods are also high in purines, which are broken down into uric acid.

Elevated levels of uric acid in the bloodstream may lead to needlelike uric acid crystals in joints, with gout as the painful outcome. In addition, kidney stones are more likely to form in someone on a high protein diet. Because diets that are excessively high in protein are acid forming after the protein is metabolized, they can lead to loss of calcium, as it is leached out of your bones and excreted through your body by urinary calcium excretion. Eating such high levels of protein, which is dense in various fats and cholesterol and takes a lot of energy to break down, also increases the risk of circulatory issues, which can hamper beauty. The percentage of protein in your diet should range from 10 to 20 percent. Again, you may have been trained to believe that you need more, but experiment with your own body and try staying within this range, noticing how your energy and beauty blossom. And later on, in Pillar 5, Beautiful Movement (page 236), we will discuss in much more detail the specific protein needs to optimize your workouts and develop muscle tone.

Your body recycles proteins, meaning that you don't have to ingest complete proteins at every meal.[45] By virtue of getting enough calories and eating a wide variety of nutrient-dense whole foods, you *will* get enough protein. Remember, the goal here is balance. You can enjoy some animal protein if you choose, but try to have more plant-based meals, which will provide you with plenty of protein but with less of a digestive burden and fewer by-products. Make it your goal to limit animal protein to a few times a week or, at the most, once a day to achieve Radical Beauty. Let your beauty shine forth with lots of nourishing, beautifying plant-based meals and foods. Here are some great plant-based sources of protein:

- Spirulina
- Hemp seeds and hemp protein powders
- Chia, sunflower, and other seeds
- Almonds and other nuts
- Green veggies (These have a surprising amount of protein, so keep having your Glowing Green Smoothie; see recipe on page 27.)
- Lentils and beans, soaked overnight for better digestion
- Quinoa, millet, teff, and other gluten-free grains
- Tempeh (a fermented, easier-to-digest form of tofu, which can be sourced organic and plain, and is relatively free from additives, unlike fake meat products that mock a type of animal food)
- Mushrooms, Brussels sprouts, and other whole veggies
- Vegan protein powders

STEAK VS. CIGARETTES

We are well aware that millions of people are attracted to popular high protein / high-fat diets, especially the Atkins diet, which advocates weight loss through the total elimination of all sugar and carbohydrate foods and a reliance on butter, cheese, eggs, poultry, meat, and fish. Paleo is a newer high protein iteration, albeit without dairy. While the human body can adapt to the special process (known as ketosis) that turns protein and fat into blood sugar, the bald fact is that our ancestors didn't evolve on such an extreme diet. Compared with us, they actually ate more nuts, fruits, berries, and vegetables than we do, and always in a whole, ripe form. It's remarkable that the human body can get its needed blood sugar (glucose) the fast, normal way, by eating natural sugars and carbohydrates, which quickly break down into glucose, or the roundabout way, by using extra calories to break down fats and proteins, the macronutrients that normally are stored and employed for cell building.

The roundabout way, or ketosis, leads to weight loss thanks to the extra calories it burns, but there are no holistic studies that tell us the overall health effect of such a diet when practiced for years at a time by adults who might have all kinds of potential disease risks. Furthermore, as mentioned previously, the buildup of ketones can cause an imbalance that leads to excessive acid production,[46] which can bring about acidosis in your body and quicken aging.

No extreme diet, especially one that excludes an entire macronutrient, is part of Radical Beauty. While these diets may be effective in helping you lose weight, at least in the short-term, the overall effect of eating steak is to deposit toxins from the meat itself—especially if it was raised under current artificial, antibiotic-laced, hormone-enhanced conditions—as well as acidic metabolic by-products into your body. This isn't the direction you want your body, or your diet, to go in.

The way you cook your meat can make it even more toxic. Grilling and barbecuing involve converting (burning) animal fats into worrisome chemical residues. The amount of benzo[a]pyrene, a cancer-stimulating agent, in barbecued meat has been pinpointed in studies to be around 4 nanograms (ng) per gram (g),[47] while the content of the benzo[a]pyrene of cigarettes is estimated to be between 4 and 30 ng per gram.[48] In restaurants, the average steak size is 8 ounces (250 g). This means that eating a steak could be the carcinogenic equivalent of smoking 33 to 250 cigarettes (depending on the exact cigarette).

Research reported in the *Proceedings of the National Academy of Sciences* shows that advanced glycation end products, or AGEs (what a fitting acronym!), occur naturally in our body in low levels but are present in high levels in heated animal products, such as grilled or roasted meats.[49] Such AGEs can cause damage to your brain[50] and destroy your collagen and elastin, which is needed to help keep your skin spongy and resilient. When your skin is damaged due to AGEs, it ages and wrinkles faster. Think of a Thanksgiving turkey after it's been roasted for a while in the oven. It's withered to a crisp, which is obviously *not* the kind of skin you'd like to have.

A study in the journal *Cell Metabolism* found that a person with high animal-protein consumption (over 20 percent of calories coming from meat) is four times more likely to die from cancer, which is a similar rate as cigarette smoking.[51] The same study found that high protein consumption led to an increased risk of diabetes and overall mortality, and that proteins derived from plant foods were associated with lower mortality levels than animal-derived proteins.[52] A contributing factor might be the heterocyclic amines (HCAs) that are produced during the cooking of meat, which might be carcinogenic,[53] as well as the carcinogenic compounds nitrosamines, which are present in processed meats[54] (yes, you read that right, carcinogenic compounds in foods you might find at your local deli or market). Yet cooking meat at higher temperatures, even if the meat is organic or nonpreserved, can still increase nitrosamine formation.[55]

You don't have to become a vegan if you choose not to be at this time in order to achieve Radical Beauty, but don't overdo the red meat and steak either. Choose more beautifying, whole-food, plant-based meals. Limit red meat eating to only occasionally—a few times a month at the very most—and choose organic meat on those occasions when you do want to eat it.

Feel a Connection to Your Food

It's easy for all of us just to stuff food into our mouths, enjoy the temporary taste, and not really think about what goes on after that. Out of sight, out of mind, right? But this approach will not help you reach your goal of building your Radical Beauty. In order to do that, you need to be able to connect with what you are eating and become conscious of how what you are eating makes you feel, both in the short- and long-term.

A good place to start is by connecting visually to what is taking place when you eat, beyond what you can see with your eyes. In other words, try visualizing what you know is taking place without literally seeing it and connecting that to the experience in your body, which you cannot help but feel. Try this now. Think of your last food binge—maybe on a "cheat" day, while on vacation, or when out with your friends. It can be any time you decided to just let loose and eat that pizza or ice cream or french fries followed by a cupcake or donut. Maybe it was on that hungover Sunday when you dug into the third serving of macaroni and cheese that you knew you really shouldn't have but were craving so badly (and you felt so crappy you didn't put up much of a defense). Imagine how the particular foods you indulged in tasted, felt, and looked.

Now try taking the visualization internally, imagining what is going on in your stomach after you binged. Picture your stomach expanding outward, trying to contend with the heavy digestive load you just burdened it with. Imagine a churning volcano. Now create the image of congestive toxicity and envision it building up on the insides of your gut.

Next, visualize inflammation striking your cells, causing friction and disharmonious aggravation. Think about diminished circulation throughout your body, the growth of the toxins, nutrients passing through but not being absorbed, your cells suffering, and ultimately your skin getting duller and wrinkling like a raisin. Sit with that for a moment, and internalize these images and imagined feeling of your digestive distress. Compare these feelings to the physical sensations you've felt in your body when indulging in a binge.

The purpose of this exercise is not to make you feel horrible or to picture disturbing images for no reason. It is to help foster a deeper mindfulness of just how much the food you are eating impacts your body, your energy, and your beauty.

Now visualize eating something healthy. Imagine eating a delicious all-vegetable ginger-squash soup, for example. The food feels warming as it goes in, and it feels grounding and filling in your stomach, but you don't feel overly stuffed. Think of this food going into your gut and various nutrients flowing into your bloodstream and circulating all around your body in a clear, healthy stream. Your skin is radiant and glowing, and you finish eating feeling great.

When you decide what to eat, it's inevitable that sometimes you'll make a less-than-ideal choice. This is perfectly fine. You are not meant to be perfect. But try to keep this imagery stored somewhere in your mind so the next time you are struggling with a food option on a menu or on the brink of going from a little treat to a full binge, you can pull this imagery back into the forefront of your mind. Hopefully this consciousness-building exercise (which can be done in as little as a few seconds) will pull you back to this side of whole, beauty-nourishing foods so that you can make the better choice more often.

Nourish Yourself As No One Else Can

Most people feel healthier and more connected to their food and energy when they cook most of their meals themselves. It's also great from a beauty perspective, because cooking your own meals puts you in control of the oils and other ingredients that you consume. You can be sure to use beauty-building organic produce and cook with coconut oil, non-irradiated spices, and fresh herbs. No matter what you choose, you always know the source of your food when you cook for yourself.

This certainly does not have to be elaborate or take up copious amounts of time. Home-cooked meals can be simple, and it's easy to rotate certain dishes you feel comfortable with over and over again, mixing and matching different vegetables and ingredients. Eating out can be social, celebratory, and a lot of fun, but it doesn't have to be your norm. Save it for special occasions, or at least try to shift into eating out less and having more meals at home, and you will feel more grounded and empowered not only with your diet but perhaps your whole life.

Radical Beauty Healthy Cooking Time-Savers

At this point, you may be feeling really inspired by all this information about how to make big shifts in your life. There truly is so much you can do to eat your way to a fuller expression of your natural beauty. And it's understandably thrilling, but then a passing dark thought may cloud your excitement: how are you actually going to have time to eat healthfully? You might feel as if you already don't have enough time to jam all your professional and personal duties into your schedule, so how are you going to possibly add the further element of eating for Radical Beauty into the mix?

Don't worry. You will not have to spend much more time preparing food to make these dietary shifts, but you will have to be a little bit strategic and take some time to plan ahead. Actually, the time you use to buy or make things in bulk and prep more at home instead of always running out to restaurants and take-out joints may actually help you save more time overall. This is especially true as you get more comfortable with simpler staple dishes and strategies.

Here are some great time-saving tricks to get you on your way to eating for Radical Beauty.

BAKE ROOT VEGETABLES

As soon as you get home from work, turn on the oven and throw some whole squash or sweet potatoes on a pan. Yes, that's right—whole! You can prick some slits in them with a knife, but don't struggle with breaking down a supertouch raw squash; it simply takes too much energy. Throwing these rock-hard root veggies into the oven whole is going to save you a lot of preious time that you would otherwise spend trying to cut them up. Let them soften up while you change, relax, and catch up with your spouse and your kids, or simply chill out. After 45 minutes or so, take them out of the oven, cube or slice them, and either sauté them with a little coconut oil or let them bake a bit longer. Sprinkle them with simple seasonings like paprika, turmeric, and a pinch of sea salt, and eat them over a salad or with some other veggies or greens. Super easy and delicious. The key is to let your oven work for you while you are getting your post-work relaxation in.

KEEP ORGANIC TEMPEH ON HAND

This is the equivalent of a fast-food health meal. It's hearty, protein dense, and fermented so it tends to digest better than other soya products. Plus, the fermentation is believed to deactivate some of the potentially less-than-great features of soya products, including digestive difficulties. And the key feature: speed. Open up a package of tempeh, cut it into squares or strips, heat it up in a pan, and you're good to go. Eat it either with some lightly cooked veggies, like courgettes or broccoli, or on top of a leafy, green salad. Play around with spices and flavorings. Tempeh goes well with everything from tamari to cayenne and paprika, cumin, or even marinara sauce. You can literally make this meal in less than 5 minutes!

TRY AN EVENING SMOOTHIE

If you get home late and are exhausted, you can always make a simple smoothie for dinner that's loaded with beauty nutrition. It doesn't get much easier than that, and if you have a Vitamix, cleanup only takes a few minutes. Eating late at night, especially when you're exhausted, isn't great for digesting heavier foods, anyway. Smoothies are great for these times because they are blended and easy to digest. With the ingredients already broken down, it's brilliantly simple for your system to absorb the nutrition. You can bulk up a smoothie to make it feel satisfying in the evening by using almond milk as the base. Other great smoothie ingredients to stock at home include bananas, coconut water, maca, spirulina, bee pollen, stevia, vanilla extract, sprouted plant-based protein powder, cinnamon, raw cacao, and acai.

MAKE A ONE-POT MEAL

One-pot cooking is popular in many parts of the world, and with good reason. If you make a soup or a stew, you can throw everything into the pot (you can even get your kids to help you!) and go do other things (change after a long day, help your kids with their homework, talk with a friend on the phone, and so on). Secondly, cooking this way instead of boiling ingredients and then throwing out the water means that the liquid in your soup or stew will retain the nutrition of the foods. Make your own vegetable broth in big batches or buy an organic variety from the market. When you get home or when you want an easy meal, heat the vegetable broth on the stove and throw in various veggies, lentils, or even beans (from cartons if you are in a rush) for an easy, nutritious, and family-friendly meal. Try pureeing everything if you like a smoother soup. You can even add brown rice or quinoa to stews, and toast up some gluten-free or whole-grain bread for extra-hungry kids and teenagers to dip into their stew. Invest in a large, good-quality soup pot, and it will be a great friend to you for years to come.

TURN YOUR FREEZER INTO YOUR LIFE RAFT

When you do have time to cook, make extra and freeze portion sizes in bisphenol A (BPA)–free containers (a chemical believed to potentially cause hormonal, developmental, and brain issues, among other health concerns). You can freeze anything from gluten-free lasagna to soups, bananas, and even dark chocolate. (Sweet-tooth emergencies are still emergencies!) When you get busy, you can rest assured that not only won't you starve, you also won't have to resort to Taco Bell or the equivalent fast-and-easy but incredibly beauty-busting option nearby. This is especially great if you have an erratic schedule that doesn't always allow for regular grocery shopping. You can grab something to thaw out in the morning before leaving for work, or stick the container in a pot of hot water when you get home if you forgot. Either way, nutritious food that you made yourself is on the way!

BUY ITEMS IN BULK

If you can find a great local (and preferably organic) market with bins, try to buy large amounts of quinoa, lentils, brown rice, steel-cut oats, and whatever other dried staples you love. Quinoa is a great one because it is mineral and nutrient dense, gluten-free, and cooks up in about 12 to 14 minutes. It's perfect for quick meals. Having these dried staples around is great when you are busy and don't have time to go out and shop. It's ideal to soak them overnight or at least during the day if you can throw them in water on the way to work. But, hey, if you forgot or are in a real time crunch and the choice is between unsoaked quinoa and takeout made with questionable oils and ingredients you aren't completely sure of, the quinoa option is the clear winner.

BE A STRATEGIC VEGGIE SHOPPER

Food shopping can take up a lot of time. Not all of us can do daily vegetable shopping like some lucky locals in the South of France. If you can only go grocery shopping once a week or so, be sure to get veggies that are heartier and can last until the end of the week. Red/purple cabbage, onions, shallots, garlic, root vegetables such as yams and spaghetti squash, carrots, and radishes are great in this regard. Use up the more perishable veggies like broccoli or watercress earlier in the week. By being strategic with your veggies' timetables, you should be able to enjoy a range of veggies over the week.

MAKE BIGGER BATCHES

In addition to freezing spare portions of entrées, it's also easier and more convenient to make large portion sizes of kale chips, courgettes hummus, and washed and chopped veggies that you can chomp on and dip when you get hungry. Keep everything in airtight glass or BPA-free containers in your fridge and you'll have a ready supply of beautifying foods even when you're exhausted or pressed for time.

MAKE A MASTER GGS

If you are a Glowing Green Smoothie (page 27) drinker, try making a master batch on Sunday (or whatever day of the week is the easiest for you), keeping some portions out for the next day or so, and freezing portion sizes that you can thaw out later in the week. This is a great time-saver and ensures you are following this all-important habit as much as possible.

CHOOSING ORGANIC

Choosing organic food is also a choice for your beauty. Organic produce contains superior nutrition—more beneficial vitamins, minerals, essential fatty acids, and antioxidants to nourish your beauty than conventional produce. By definition, organic produce does not include genetically modified organisms (GMO) and is produced without the use of artificial pesticides, antibiotics, synthetic fertilizers, and hormones that can tax and age your body, cumulatively destroying your beauty over time.

Going organic is definitely worth the extra cost for your health and beauty's sake. If budget is an issue, check out the latest list of the "Dirty Dozen" from the Environmental Working Group to determine which twelve produce items are the most important to buy organic. If you can put your budget toward organic versions of the crops that are sprayed most often with pesticides, you can avoid a lot of pesticide contamination. Check out local farmer's markets and talk to local sources, which may or may not have organic certifications but still use organic farming practices.

It's especially important to buy organic meat, which we'll discuss more in a moment. It's important to know that the label *free-range* doesn't necessarily mean organic or that the animals were fed a natural-food diet. Always look for the term *organic* or *organic and free-range* on the label. According to the National Organic Program under the United States Department of Agriculture (USDA), to be labeled organic meat, the animals must be raised on certified organic land; fed organic feed without growth hormones, antibiotics, GM feed, or animal by-products; and can't be grown using persistent pesticides or chemical fertilizers.[1]

Don't be fooled by the generic word *natural*. Natural foods are not necessarily organic. They may contain some organic ingredients—or they may not. If you are buying packaged products, look for the USDA *certified organic* seal, which signifies that a product contains at least 95 percent organically grown ingredients. You vote with your food choices! Choosing organic for the recipes in this book and in general will help increase the demand for organic. This will eventually help lower organic prices, support the environment, and build and sustain your precious beauty and health.

Reality Check: You Eat
What Your Food Eats

The fact that you ultimately ingest whatever the animals you eat ingest is an uncomfortable reality for many of us, but getting in touch with your food means really understanding what it is composed of and facing the good, the bad, and the ugly. The harsh truth is that compounds in an animal's diet *bio-accumulate*, meaning they become concentrated in the animal's tissues[2] and end up on your fork whether you're eating a piece of roast chicken or digging into a steak. Upon close examination of what commercially raised animals are fed, this fact is not only uncomfortable, it's frightening and downright ugly.

First of all, if you eat factory-farmed animals, which means pretty much any animal product that isn't labeled organic and grass-fed, you're most likely ingesting genetically modified corn and soya along with that seemingly innocent grilled chicken or hamburger at your weekend barbecue. The United States currently provides subsidies to farmers who grow corn and soyabeans, and currently around 90 percent of these crops in the United States are now genetically modified. Livestock producers choose to use corn and soya as the basis of their animal feed not only because it's cheaper but also because these foods help the animals gain weight faster.[3]

Genetically modified crops weren't released until 1996 and started with soya, corn, and cotton (cottonseed oil is commonly used in products like salad dressings and mayonnaise) before spreading into other foods. There hasn't been enough time to assess the full health ramifications for humans, but research on the effects of genetically modified organism (GMO) consumption in animals (with a much shorter life span than humans) has revealed frightening effects, including reproductive issues, liver and kidney toxicity, sperm damage, and infant mortality.[4,5] Researchers at Baylor College of Medicine accidentally discovered that rats that were fed GMO corn material had reproductive issues, and tests on the feed revealed two compounds that "stopped the sexual cycle in females at concentrations approximately two-hundredfold lower than classical phytoestrogens."[6] Both of these substances were also found to contribute to the growth of breast and prostate cancer in cell cultures.[7]

GMO corn and soya crops rely heavily on pesticides and herbicides (such as

Roundup, an herbicide produced by Monsanto that is designed to work with their GMO crop seeds) that build up in animals' tissues after being consumed, and the meat from these animals therefore contains these residues.[8] Exposure to pesticides has been shown to have a negative impact on reproductive, nervous, and immune system functions and increases the risk of cancer.[9]

But wait, there's more—much, much more.

On a global scale, commercial animal feed is laced with a cornucopia of toxins, including mycotoxins, antibiotics, prion proteins, pesticides, heavy metals, and bacterial pathogens.[10] These toxins can cause a variety of problems, including reproductive dysfunction, bacterial infections, imbalanced gut flora, and reduced immunity. You obviously want to avoid consuming these toxins, but unfortunately that's not always simple. Comprehensive legislation is already in place to restrict several of the chemical compounds and pathogens in feed, but as we've seen from outbreaks of contaminated meat in the past, complete bacterial monitoring is impossible to enforce.

Here is a breakdown of some of the most harmful toxins found in commercial animal feed:

Dioxins and polychlorinated biphenyls (PCBs) are industrial pollutants that may contaminate feeds and have been detected in milk and dairy products in particular. Dioxins are highly dangerous toxins that are linked to reproductive, developmental, and hormonal problems as well as cancer.[11] According to the World Health Organization, "More than 90 percent of human exposure to dioxins is through the food supply, mainly meat and dairy products, fish, and shellfish. . . . Contaminated animal feed is often the root-cause of food contamination."[12]

Mercury has been found to contaminate the fishmeal that is used to feed certain animals.[13] Mercury is a heavy metal that causes slow but steady damage in your body in a sneaky way. It causes your cell membranes to become leaky, inhibits key enzymes your body needs for energy production and toxin removal, and creates oxidation in your tissues. Oxidation is one of the main reasons you develop disease, as well as the primary reason you age.

Some feed studied revealed samples of bacterial *E. coli* (short for *Escherichia coli*) variations (though not strain 0157:H7)[14] as well as *Salmonella enterica* bacteria.[15] We *have* seen *E. coli* O157:H7 rear its ugly head from time to time in outbreaks, which have unfortunately caused fatalities. Not only potentially deadly, it also can cause bloody diarrhea, dehydration, and kidney failure. There have been numerous beef recalls in recent history, including one of over 50,000 pounds of meat sold by the National Beef Packing Company in 2013.[16]

There are consistent reports of worldwide feed contamination with fungi and their spores.[17,18] Mycotoxins are secondary metabolites of fungi that have the capacity to impair health[19] and lead to a range of illnesses and diseases. One German study found that 94 percent of feed samples analyzed were contaminated by two to six different *Fusarium* mycotoxins.[20] Forms of the extremely dangerous toxin aflatoxin have also been identified in contaminated feed.[21] This is of particularly grave concern, as chronic aflatoxin exposure has been linked to cancer in humans.[22]

Another ugly ingredient in animal products is . . . well, other animals. These include members of the same species that have died in the factory farm. Some commercial feed even includes meat and bonemeal, containing prion proteins. These components of animal tissue have the capacity to transform into agents that cause fatal neurological lesions in a wide range of species.[23] Cows were not meant to eat other cows. Period.

Then there are the copious amounts of antibiotics that are added to commercial animal feed on purpose. Animal products are frequently contaminated with residues from drugs that were purposely added to the feed to control disease and enhance livestock performance. In other words, they're meant to keep the animals alive and healthy enough to grow hefty before being slaughtered. Many of the drugs added to animal feed are undeclared, and residues of these drugs can be found in the meat. One study that examined animal feed in Northern Ireland showed that out of 247 medicated feeds, 35 percent contained undeclared antimicrobials. Even worse, out of 161 "un-medicated" feeds, 44 percent were found to contain antimicrobials. The contaminants most frequently identified included chlortetracycline, sulfonamides, penicillin, and ionophores.[24] Yes, you read that right—*penicillin*. Who knew you were eating one of the strongest antibiotics available with your Sunday morning bacon and eggs?

Farms also use a range of antibiotics to get their chickens to market weight faster, and low-dose-antibiotic use in animals has been linked to the development of antibiotic-resistant bacterial strains. This can also wipe out your gut flora—and your whole health, really.[25] In 2011, the pharmaceutical company Pfizer temporarily suspended use of the poultry drug Roxarsone after US Food and Drug Administration (FDA) reports showed that compounds in the drug could break down into inorganic arsenic, a toxin that can produce skin lesions, respiratory irritation, and several types of cancer. Inorganic arsenic was leaching into local water supplies and remaining in chicken tissue after slaughter.[26]

The effects of chronic low-arsenic exposure are not well known, but studies have indicated that even low-level exposure may contribute to endocrine and cognitive deficits.[27] Although use of Roxarsone has been suspended, there are several other similar drugs being used in animal production that have the possibility of exposing consumers to toxic forms of arsenic. Some have even hypothesized that arsenic can be linked to the rise in autism rates.[28]

Clearly, there is nothing pretty about commercial meat. If and when you choose to eat animal products, look for items that are organic, grass-fed, and free of steroids and hormones. Ideally, try to find someone who sells these products at a local farmer's market and talk to him or her about how the animals are fed and treated in general.

THE ENVIRONMENTAL IMPACT OF ANIMAL AGRICULTURE

Eating organic meat will still not solve the major detrimental environmental issues of animal agriculture, which is the leading cause of deforestation, water consumption, and pollution; it is also responsible for more greenhouse gases than the transportation industry. Animal agriculture from producing meat, chicken, eggs, and fish is a primary driver of rainforest destruction, species extinction, habitat loss, topsoil erosion, ocean "dead zones," and more.[29] It's shocking that this is not discussed more, but hopefully that will start to change.

If we truly care about the environment, the most impactful thing we can do is to be conscious of our food choices and the impact they have on the earth. The choice to give up meat, or to at least greatly reduce your consumption, will make for a healthier and more beautiful you *and* a healthier and more beautiful planet.

Incorporate Top Radical Beauty Foods and Routines

Routines and daily rhythms are stabilizing forces that have a balancing effect on your life. Routine in a dietary sense is important for establishing excellent digestion and patterns. Having a structure makes it easier to maintain your beneficial eating habits. Such daily rhythms provide a sense of steadiness, like counting on the sun to rise as we get up and start our day and to set every evening as we settle toward rest. This steadiness creates an environment of safety for your mind, helping to reduce stress and anxiety. A more calm, peaceful mind manifests outwardly in a body that does not age as quickly and is more naturally beautiful.

Now that you have information about general shifts, here you'll learn some very specific daily routines that will give you the most Radically Beautiful results to enhance your authentic expression. Here are some things to remember and some new ideas as well.

Start the Day with Hot Water with Lemon

You already know how great this is for your digestive system and liver and to support cleansing. Keep lemons stocked at home and make this a daily habit! For even more digestive benefits, especially if you live in a place with cold winters, add some sliced ginger to this nourishing morning beverage.

Drink a Glowing Green Smoothie Daily

This is a big component of Kimberly's Beauty Detox program and is outlined in great detail in the Beauty Detox books. Smoothies are a really efficient way to get nutrients, and blending abundant amounts of beauty greens and fruit makes it easy for you to digest and absorb all those minerals, vitamins, and antioxidants while loading up your system with fiber. Start making it part of your morning routine (see recipe on page 27) after you drink your hot water with lemon.

Take an Excellent Probiotic Supplement Every Day

Probiotics support optimal digestion, leading to better nutrient absorption and more efficient expulsion of waste. This is an incredibly important beauty supplement. See the authors' websites for recommendations (deepakchopra.com, kimberlysnyder.com).

Become Veggie-Centric

Make it part of your rhythm to include these key, fiber-filled components into every meal, whether a salad, some cooked or chopped greens, or greens topped on whatever you are eating. No more meals of just bread and cold cuts or eggs and toast. Get your veggies in at every meal for alkalizing balance.

Eat Seeds Daily

Sprinkle some freshly ground flaxseeds onto your salads or have some soaked chia seeds (in puddings, salad dressings, or smoothies) every day. You can also take an algae-based DHA and EPA supplement. This will ensure you're getting the proper level of beautifying omega-3 fats for beautiful skin, a balanced mood, and a healthy heart.

Make Turmeric Part of Your Life

If you are new to turmeric, it's time to start befriending it. Pick up some organic, powdered turmeric and add a bit to your evening tea, hot soups, veggie dishes, or blended into salad dressings (see the Creamy Masala Vegetable Stew recipe on page 298).

Break Before Meals

Take time before lunch and dinner and pause to ask yourself what your body truly needs at that meal. At first it might be hard to listen to yourself. You may feel like you should just go for what you've normally eaten in the past, but as you stay receptive and practice asking and listening to your body, you will be able to "hear" more intuitively from your body what you need, and you will feel more satisfied after eating.

Eat More Slowly

Take time just to eat. Don't eat while reading or writing e-mails or during a conference call. Treat eating as sacred for better beauty digestion. Even if it's just a few minutes, take the time for yourself.

Practice Gratitude

Take a moment for gratitude before each meal and even snack. Creating that feeling of gratitude puts your body and mind in a calmer, happier state, which paves the path for optimal digestion.

Sip Hot Herbal Tea in the Evenings

This is soothing, good for digestion, and signals to your mind that it's time to start preparing for sleep and rejuvenation. Tulsi (also known as holy basil) tea is a particularly excellent choice. It's an important herb in Ayurveda, which has been used in India for over 5,000 years, and is said to help reduce stress and anxiety. It's also an adaptogen, helping to balance the body and protect it from the effects of different kinds of stressors.

Try a Daily Fast: Alkalizing Foods Until Lunch

Some research on intermittent fasting, which means going for prolonged periods of time without eating, shows that it may help extend life span and ameliorate aging-related diseases[1] by allowing more time for your body to repair and rejuvenate itself. This backs up the plan proposed in *The Beauty Detox Solution,* which encourages consuming the Glowing Green Smoothie (page 27) and hot water with lemon in the mornings. This is essentially a type of "fast," consisting of only alkalizing foods that are very easy to digest, until noon. By restricting heavier foods for a few hours in the morning you're adding to the hours since dinner the night before, giving your body longer periods of digestive rest. This is easier on your body than some types of traditional intermittent fasting that prescribe alternating normal eating days with whole fasting days on a weekly basis.

Although some schools of thought favor frequent eating, the problem with that approach is that your stomach doesn't have time to properly empty and break down a given food or meal before you give it something else to digest. This can contribute to digestive overload. Give your body more of a rest, and keep your mornings full of alkalizing smoothies, juices, fruit, and maybe some porridge oats, without the digestive burden of very heavy or acidic foods right at the start of your day.

While a late morning or late afternoon snack might be warranted, depending on your constitution, try not to eat constantly all day long (unless you have a specific medical condition like hypoglycemia). Be sure to eat dinner at least 3 hours (ideally) before bed. You want to be sure to digest your food thoroughly before hitting the sack.

Eat in Order

If you have a thin soup, it's best to have it at the beginning of the meal. The stomach will first process and remove liquids before it can really work to break down the solid food items. Drinking a lot of liquids with solid foods is not good for digestion and can cause bloating, as liquids can dilute digestive enzymes and slow digestion. Come into meals hydrated and sip on liquids as needed while eating. Start your meals with fiber-filled, enzyme-rich raw foods such as salads and then move into other items. Avoid eating fast-digesting fruit at the end of your meals or for dessert. For more on this, check out *The Beauty Detox Solution*.

Keep Meals Simple

Instead of having a lot of different elements on your plate, try using fewer types of foods and larger portions of each. It's easier for your body to digest simpler meals, and more efficient digestion promotes your beauty.

How the Temperature of Foods and Beverages Affects Your Beauty

The temperature of what you eat and drink, not just *what* you eat and drink, has an impact on your beauty. Let's talk about beverages first. In Western culture, ice has become ubiquitous. Go to a restaurant and tap water loaded with ice will automatically be plunked down in front of you. We've become so used to drinking only extremely cold beverages that most of us keep or purchase bottled water and other beverages in icy cold refrigerators. Some people even add ice to white wine!

Historically, ice was never as readily available as it is today. This hyper infusion of very cold temperatures into our beverages—and bodies—is a modern phenomenon. If you stick your feet in cold ocean water or your hand into the freezer, it doesn't take long to feel a numbing effect. Think about that happening inside your body. The excessive cold can contract your stomach, impairing it from properly secreting proper enzymes and inducing a contracting or almost "shrinking" effect throughout your digestive system.

The ancient medicinal systems of both Traditional Chinese Medicine (TCM) and Ayurveda both heavily frown on ice-cold water and beverages. TCM holds that cold beverages have a negative effect on metabolism and digestion and that consumption of them over many years can exert a negative effect on the health of other organ systems as well, creating an environment where pain and chronic diseases can develop.

According to the TCM belief system, drinking cold beverages blocks meridian channels (or pathways through which energy flows), slows and even congests blood circulation, and diminishes organ functioning.[2] From a beauty standpoint, this ancient Asian medical system also believes that chronic cold-water drinking can lead to bloating, weight gain, fatigue, chronic pain, varicose veins, poor digestion, and even painful PMS.[3]

From the Ayurvedic perspective, iced and very cold beverages, as well as cold foods, can put out your *agni,* or digestive fire. This can reduce your immunity, lower your resistance to disease, and allow for the buildup of *ama,* or toxins, in the body. These all diminish your beauty potential.

Your internal body temperature is 98.6 degrees Fahrenheit, or 37 degrees Celsius. Cold water is close to freezing temperature, so it is about 33 to 35 degrees Fahrenheit or just above 0 degrees Celsius. A cold beverage shocks your system. Your body is then forced to work harder, wasting precious energy in order to make cold drinks warm enough for the body to actually use. This takes away from energy that could otherwise be directed to repairing your skin's collagen, boosting your energy and immunity, and taking on a multitude of other beauty functions.

From a Western perspective, a popular idea that's promoted in certain diets is that drinking ice water helps you burn calories. But as information from the University of Washington points out, this is essentially a myth. When you drink a cup of ice water, you burn about a measly 8 more calories than downing a cup of room temperature water, as your body raises the temperature of the ice water to normal body temperature.[4] This tiny caloric pittance is hardly significant for any aid in weight loss. Plus, what truly matters is optimizing your health and beauty for the long-term.

RADICAL BEAUTY ACTION STEPS

- Stop adding ice to your water and other beverages and get in the habit of asking the waitstaff at restaurants not to add any ice to your water.

- Over time, transition to drinking water and other liquids at room temperature or sipping on warm herbal teas during the day to stay hydrated.

- If you do drink bottled water when out and about or traveling (versus at home, where it is better to invest in a good water filter), start keeping the bottles out on the counter or in a cupboard instead of in a very cold fridge.

- Let your Glowing Green Smoothie or cold-pressed juices warm up slightly to room temperature before drinking them. When you're getting used to drinking green drinks in the first place, colder temperatures can help them taste more palatable, but over time you will adjust to them being a bit closer to room temperature. These drinks certainly don't have to feel warm, which would be unappetizing, but if they are cool rather than icy cold, they will still be delicious.

- It's important to support your digestion with something warm in the morning, which is why the Beauty Detox program has always recommended drinking hot water with lemon upon rising. While you are sipping on this, you can get into the habit of making or taking your green drinks out of the fridge so they have time to warm up slightly.

Cooked Versus Cold Raw Foods

What about food? There are vastly conflicting ideas on this topic. TCM and Ayurveda heavily disfavor consuming too many cold or raw foods, believing that the overconsumption of them can predispose you to disease and excessive internal "dampness," and that cooked foods actually digest more easily. On the opposite end of the spectrum is the raw food theory, which maintains that food should be eaten unheated to conserve vitamins and also food's natural enzymes, which can be destroyed during the cooking process.

A combination of both raw and cooked foods is best to preserve your beautiful balance. Consume warm liquids throughout the day: hot water with lemon in the mornings and herbal teas during the day or evening. Get your raw enzymes and vitamins from fresh fruits and veggies in green smoothies, salads, and plain whole fruit. Mix in hot soups; baked, steamed, or roasted vegetables; veggie stir-fries; and other hot entrées. It's also a good idea to take digestive enzymes before eating heavier or cooked foods to aid in digestion.

It's also important to adjust your diet naturally for each season (see Pillar

4 for more detail on seasonal tips). Just as your clothes change for the seasons, so should your foods. For instance, you'll probably naturally favor lighter, raw foods in the spring after a long winter of eating heavier foods. When it's freezing out, hot meals are going to help keep that internal digestive *agni* fire burning, and you'll intuitively feel better eating heartier fare. In the midst of a hot summer, you will be more apt to naturally reach for cooling, juicy fruits and coconut water. Cooler drinks are okay in the summer, but we still want to avoid very icy ones year-round for the reasons listed above.

Keep listening to yourself, and you will stay beautifully balanced. You are a dynamic being who is experiencing constant shifts and movement down to the cellular level. Your emotions and everything that is going on in your life, as well as environmental factors and geographic placement, are all important influences on your dietary shifts. It becomes imperative to listen to your natural instinct and to be aware of changes and influences in your body's energies and develop a greater and greater sensitivity to taking better care of yourself as you become more receptive to your own body's needs.

Top Foods for Radical Beauty

While all whole foods build beauty, there are some specific foods that particularly help your beauty shine through. This is not meant to be an exhaustive list— just some stellar foods to work into your rotation.

BITTER FOODS

According to Ayurvedic principles, bitter foods, which are lacking in most American diets, help tone skin and purify the body. Foods that taste bitter typically contain potent antioxidants and other phytochemicals like flavonoids and polyphenols, which are responsible not only for their bitter taste but also their phenomenal health and beauty benefits. Bitter foods also help to stimulate and improve digestion and support liver function. Beneficial bitter foods include dandelion greens, parsley, cranberry, spring greens, and bitter melon.

Incorporating bitter foods for beauty:

Add bitter melon to your next curry or stir-fry. (Look for it at the Asian grocery or section of your local market.)

Use spring greens as a natural wrap for veggie burgers or hummus or veggie wraps.

Add parsley to your green smoothies.

Sip on unsweetened, diluted cranberry juice with water as a refreshing beverage.

Chop and throw some dandelion greens into your green salads.

SOUR FOODS

Sour foods are another important group that, according to Ayurveda, can help cleanse the liver. Sour foods such as tomatoes, lemons, star fruit, tamarind, and fermented cabbage often include important vitamins like A and C.

Incorporating sour foods for beauty:

Squeeze lemon juice into water.

Use lemon juice as a primary base for your salad dressings.

Add tamarind paste to soups.

Eat half a cup or so of fermented cabbage (aka raw sauerkraut) with your dinner.

MUSHROOMS

In ancient Chinese medicine, mushrooms are regarded as tonics, which means they have nonspecific benefits across several systems of the body. Mushrooms are one of the few food sources of vitamin D, which is important to keep your bones and muscles beautifully strong. Certain varieties, such as shiitake, help improve immunity.[5] Himematsutake mushrooms are relatives of the common button mushroom that is found at nearly every grocery store. Very popular in Japan, himematsutakes are believed to help improve your skin and hair.[6] Eating button mushrooms may impart the same benefits!

Incorporating mushrooms for beauty:

Slice raw mushrooms into salads (be sure to source organic varieties).

Bake, steam, or sauté mushrooms or stuff and roast Portobello mushrooms as the main protein in your meal, or as a side dish.

Add freshly sliced or dried mushrooms to your soups.

Try some of the many Beauty Detox mushroom-based recipes (see Kimberly's blog, kimberlysnyder.com).

BLACK RICE

Like brown rice, black rice offers various beauty benefits, such as fiber and minerals, including manganese and iron. It is sometimes referred to as "purple" rice or even "forbidden rice," because in ancient China it was reserved for the emperors and nobles, and the commoners were prohibited from eating it. Thankfully, now all of us "commoners" have access to this fantastic food. It really is delicious, and it has some striking properties. You might never think to compare black rice to blueberries or blackberries, but if you put them side by side, they are actually nearly the same gorgeous purple color. That's because the bran of black rice contains the same anthocyanin antioxidants as these berries. Research from the Department of Food Science at Louisiana State University reported that a spoonful of black rice bran contains more health-promoting anthocyanin antioxidants than a spoonful of blueberries, but with even more fiber and vitamin E antioxidants.[7] This makes black rice wonderful for boosting your skin's natural beauty. As with all rice, be sure to soak it overnight; this will make it easier to cook and also make its nutritional benefits more readily absorbed by the body.

Incorporating black rice for beauty:

Add black rice to bean, lentil, veggie, or other vegetarian soups, making an easy and delicious entrée with just these two nutritious components.

Stir-fry black rice with some coconut oil and veggies for a healthy "fried rice."

MICROGREENS

These tiny powerhouse greens not only help you look more beautiful but also make any dish, however simple, look more beautiful. Just sprinkle them on top of any meal. They're one of the healthiest and most beautiful garnishes you could use. These young greens, including red cabbage, coriander, and broccoli, are harvested less than fourteen days after germination and are about 1 to 3 inches long. They contain up to forty times higher levels of vital nutrients than their mature counterparts. For example, red cabbage microgreens have forty times more vitamin E and six times more vitamin C than mature red cabbage. Want one of the easiest, most space-effective ways to nourish your beauty? Add a handful of microgreens into your diet and watch your skin glow.

Incorporating microgreens for beauty:

Toss microgreens into your salads.

Add them to wraps and veggie burgers rather than regular lettuce.

Top soups and just about any entrée you serve with them, right before serving.

Blend a quarter or half cup or so into your Glowing Green Smoothies!

ALOE VERA JUICE

New York City's Memorial Sloan Kettering Cancer Center has studied aloe, including the plant's extracted juice, for potential effects on dry skin, psoriasis, and other skin issues, along with internal issues like constipation and diabetes.[8] The center also notes studies indicating aloe's potential anti-inflammatory and antioxidant effects. Aloe vera juice is quite different from topical gel versions, so make sure the label specifies use as a dietary supplement or juice. Some side effects have been reported, such as gastrointestinal upset with long-term consumption, so, as with any new supplement or food you are unsure of, be sure to check with your doctor first.

Incorporating aloe vera juice for beauty:

Dilute it into water along with some freshly squeezed lemon and sip.

Add small amounts of it into smoothies.

MACA ROOT

Packed with minerals such as calcium and magnesium, B vitamins, enzymes, and all of the essential amino acids, maca is a Peruvian root that has been used for more than 2,000 years. It can help balance hormones and stimulate and nourish the hypothalamus and pituitary glands (the "master glands" of the body), bringing beautiful balance throughout your entire system. Working as an adaptogen, maca is a "responsive" food that helps regulate the production of your hormones downward or upward, depending on your body's individual needs. Hormones are important for so many things in your body, including your mood and tissue function. Balancing them is crucial for your overall beauty. Maca has anecdotally been known to help improve skin, increase fertility, and even help with premenstrual syndrome (PMS) symptoms and libido. Start with $1/2$ teaspoon or less to see how your body reacts to maca if you are new to it, working up to 1 teaspoon or more over the next few weeks.

Incorporating maca for beauty:

Enjoy a delicious smoothie of maca blended with banana and almond milk or coconut water.

Stir into your herbal teas.

Sprinkle over porridge oats.

EDIBLE WEEDS

Believe it or not, weeds can help you look and feel more beautiful. They are the perfect demonstration of the abundance of nature's beauty foods: they literally are everywhere you turn. You can find weeds in your backyard and at your local farmer's market. If you are unsure of exactly what weeds you are looking for, it's always a better bet to get them from the market. Purslane, dandelion greens, and fat-hen are all particularly beauty-boosting weeds. Weeds are hearty plants that tend to be especially high in nutrients and antioxidants. Purslane is an exceptionally high source of omega-3 fatty acids, while dandelion (also a bitter food) and fat-hen (which tastes like a combination between spinach and Swiss chard) contain large amounts of vitamins A, C, and K and minerals such as calcium, iron, manganese, and potassium.

Incorporating edible weeds for beauty:

Add to smoothies.

Lightly steam or sauté.

Add to soups.

MSM-RICH FOODS

Methylsulfonylmethane, also known as MSM, has a lot of health- and beauty-enriching properties. It contains sulfur, which helps with the proper functioning of proteins in your body. MSM is revered for joint health and helping to promote beautiful skin. It has anti-inflammatory and antioxidant effects and is even said to aid with circulation. Some of the richest natural sources of MSM include tomatoes, raspberries, apples, Swiss chard, and alfalfa sprouts.

Incorporating MSM-rich foods for beauty:

When they're in season, snack on lots of fresh raspberries and apples.

Slice up tomatoes and eat them plain.

Add chopped tomatoes to your soups or stews.

Blend Swiss chard into your smoothies.

WHITE TEA

White tea may be very helpful in maintaining your weight, and some have even anecdotally claimed that it protects against acne. A series of experiments on human fat cells (adipocytes) demonstrate that white tea can help inhibit new fat cells while stimulating the fat mobilization from mature fat cells.[9] This may even be useful in combating cellulite. Green tea has received great press, but it contains a fairly high level of caffeine. We all know this can feel temporarily energizing but is still irritating to your nervous system. While actual caffeine levels depend on the specific buds and brewing methods used, green tea generally contains more caffeine than white tea. White tea undergoes less processing than green or black tea, even though they derive from the same plant (*Camellia sinensis*). Because it is less processed, white tea also contains more antioxidants, which are great for keeping your skin youthful and protecting your vitality.

Incorporating white tea for beauty:

Source some excellent organic white tea and drink it during the day, stopping by late afternoon, as it does contain some caffeine. For added benefits, add some sliced ginger, turmeric, or lemon.

A Word About Supplements

You certainly do not have to take a dozen supplement pills every day to be healthy. And you will never achieve the beauty and health results you are after by trying to rely on pills in lieu of eating a superior, nutrition-packed diet made up mostly of whole foods. Unfortunately, most supplements out there are synthetically created, which makes them cheaper to produce and more stable.

The problem is that with vitamins, more is most definitely *not* more. Synthetic vitamins are not remotely similar to the forms of these nutrients found in nature, which you would obtain from eating natural foods. Our bodies evolved for millions of years getting these nutrients in unison with countless other nutritional cofactors that are present in real food. Vitamin supplements may not be bioavailable, usable, or absorbable by your body, and even worse, they can be recognized and treated as a toxin, which then has to be processed and expelled by your eliminative organs. One study even found synthetic vitamin supplementation can actually increase mortality rates![10]

One supplement that is a must is an excellent probiotic supplement, which is not an isolated micronutrient but rather helps your entire body function more efficiently. Remember that the best probiotics are not necessarily those with the highest culture counts but ones that have the most effective and diverse strains that can actually be assimilated into your body (please see authors' websites for resources and recommendations: deepakchopra.com, kimberlysnyder.com).

What's the best way to get the nutrients you need? Be sure to eat from a wide variety of plant foods, preferably organic, as the first step. You can also source specific superfoods rich in certain vitamins (bee pollen is rich in B vitamins, for instance). If you still are worried you aren't eating as well as you should, you can also source a high-quality, whole-food-based and nonsynthetic multivitamin or multimineral supplement from a reputable company that has done the necessary work and research to ensure optimal nutritional absorption. It should include vitamin D_3 (which many people do need to supplement, especially if you aren't getting an adequate dosage of regular sunshine) and the spectrum of B vitamins, including vitamin B_{12}. If you're vegan, you should definitely supplement vitamin B_{12}.

A magnesium-oxygen supplement is great for promoting ongoing cleansing (see page 37). As recommended in Pillar 1, be sure to consume chia, hemp, or flaxseeds daily for daily omega-3 fats. An algae-based DHA and EPA supplement can be good insurance, as some people don't convert omega-3 fats adequately into longer-chain DHA fats. Algae is the primary source from which fish their DHA, and scientists from Harvard and the Cleveland Clinic also report in *The Journal of Nutrition* that algae-based DHA can boost levels of good cholesterol and cut levels of triglycerides.[11] Fish oil pills as a source of omega-3 fats are not recommended, as they can often become rancid and contaminated with toxins.

How Does Salt Fit In with Beauty?

Sodium, found in salt, is an element our bodies need to function properly. It helps to control our blood pressure and blood volume, as well as ensuring proper muscle and nerve function. The best beauty forms of salt to use are small amounts of high-quality sea salt, such as Celtic or Himalayan sea salt. These sea salts also have trace minerals and elements. Sea salts are obtained from the evaporation of saltwater bodies, rather than the heavy processing that produces table salt; this includes bleaching and diluting the salt after harvesting with anticaking agents and other chemicals. For these reasons, stick to sea salt in your cooking.

But too much salt is definitely a beauty and health no-no. Excessive salt intake can increase the risk for heart disease, hypertension, high blood pressure, and kidney disease. It can also make your skin look dehydrated.

Excessive sodium can also create "false fat," making you look bloated and pounds heavier than you truly weigh.

An average daily guideline is 1,000 to 1,500 milligrams (mg) of sodium per day or less. If you are at risk for a medical condition, such as those listed above, you can certainly omit salt from your cooking altogether. Most of us, accustomed to so many processed and restaurant foods that contain loads of sodium, are used to a very salty flavor. Shifting into eating more natural foods and preparing simpler food will help you become more sensitive to the taste of salt. It's also a good idea to add sea salt to your food right before you eat it, so it tastes more salty without using more actual salt!

External Nourishment

Now that you know how to lay the foundation for your beauty with your diet, we are going to talk about the best forms for the outer care of your skin. This includes the safest and most effective skin-care products and ingredients as well as self-care practices that will help you grow strong nails; healthy, shiny hair; and clear, glowing skin. Incorporating superior inner and outer care will nourish your whole body from the outside in and let your natural beauty shine through to the highest degree possible. In this pillar we'll cover the best—as well as the worst—ingredients and practices so you can allow your most beautiful self to be authentically reflected.

Incorporate Natural Skin-Care Ingredients

Your Amazing Skin

Our largest organ, the skin, is a fascinating one. It is an elimination organ, meaning it helps dispel wastes from your body through sweat. Your skin receives roughly a third of all the blood that is circulated throughout the body. It makes sense that if the blood is congested, this is reflected in your skin. Your skin is the last organ to receive nutrition in the body, yet is among the first organs to show signs of an imbalance or deficiency.

But skin does also work in the opposite way, absorbing what is applied to it on the outside. It is therefore critical to be strategic about putting the best ingredients on the surface of your skin to help repair and support its health from the outside in. This seems obvious, but there is a great deal of marketing hype to weed through to determine what works and what is merely an empty claim. It's also critical to avoid the numerous toxic ingredients that can be absorbed and not only tax your skin but also enter your bloodstream and burden your liver.

Your skin is also influenced by your emotions and mental state. Research shows that stress can cause visible aging at the cellular level, including a study published in the *Proceedings of the National Academy of Sciences*.[1] Elissa Epel, one of the researchers for this study, states, "This is the first time that psychological stress has been linked to a cellular indicator of aging in healthy people."[2] Luckily, many of the techniques in this pillar will help relax your mind and body while nurturing your skin from the outside in.

Healthy, smooth, and radiant skin is considered the holy grail of beauty. If you survey any woman (and most men, even though they might not discuss it as openly!), you will find that beautiful skin is at the very top of her beauty wish list. Well, the time has come for you to get your wish. By working with your skin and incorporating ingredients into your routine that will help nourish your skin, you'll create an optimal environment for your skin to grow, repair, and heal itself. The result will be skin that glows, reflecting your highest beauty.

Natural vs. Chemical Ingredients

Some may think that the expensive, scientifically created, cutting-edge products on the market are automatically the most effective choices out there, but this is not necessarily the case. The antioxidants found in natural plant ingredients are still widely considered to be among the most powerful skin-care ingredients, and this is consistently proven in research.

As Richard Baxter, MD, of the University of Washington School of Medicine, states, "There is enough published work to convince me that the antioxidant botanicals will be the next big thing in skin care."[3] They may be the "next big thing," but they have also been around for thousands of years—much like ancient practices like yoga and meditation are tagged as "new age." (Ironic and illogical, right?) Synthetic ingredients may have properties to help boost your skin, but some may tax your skin and even be toxic.[4] That toxicity can be absorbed right from your skin into your system.[5]

As with your diet, the best approach to skin care is to understand the power of nature. Nature's beauty is unparalleled, and if you live closer to nature in all aspects of your lifestyle, your natural beauty will increase. Choose nontoxic products that contain natural, plant-based ingredients. As long as they aren't toxic, scientifically created ingredients, like concentrated, isolated peptides, that are aimed at a specific purpose such as minimizing the appearance of fine lines and wrinkles can work together with natural ingredients to create powerful combinations. Nature and science can most certainly work together in a balanced way.

Organic ingredients are, by definition, pesticide- and GMO-free. But keep in mind that products may contain some organic ingredients but may not be *100 percent* organic if other ingredients are processed in some way to make them usable or if they are actually lab created. Natural minerals such as mica are not considered organic because they are not plant based. Also, water and salts are excluded when determining a product's percentage of organic ingredients. This means that some great products may be an effective blend of nontoxic ingredients derived from nature and science, but may not be necessarily labeled 100 percent organic.

There are literally tens of thousands of beauty products on the market, all virtually screaming at you from store aisles with their bold, brightly colored packages. If you glance at magazines, you'll see the latest, hottest new skin-care ingredients pop up every month. It can be very confusing to determine the best (and worse) choices for your skin.

HOW TO READ SKIN-CARE PRODUCT LABELS (IT'S NOT WHAT YOU'VE HEARD)

The FDA requires that ingredients be listed in INCI (International Nomenclature of Cosmetic Ingredients) language. These labels often are not easily read and usually contain long words and names. An overly simplified and false statement you hear a lot is that if you can't pronounce it, you should not eat it or use it on your skin. But if you look at the INCI language required for a natural ingredient like shea butter, you would see *Butyrospermum parkii,* and for avocado you would see *Persea gratissima.* These hard-to-pronounce words (which are the binomial plant names) would scare anyone who tried to follow this rule! If you are unsure of an ingredient or INCI language name, you can search the INCI directory.

Best Radical Beauty Skin-Care Ingredients

Despite the "breakthrough" ingredients that are constantly being introduced by skin-care companies, there are some important staples that should be included in your external beauty skin-care routine. Over time, these have held up as being the most effective, from both a clinical research and an anecdotal point of view. They are among the most important beauty ingredients to include in your personal external skin-care beauty arsenal.

Antioxidants

Unless you haven't opened a beauty or health magazine in the last two decades, you have surely heard of antioxidants. Antioxidants, naturally present in most plant foods in varying degrees, can help counter skin-aging free radicals and prevent damaged skin cells. This means slowing down those pesky skin issues we all want to avoid, such as wrinkles, dry or dull skin, dark under-eye circles, and crow's feet.

You'll find a very wide range of antioxidants and corresponding plant ingredients touted in various skin-care products. These can range from coffee berry to acai and a range of other berries and fruits. Some of the most powerful antioxidant ingredients are listed below.

Vitamin C

Vitamin C is so powerful and produces such great results that no skin-care routine should be without it. It's present in many fruits and vegetables and is added into skin-care products in a concentrated form. Vitamin C has long been considered a workhorse ingredient, and its effectiveness has been backed up by clinical research.[6] It increases collagen production, which creates firm, beautiful, and thicker skin over time, helps to keep skin hydrated, and diminishes fine lines and wrinkles. As an antioxidant vitamin, it helps squash skin damage caused by unstable free radicals and sun exposure[7] and also boosts the efficacy of vitamin E. On a label, concentrated forms of vitamin C often read as L-ascorbic acid.

Vitamin E

Vitamin E, made up of tocopherols and tocotrienols, is another great antioxidant vitamin that is highly protective of your cells and helps your skin retain moisture to stay supple and beautiful. Vitamin E also helps reverse existing damage to your skin, including scarring from acne and blemishes and age spots. Used in a skin-care product formulation, vitamin E also helps stabilize other ingredients as well as oils, preventing them from going rancid. Tocopherol acetate is an artificial form of vitamin E that is often seen on product labels. It's made from a combination of naturally derived vitamin E and other chemical compounds, such as acetic acid. The natural vitamin E is generally considered preferable.

Vitamin A and Its Derivatives

There has been a lot of research on this ingredient dating back to the 1980s, proving it to be a highly effective anti-aging treatment. It helps improve cell communication, in effect "telling" your skin cells to correct themselves. This improves the look of wrinkles and promotes firmness so your skin appears more healthy and youthful. Vitamin A is the precursor to retinoids, which can be applied topically or ingested; they cannot be made in the human body. These retinoids, or retinoic acids, come in various forms, including retinol, retinyl palmitate, tretinoin, and tazarotene. Some of these require a prescription, while retinol and retinyl palmitate can be found in various over-the-counter products. This category of ingredients has been shown to help promote smoother skin and overall brighter skin tone, while reversing discoloration and repairing cellular structure damage, such as scars, lines and wrinkles, and even acne.

This is all great, but—and there's a big "but" here—retinoids are considered by some to be toxic. This is largely due to their ability to make you more sensitive to sunlight and because of pregnancy concerns. The Environmental Working Group states, "Data from an FDA study indicate that retinyl palmitate, when applied to the skin in the presence of sunlight, may speed the development of skin tumors and lesions. The FDA and Norwegian and German health agencies have raised a concern that daily skin application of vitamin A creams may contribute to excessive vitamin A intake for pregnant women and other populations."[8]

Retinoids can also be irritating and intolerable, so be sure to check with your dermatologist and evaluate whether or not retinoids in any form are right for you. They are considered a highly effective ingredient, but from a toxicity standpoint they are not completely in the clear. Again, evaluate for yourself and see what is right for you and your skin. If you do choose to go this route and use some vitamin A derivatives, be sure to use strong protection from the sun or avoid sunlight altogether. And remember that all women trying to conceive or who are pregnant must completely avoid retinoids.

Alpha Hydroxy Acids (AHAs)

Exfoliation helps your skin shed old, damaged surface skin cells to allow new, fresh cells to grow in their place. If you don't slough old cells, it's harder for your body to absorb the ingredients from your skin-care products; they will more likely just sit on the surface of the older, dead skin cells and not do you any real good. What a waste! This is similar to the concept of internal detoxification. You have to make space for the new raw materials to come in and be absorbed and assimilated so they can be used to fuel your beauty.

AHAs exfoliate without scrubbing with physically dense abrasives such as grains, granules, apricot pits, and the like, which can lead to broken capillaries and damaged pores. However, if your skin is dark or particularly sensitive, be very careful to avoid irritation. There are various kinds of AHAs and different strengths to choose from, including malic, mandelic, lactic, and glycolic acids. The mandelic and malic acids tend to be much safer for dark skin, though be sure to ask your dermatologist if you are unsure which AHAs are right for your skin, and ask what strength to use. AHAs can also make your skin more sensitive to sunlight, so be sure to protect yourself properly.

Green Tea

Green tea is a fantastic ingredient to include in your skin-care routine due to its polyphenols, a type of flavonoid that enacts powerful antioxidant activity. Topically applied, green tea can help reduce inflammation in your skin, thereby preventing or slowing the formation of lines and wrinkles and reducing sagging skin. Some studies have shown that green tea can also reduce damage from environmental pollution and sun damage.[9]

Peptides

Peptides are protein fragments that have been shown to have some beneficial effects on skin. In particular, they help heal damaged tissue from scars and wrinkles and stimulate the production of healthy normal skin. Some research has shown that peptides can help enhance cell communication,[10] regulating the exchange and growth rates between layers of skin cells. Peptides can also prevent harmful oxidation that damages the skin, and they have anti-inflammatory properties that can better set up your skin to heal itself.

Essential Fatty Acids (EFAs)

EFAs reduce the amount of moisture lost through your epidermis, the top layer of your skin, thereby keeping your skin soft and elastic instead of dried out. They are particularly protective in cold or windy weather, which can strip away the skin's lipid barrier and contribute to skin conditions such as eczema. The anti-inflammatory properties of these essential fats are also helpful for eczema and psoriasis, and in preventing inflammation that can contribute to aging.

There are many natural sources for these essential fatty acids, such as shea butter, kukui nut, jojoba, rosehip, sesame seed, black currant, evening primrose, camellia seed, almond, apricot kernel, argan, hemp seed, manuka, kokum, pumpkin seed, olive, black cumin seed, coconut, sea buckthorn, avocado, borage, tamanu, and walnut oils.

Hyaluronic Acid (HA)

The body uses hyaluronic acid to make new cells, and it is a natural compound found in the skin. As we age, we produce less of this acid, so adding it back helps repair the skin and reduce inflammation. As a skin-care product ingredient, it helps not only to deliver moisture to the skin but also to hold it there, preventing moisture loss for continued smooth skin while protecting the skin from dirt, debris, and pollutants. It doesn't penetrate too deeply, staying near the surface of your skin. Hyaluronic acid was once produced largely from the comb of a rooster, but thankfully it is now produced in a lab from a fermentation process that involves plant materials.

Clay

There are different kinds of clays, which are a highly beneficial ingredient to include in skin masks. Sometimes masks are pushed to the side in a skin-care routine, but applying masks is an ancient beauty tool that can be very beneficial to use at least once a week (depending on your skin type) to help you maintain beautiful skin for the long-term.

Clay is a unique ingredient with the ability to absorb excess oils, dirt, and harmful toxins from the skin. Clays are made up of different mineral contents, which are unique to different types of clays, and these minerals help rejuvenate the skin as the clay simultaneously exfoliates and stimulates blood circulation to the skin. The more regularly you use clays, the fresher your skin will look. Improved circulation and the removal of debris from your pores instantly improve the brightness of your skin.

Rose clay is mild kaolin clay that is great for normal to dry skin and gently helps cleanse, exfoliate, and improve skin's condition. It gets its delicate pink color from the iron oxides it contains. White clay, also known as China clay, is

ANCIENT BEAUTY INGREDIENT: ROSE WATER

Roses are one of the most universally revered flowers for their beauty and sweet fragrance, but what can they do for your skin? In ancient Rome, rose water was allegedly used as a cleanser. Some even bathed in it. Rose water has also been a part of Indian skin care for millennia. Just like natural foods, natural skin-care ingredients can impart their beautifying properties onto you. Pure, true rose water is created from steam distillation of damask rose petals. It smells delicate and delicious and nothing like the synthetic and sickeningly strong fragrances that are used in toxic sprays and car air fresheners.

Rose water is said to have some antibacterial and antiseptic properties and is believed to help restore the skin's pH levels and tighten pores. It's also considered to be anti-inflammatory and to help regenerate skin tissue. The sugars and natural oils found in rose petals trap moisture in your skin, making your skin look smoother and softer—just like the beautiful rose petals themselves. Plus rose water's natural fragrance can help soothe your nervous system. This will help destress you, another key factor in keeping your skin youthful and healthy.

Try to find some pure rose water at a health store and add a few drops to your cleanser or moisturizer. You can also try using it as a toner, either pure or mixed with a bit of witch hazel, gently brushing it over your skin with a cotton pad after cleansing.

basically kaolinite and is the mildest of all clays. It helps stimulate circulation to the skin while gently exfoliating and cleansing. French green clay consists mostly of montmorillonite and is highly efficient at drawing oils and toxins from the skin. It also helps nourish the skin with minerals and phytonutrients. It is great for oily skin and is commonly included in spa body wraps. It's not recommended for sensitive or dry skin. Yellow kaolin clay is mild and stimulates circulation to the skin; it is suitable for use on sensitive skin as well as dry skin.

Bentonite clay is derived from deposits of weathered volcanic ash. It absorbs toxins such as heavy metals and other pollutants from the surface of your skin like a kitchen sponge. There is also an electrical aspect to bentonite clay's ability to bind and absorb toxins. Bentonite clay has a negative electrical charge, attracting positively charged molecules. As most toxins are positively charged, clay naturally rids the body of toxins as it pulls and holds the toxins in its core.[11]

Cosmetics Safety: Critical for Your Overall Beauty

Just because a cosmetic is sitting innocuously on the shelf at your local pharmacy, there's no guarantee that it is safe and will not have toxic ramifications on your body. The US Food and Drug Administration (FDA) has no authority to require companies to test cosmetic products for safety, and most products and ingredients are not approved or reviewed before they are placed on shelves. The FDA conducts premarket reviews only of certain cosmetics' color additives and active ingredients that are classified as over-the-counter drugs.[12,13] It also has no authority to require recalls of harmful cosmetics, and manufacturers are not required to report cosmetics-related injuries to the agency. The FDA relies on companies to report injuries voluntarily[14] (yes, you read that right—*voluntarily*!).

Cosmetics in the European Union are far more strictly regulated. There, over 1,000 ingredients have been banned from use. In contrast, the FDA has only prohibited a fraction of those ingredients, including some color additives and other prohibited substances.[15] Another scary fact is that federal law allows companies to leave some chemical ingredients off their product labels, including those considered to be trade secrets and some components of fragrance and nanomaterials.[16]

Since the FDA does not play a big role in regulating the safety of ingredients, it has authorized the cosmetics industry to police itself with the Cosmetic Ingredient Review panel. To date, in its thirty-plus-year history, the industry panel has declared only eleven ingredients or chemical groups to be unsafe,[17] and its recommendations on restricting ingredients are not binding on companies.[18] So it doesn't sound like much real "policing" is going on. Where does that leave us, as consumers?

Ingredients from cosmetics not only are absorbed through the skin but are also often swallowed and inhaled from sprays and powders. Many of them are hormone disruptors that can create developmental and reproductive damage and allergic reactions, act as carcinogens, and create other kinds of damage in the body.[19,20] It's ultra-important to understand labels and ingredients, as the FDA says that descriptions such as "hypoallergenic" or "natural" can "mean anything or nothing at all."[21] Don't assume that companies or any prevailing organizations—governmental or otherwise—are necessarily looking out for your best interests. It's important to scan labels and look into the ethos of brands that you choose to use in and on your body. Ultimately, we have to look out for our families and ourselves and not leave our safety in the hands of anyone else.

Toxic Skin-Care Ingredients to Avoid

There are countless toxins and additives in commercial skin-care, makeup, body-care, and other personal-care products. It would fill this entire book (and more) to list and describe them all. But there are some common offenders that are worse than others. For more information, the Campaign for Safe Cosmetics (safecosmetics.org/) and the Environmental Working Group Skin Deep Cosmetics Database (ewg.org/skindeep/) are two great resources to consult about the toxicity of specific products and ingredients. These organizations, as well as certain reports, believe that toxic ingredients can create DNA damage; act as carcinogens; create brain, liver, kidney, and other organ abnormalities; produce allergic or other reactions; and cause eye damage, nervous system damage, reproductive damage, and birth defects.[22] The list of these possible dangers continues to grow as more chemicals are introduced and studied.

Here are some of the most glaringly toxic ingredients to avoid. Again, this is like a drop in the ocean, *not* an exhaustive list:

- Benzoyl peroxide
- Synthetic (or artificial) FD&C colors and dyes
- Propylene glycol (PG) and butylene glycol
- Diethanolamine (DEA), monoethanolamine (MEA), and triethanolamine (TEA)

- Methyl-, butyl-, ethyl-, and propylparabens
- Sodium lauryl sulfate (SLS) and sodium laureth sulfate (SLES)
- Dioxin
- Polyethylene glycol (PEG)
- Avobenzone
- Phthalates
- Triclosan
- DMDM hydantoin and imidazolidinyl urea

RADICALLY TIMELESS BEAUTY MASK

This nourishing mask will leave your skin feeling moisturized, smooth, and radiant. Used regularly, it can help ward off wrinkles and puffiness. These ingredients are rich in nourishing enzymes, vitamin E, and beauty fats and oils.

1 tablespoon raw, organic honey 1 teaspoon rose water
1 teaspoon almond oil

Combine the ingredients in a small bowl. Apply to your face and neck for about 15 to 20 minutes. Rinse well.

Sunscreen Ingredients: Wading Through the Toxic and the Safe

It's well established that sunscreen can help protect against skin cancers and sun damage. The risk isn't entirely related to how much sun hits your unprotected skin, since exposure when you were a child can lead to a higher risk of skin cancer as an adult, and the exposure doesn't need to be drastic. The best rule, however, is to protect yourself from the sun's ultraviolet (UV) radiation as much as you can. Best medical advice also holds that you use a higher sunblock number. Simple measures like wearing a sun hat with a wide brim help remove the burden from sunblocks, along with sitting in the shade and wearing sunglasses that are UV resistant.

Also be aware that there are a multitude of toxic ingredients in most sunscreens. When choosing a sunscreen, look for products with the active ingredient zinc oxide or titanium dioxide. These are physical protectants, which reflect UV rays off your skin, rather than chemical products.

Here are some toxic skin-care ingredients to look out for and avoid.

OXYBENZONE (AKA BENZOPHENONE-3)

While the American Academy of Dermatology says oxybenzone is safe, the Environmental Working Group (EWG) and other toxicology experts believe that oxybenzone is linked to hormone disruption and potentially to cell damage that may lead to skin cancer.[23] Some studies have linked oxybenzone use in pregnant women to low birth weight,[24] which can lead to serious health problems later in life; it also may impact the adrenal system[25] and may also reduce testosterone levels in men.[26]

NANOPARTICLES

These are extremely tiny particles added to sunscreen that are easily absorbed by the skin. About 100,000 times smaller than the width of a human hair, these tiny particles can penetrate the blood-brain barrier, leading to damage or genetic changes in the brain cells.[27] Be sure that the ingredients on your sunscreen are in a non-nano form. This even goes for safer sunscreen ingredients such as zinc oxide and titanium dioxide, as micronized titanium dioxide has been associated with cellular damage.[28]

RETINYL PALMITATE

In a National Toxicology Program study on lab animals, it was found that when skin is treated with a mix of retinyl palmitate (RP), a vitamin A derivative, and skin cream and exposed to ultraviolet light, the cream with retinyl palmitate stimulated lesion and tumor growth.[29] As discussed earlier, while vitamin A may be considered a wonderful skin-care ingredient in its natural state, it should be restricted to night creams for those that choose to use it—and never used in sunscreen.

OCTYL METHOXYCINNAMATE (AKA OCTINOXATE, EUSOLEX 2292, AND UVINUL MC80)

This is an ingredient that is believed to create free radicals inside the skin, which can create cellular and DNA damage. Similar to oxybenzone, it works with other penetration enhancers to enter through the skin and accumulate in the body. It has the potential to possibly create phototoxic effects, meaning that toxic reactions are provoked by light.[30]

PADIMATE O (AKA PARA-AMINOBENZOIC ACID, OR PABA)

Because this can be very irritating to the skin, it has largely been phased out of most sunscreens. But it's worth looking out for, just in case it's still lurking around in some brands. According to the EWG, PABA can release free radicals, create allergic reactions, damage DNA, and induce estrogenic activity; and they implicated padimate O as a nitrosamine, a class of compounds that may be carcinogenic.[31]

SOLAR BEAUTY SMOOTHER TREATMENT

Almond, argan, and olive oils are particularly good for replenishing the moisture in dry skin and contain vitamin E and nourishing minerals. Sweet orange oil is believed to be particularly effective in helping rejuvenate and revitalize the skin against sun damage.

2 teaspoons almond oil
1 teaspoon argan or avocado oil

8 drops sweet orange essential oil

Combine all ingredients until mixed well. Rub onto sun-exposed areas, reapplying two or three times per day. For a firmer, more cream-like consistency, store in a glass or BPA-free container in the refrigerator.

Beautiful Underarms: Toxic Versus Safe Deodorants and Antiperspirants

One beautiful way your body was designed for detoxification is to allow wastes to evaporate through the pores of your skin. A key area where your body detoxes itself is under your arms, where sweat glands and lymph nodes are located. The modern concept of using antiperspirants to stop your underarms from sweating can hold toxicity in. This is not natural or recommended.

Clogging your body's normal channels for waste removal is not a good idea. You can wipe or cleanse your underarms during the day if you are concerned about excessive moisture, and there are natural solutions to prevent underarm odor. Keep in mind that as you clean up your diet and improve your digestion and the elimination of wastes in your system, your level of offensive bodily odors may naturally decrease. But you will probably still want to use something to ensure that you always smell fresh and clean. When you do, it's important to choose your deodorant wisely. Commercial deodorants contain some potentially toxic materials that you should try to avoid. Some of these ingredients include aluminum, parabens, propylene glycol, triclosan, TEA, DEA, FD&C, phthalates, and talc.

Aluminum has been linked to Alzheimer's, cancer, and allergic reactions. Some people dispute the link between the type of aluminum used in deodorants and these diseases,[32] but others believe it is worth avoiding. Some have suggested that aluminum-based compounds in antiperspirants may be absorbed through the skin and can be a health risk factor, though much more research is needed to show a definite link. With all the alternatives out there nowadays in various deodorants, you can certainly avoid aluminum if you choose.

Parabens mimic the activity of estrogen in the body. Since estrogen promotes the growth of breast cancer cells, and a woman is eight times more likely to develop breast cancer in the part of the breast closest to the underarm, scientists are studying the connection, though further studies and research are needed.

RADICALLY SAFE DEODORANT

It is easy to make your own deodorant that is safe and effective in eliminating unpleasant underarm odor! The coconut oil and baking powder in this DIY version both have antibacterial properties and help prevent odor, while the grapefruit extract smells bright and fresh and has antibacterial and antiseptic qualities as well. The arrowroot helps thicken your deodorant into a somewhat solid form that is easy to apply.

3 tablespoons coconut oil

3 tablespoons baking powder

1¹/₂ tablespoons ground arrowroot

40 (or so) drops grapefruit extract

In a bowl, mix together all the ingredients until well combined into a thick, paste-like consistency. Store in the refrigerator for 20 to 30 minutes to let the coconut oil resolidify if it liquefied during the mixing process. Place the mixture into a small glass or BPA-free container. Dip your fingers into the mixture and apply it directly to your underarms. To keep your deodorant solid, be sure to store it in a cool place, but even if it liquefies a bit, it will still work just as well!

Practices to Nourish Your Skin from the Outside In

In Pillar 1, you learned to boost your beauty from the inside out by eating foods with unique properties that help boost circulation and support your body's natural processes. Many people don't realize that in addition to using the right skin-care products, there are also many things you can do to improve the body's functions from the outside in.

Supporting Your Lymphatic Circulation for Enhanced Detoxification and Slowed Aging

Most people don't think about it that much, but we have a second circulatory system devoted to healing and immunity known as the lymphatic system. Composed of your spleen, thymus, lymph, lymph nodes, and lymph channels as well as your tonsils and adenoids, your lymphatic system works directly with your cardiovascular circulatory system to keep blood and lymphatic fluid levels in balance and flush toxins out of the body. Fluid squeezed from the blood, called interstitial fluid or "lymph," transports waste to your lymph nodes through a series of vessels similar to veins. There, the fluid is neutralized, filtered, and eventually returned to the bloodstream. These vessels also carry immune cells throughout the body to help defend against infections.

Called *rasa* in Ayurveda, your lymph is part of the plasma that is considered part of the primary *dhatu,* or structure of the body. Healthy *rasa* is key in order to give rise to the next *dhatu,* healthy *rakta,* or blood, and consequently the other *dhatus* in the body. *Rasa* is said to govern your emotional and hunger responses, which is another good reason to keep it flowing.

Unlike the cardiovascular system, the heart does not pump the lymphatic system, which is basically self-circulating. Gravity, muscle contractions, and certain forms of movement and manipulation stimulate this system. If your lymphatic circulation gets sluggish, toxins build up, which is the precursor to accelerated aging.[1] Aches and pains can also appear, and your immunity is lowered. This can adversely affect your thymus gland, tonsils, and spleen, which in turn can weaken your body against sickness and diseases. Traditional Chinese Medicine believes that your spleen plays a central part in your vitality and strength.

Because the two systems work together, incorporating the foods recommended in Pillar 1 for your cardiovascular system will also be beneficial for your lymphatic system. However, since your almighty heart does not pump the lymphatic system, there are specific methods to support this system that are applied to the outside of the body. Here are some great methods you can incorporate to support your lymph system and nourish glowing, healthy skin from the outside in.

GET A MASSAGE

Massages are incredibly beneficial for detoxification. Stimulating the blood and lymph vessels helps move the fluids and enhance circulation. Professional massages are wonderful, as well as a regular practice of self-massage.

PRACTICE ABHYANGA

This ancient form of self-massage is a powerful anti-aging practice that can easily be incorporated into your daily routine. *Abhyanga* will make you feel rejuvenated, soften your skin, and contribute to a better overall skin tone while also fostering muscle tone. There is a belief in Ayurveda that working manually on the surface of the skin helps support the structure and health of your muscles, as there is a connection between your skin and muscle health. Some of *abhyanga's* deeper, detoxifying properties are meant to be cumulative and long-term, so you may not witness immediate benefits, but you will likely feel invigorated by the movement while you trust that deeper support for detoxification is taking place beneath the surface! As you know, the importance of improving circulation and detoxification (which is part of what *abhyanga* is all about) cannot be overestimated for its long-term role in maintaining your health and beauty.

Abhyanga has been part of Ayurveda for thousands of years and is perhaps the foremost anti-aging practice you can incorporate into your daily life. That is a pretty strong statement, but *abhyanga* can help balance your entire mind and body, relieve fatigue, provide stamina, enhance sleep, promote a better complexion, improve the luster of your skin, increase longevity, and foster all-around body nourishment. You may be skeptical that a simple self-massage practice can really reap all those benefits, but as you progress in your understanding of the circulation and lymphatic system, you'll surely realize these benefits and appreciate how anti-aging *abhyanga* truly is.

First, it's important to learn more about your skin. Besides being a major elimination organ, your skin is the largest organ of sensory perception. Your skin takes in a great deal of information from the outside world and is connected to every part of the body by thousands of nerves throughout your entire nervous system. As such, Ayurveda believes that touching the outside of your skin has a big impact on your nervous system, while your nervous system further impacts your endocrine system and immunity. An imbalanced nervous system can manifest in excessive worry, decreased energy, imbalanced digestion, and can eventually contribute to deeper and more plentiful wrinkles, as you generally age at a much faster rate when your nervous system is imbalanced.

Stress and toxins constantly accumulate in the mind and body, but thankfully *abhyanga* can help dissolve them on a daily basis. By manually working with skin, Ayurveda claims you can help bring yourself back to the present moment and reduce excessive *Vata* energy, or an overabundance of the air element that can make you feel flighty, anxious, and ungrounded. In other words, the sense of touch can help settle your overactive, restless mind as it recharges and rejuvenates you.

On a physical level, according to Ayurvedic texts, *abhyanga* prevents the accumulation of physiological toxins, known as *ama,* and lubricates muscles, tissues, and joints, promoting flexibility. Ancient Ayurvedic texts claim that it also improves the softness and luster of the skin. Exercising or taking a hot shower after practicing *abhyanga* helps the oil penetrate the dermis, which further nourishes the collagen and elastin. The penetration of the oil into the skin can also help to remove toxins and debris while improving the health of blood vessels.

For your oil, sesame oil is best to use in the winter because it is considered warming, while coconut oil is considered cooling and therefore recommended for the warmer summer months. You can also try special Ayurvedic herbal oils that you can source from a reputable Ayurvedic purveyor or find online, or make your own massage oil. Be sure any oil you use is organic, unrefined, and cold-pressed.

Ideally, do your *abhyanga* practice in the morning. This will help release the toxins that have accumulated during the night and rejuvenate you for the day. To avoid slipping, we recommend sitting on the floor or a chair near your shower. Start by warming the chosen oil slightly by holding it under hot water for a few minutes. Then apply some of the warmed oil to your hands and massage your entire body for 5 to 10 minutes, applying even pressure with your palm and fingers. Apply lighter pressure to sensitive areas such as your upper torso, breasts, heart, and abdominal area. When you are massaging your abdomen, start on the right side (from your perspective when looking down) and then make a circular motion up, across, and down the left side. This supports the natural pathway of digestion. Spend a few moments conducting this circular pathway.

Next, take more oil and spend time massaging the soles of your feet, the palms of your hands, and the base of your fingernails, where there are many nerve endings. Don't forget about your face, ears, and neck. Be sure to give them some love, too! Don't worry; pure, organic oils should not make you break out. (If you have excessively oily skin and are worried about breakouts, you can always avoid your face.) On days when you are going to wash your hair (which could be one to five times a week, depending on your hair type), spend some time massaging your entire scalp. Use circular motions over rounded areas such as your feet and scalp and straight, longer strokes on your limbs. If you don't have much time, focus on your feet and scalp; Ayurveda teaches that these are the most important areas to stimulate with touch.

When you're done, make sure you've rubbed the oil in as much as possible, especially on your feet; be very careful to rub in all oils on the bottom of your feet before attempting walking or showering! It's common to use too much oil at first, but you will soon reach the right amount. Towel off with a fresh towel. Then you can choose to work out or go straight into a hot shower. The heat from your workout (or the shower) will help the oil penetrate transdermally. This will strengthen the connective skin tissues and help your skin stay supple and healthily beautiful. In the shower, only use soap on your private parts and underarms. Excessive use of soap can strip your skin of moisture, and coconut and other oils have antibacterial, cleansing properties. If you still feel oily or greasy, use a natural soap sparingly. After you towel off, you'll find a thin film of oil on your skin. This will help your skin stay moisturized and protected, while keeping your muscles warm throughout the day.

BEAUTY SECRET IN A TINY SEED: SESAME OIL

Coconut oil is all the rage right now (and for good reason), but sesame oil is another great natural, nongreasy moisturizing oil. Don't worry; you don't have to smell like your neighborhood Chinese take-out joint. In fact, Asian cooking oils are not the right kind. Pure, cold-pressed sesame oil is what you want; it has a mild, pleasant scent and is absorbed readily into your skin. If you purchase sesame oil that has a strong odor, it's probably roasted or toasted sesame oil. Unroasted, cold-pressed sesame oil, on the other hand, is highly lubricating and fantastic for both your skin and scalp, promoting vitality and healthy hair growth. Keep it refrigerated except for the daily amounts you set aside for your massage.

Sesame oil is highly nourishing and healing and contains vitamin E and B vitamins, amino acids, and minerals such as magnesium, calcium, and phosphorus. It helps soften your skin and hair, keeping them hydrated by locking moisture in. Sesame oil will effectively penetrate deeper into the epidermis to moisturize and repair skin, especially if heat is applied after sesame oil application (as from a hot shower after *abhyanga*). Sesame oil is particularly protective against pollution and effective at revitalizing damaged hair from deep within.

DRY BRUSHING

Like *abhyanga*, dry brushing is a manual treatment that is great for improving circulation and rejuvenating your skin. You can actually integrate dry brushing into your *abhyanga* routine by dry brushing for just a few minutes right before applying the oil and starting the self-massage. This heightens the benefits of *abhyanga* even more.

Like other forms of sloughing the skin to exfoliate, dry brushing has been practiced widely around the world, from Japan to Sweden. Manually working with the skin—our largest organ of sensory perception made of multiple cell layers, glands, and densely packed nerve cells—has amazing whole body benefits. It helps remove dead skin cells and clear out clogged pores, allowing your body to eliminate wastes and toxins more efficiently. This also activates waste removal via your lymphatic system, draining wastes through your lymph nodes and lymphatic drainage. Increasing circulation to your skin allows metabolic wastes to clear from your body more efficiently, making dry brushing a great detoxifying aid.

Like a light massage, dry brushing also provides some anti-stress benefits and may even help with bloating. Massaging the lymph nodes can help the body shed excess water and toxins, improving kidney function and flushing out your system. Dry skin brushing rejuvenates the nervous system by stimulating nerve endings in the skin, and it feels pretty great, too! (Well, it can feel a little rough at first when you are getting used to it, but it will leave you feeling revitalized and with a great memory of the experience.) Last but not least, dry brushing will almost certainly help make your skin glow and become tighter. Try it for yourself and see what kinds of benefits you experience!

To do it yourself, all you need is about 2 to 3 minutes a day (ideally layered into your *abhyanga* practice) and a long-handled brush made from dry bristles, which you can generally purchase for under $20 online or at a health market. Starting at your feet, brush your skin in long strokes toward your heart. Be sure to brush your legs, arms, chest, back, and stomach. Avoid sensitive areas, such as your face, and be very careful with delicate areas like varicose veins (though gentle dry brushing can be great for flat spider veins). Be firm, but don't press too hard. Your skin should be pink when you're done but certainly not red or irritated. Afterward, be sure to engage in your *abhyanga* practice or apply a natural moisturizer or emollient oil, such as shea butter or coconut or sesame oil. Since dry brushing helps slough off the dead, outer cells, your skin will be able to hydrate more efficiently and absorb more moisture.

Kelp is seaweed that is rich in minerals and vitamins. Used in a mask form, it will draw impurities out of your skin as it also helps restore nutrition to your complexion.

2 tablespoons kelp powder   2 teaspoons filtered water
4 fl oz (125 ml) aloe vera gel

Combine the kelp and aloe vera in a small bowl. Slowly mix in the water until you create a thick paste. Apply to your face and neck for about 15 to 20 minutes. Rinse well.

JUMP ON A TRAMPOLINE

This type of movement is particularly good for increasing lymph flow, as the up-and-down rhythmic gravitational force created by bouncing encourages the lymph system's one-way valves to open and close.

GO FOR A WALK OR HIKE

In addition to all the other benefits of getting out into nature (not to mention exercise), walking is a great way to help move your lymphatic system and improve circulation.

CLEANSE

Try a properly administered cleanse, especially in the springtime. If well designed and followed, this can be a great way to detox your whole system and let your lymph system flush out accumulated wastes and toxins. If you are interested, check out Kimberly's organic smoothie and juice company (myglowbio.com) for cleanses she designs that ship nationally.

WEAR LOOSE CLOTHING

Tight clothing can restrict your body's natural circulation, so peel yourself out of your skinny jeans (at least part of the time) and incorporate more flowing skirts and maxi dresses into your wardrobe. You'll be more comfy—and more detoxed. After detoxing your lymphatic system with looser clothes on most days, you'll look even better on those nights when you do want to wear a tight, slinky dress.

PRACTICE HYDROTHERAPY

If you've ever been to a traditional Korean spa, you'll find a cold plunge pool next to a hot pool. Experiencing side-by-side temperature shifts externally to the outer surface of your skin (again, *not* by saturating your internal organs with icy liquids!) is believed to be invigorating in some Eastern traditions, as it promotes enhanced blood flow and great circulation throughout your whole body. You can do this at home by simply alternating warm and cold water in the shower. Start your shower with a few minutes of warm water, and then shift the dial for 2 minutes of cold water. Make it as cold as you can stand it! Then continue alternating, ending your shower with cold water. You will feel refreshed and energized, and your hair will look shinier (on the days you wash it). What an excellent way to start the day—your skin will also be glowing all over!

NERVOUS SYSTEM SOOTHING MASSAGE OIL

Jojoba oil is a great carrier oil for most essential oils because it is easily absorbed into your skin and is rich in vitamin E. Neroli essential oil is a great choice for this skin recipe, as research has found neroli helps reduce anxiety and improve sleep quality.[2] Besides its calming, grounding properties, it has a lovely sweet and spicy aroma.

Combine 4 fl oz (125 ml) jojoba oil and 40 drops neroli essential oil, using it in your *abhyanga* practice or with just a quick, modified hand or foot massage at the end of the day—or whenever you feel you need some soothing.

Address Specific Skin Issues

While the ingredients we discussed earlier will naturally boost your skin's glow and vitality, there are some common skin issues that respond well to particular ingredients. In this shift, you'll learn tips to overcome any issues that might be plaguing your skin. We've also included recipes for masks and tonics that were designed specifically for each individual concern.

Acne

Acne is an all too common skin condition that can be exacerbated by impurities in your blood that push out through your skin, causing breakouts. Here are some of the best ways to cut down on these impurities and create clear, radiant skin:

- Reduce consumption of oils in general and high fat, heavy foods. Excessive oils in the system can aggravate your moisture balance and clog the pores.
- Incorporate cumin, turmeric, and ginger when cooking to boost digestion and help promote pure, healthy blood.
- Eliminate dairy from your diet, which some research has linked to acne.[1]
- Take an excellent probiotic supplement (see page 33) and an oxygen-magnesium supplement, which is a nonlaxative, non-habit-forming, and nonirritating internal cleanser that is free of gluten, animal products, and corn.

Here are a few good skin-care ingredients to target acne:

TEA TREE OIL

This has antibacterial and soothing properties and is a great alternative to benzoyl peroxide, which can be drying and irritating.

CLAY

This is great, especially in face masks, as it helps to calm the skin and balance sebum production (see page 111 for more details).

RADICALLY CLEAR SKIN MASK

The bentonite clay in this mask will help draw out impurities in your skin and balance oils, while raw honey has both antibacterial and antiseptic properties.

1 tablespoon water $1^1/2$ teaspoons bentonite clay
1 teaspoon raw, organic honey

Mix the water with the honey first, then stir in the clay and mix well to form a paste. Apply to your entire face, being careful to avoid contact with your eyes. Leave on for about 20 minutes, then rinse well. Try using this mask once or twice a week for problematic skin.

ALPHA HYDROXY ACIDS (AHAs)

These help to exfoliate dead skin cells, prevent clogged pores, and leave your skin smoother (see page 109 for more details).

Used externally, cranberries and oregano both have some astringent properties, which helps cleanse the skin and balance its oils.

2 to 3 tablespoons filtered water
plus a bit more as needed
1 tablespoon dried oregano

$3^1/_2$ oz (100 g) cranberries
(dried is okay)

Boil the water and stir in the oregano. Turn off the heat, cover, and allow the oregano to steep for 15 minutes. Strain and set aside. Next, puree the cranberries in a food processor or blender (adding a few tablespoons of filtered water as needed for dried cranberries). Strain through a cheesecloth. Combine the cranberry puree with the oregano liquid. Soak a washcloth in the liquid, place it on your face, and relax for 15 minutes. (Listen to some calming music so you aren't tempted to move around!) Rinse with warm water.

Bags Under the Eyes

Poor drainage of fluids can contribute to puffy, baggy under-eye circles. It's important to keep your circulation working optimally and prevent a buildup of fluids, which can be done by eating foods with balanced electrolytes (essential minerals that affect your body-fluid balance, among other critical processes) and avoiding too much sodium. Bags under the eyes can also mean you have a buildup of impurities from sluggish digestion or overtaxed adrenals, so be sure to incorporate lots of lemons and lemon water to flush out your system and to supply your body with vitamin C. Before we talk about some of the remedies for the skin around your eyes, here are some more tips to avoid or improve the existence of bags under your eyes:

- Increase your rest and sleep, especially if you're a woman on your moon, or menstrual, cycle; a lack of sleep can exacerbate the visibility of under-eye issues.

- Avoid (or at least cut down as much as possible) on caffeine and alcohol, which can leach minerals from your system and tax your adrenals, contributing to under-eye bags and circles.
- Avoid smoked, grilled, or barbecued foods, which tend to be excessively high in sodium (as well as nitrosamines, which are considered carcinogenic).
- Incorporate coconut water, which helps balance electrolytes such as potassium and sodium.
- Hydrate more in general, as some research out of Oxford University has shown the appearance of the skin under the eyes is linked to kidney health,[2] and your kidneys function best in the presence of abundant hydration.
- Make sure to incorporate banana into your Glowing Green Smoothie (see page 27 for recipe), which is high in B vitamins and potassium; these are great for helping to keep your skin smooth and puffiness at bay.
- Cut out refined sugars and use only stevia or raw coconut nectar as your go-to sweeteners. Unlike refined white or artificial sugars, stevia and raw coconut nectar won't tax your adrenals and cause inflammation, a by-product of which can be under-eye bags and puffiness.
- Avoid consuming other foods with high sodium, such as soya sauce, close to bedtime. This can contribute to greater dehydration throughout the night and can cause you to wake up sporting prominently pronounced under-eye bags.

Here are a few good skin-care ingredients to target under-eye bags:

Peptides
Look for this on ingredient lists. They are great for supporting healthy collagen and elastin in the structure of your skin, which will help it stay taut and less prone to bagginess.

Topical Coenzyme Q10
This can support the amount of adenosine triphosphate (ATP), which transports chemical energy between skin cells for improved overall function and enhanced skin repair and regeneration.

Almond milk is full of vitamin E and is believed to be anti-inflammatory,[3] while rose water also possesses anti-inflammatory properties and is soothing to the skin, helping to make it soft and smooth.

1 tablespoon rose water   1 tablespoon cold almond milk

Mix the two ingredients together. Dip a washcloth into the mixture and place over your eyes for 10 minutes in the evening while you lie down and relax.

Cellulite

Beyond just a simple accumulation of fat, cellulite can involve the breakdown of collagen and the buildup of heavy metals and toxins in fat cells. Many of us believe that cellulite is something they just have to live with, and it's true that it's a natural phenomenon in at least 70 percent of people, but there are things you can do to cut down on the appearance of it. Here are some of the most effective methods:

- Infrared sauna sessions help penetrate tissues and fat cells and encourage your body to let go of heavy metals that can expand fat cells.
- Perform dry brushing (see page 124) on a regular basis over the cellulite-infected areas to move stagnant lymph.
- Cook only with coconut oil and avoid cooking with vegetable oils that become rancid at higher temperatures. Rancid oils can be very difficult for your body to break down, so they may contribute to excess storage in your fat cells that can amplify the appearance of cellulite.

There is limited to no scientific proof that cellulite creams actually work, but if you want to try using a cream on top of your other efforts, here are a few ingredients to look into:

VITAMIN A

This has been proven to thicken the uppermost skin-cell layer, thereby reducing the appearance of lumpy cellulite. However, refer back to page 109 for more information on potential toxicity precautions about vitamin A ingredients. And if you are trying to conceive or you're pregnant or nursing, it's important to forgo vitamin A products altogether.

CAFFEINE

Used topically, caffeine can improve blood flow to the skin and is purported to help reduce the appearance of cellulite.

RADICAL ENZYME MASK

Pineapple has potent detoxifying properties and contains bromelain, a protein-digesting enzyme that helps exfoliate dead cells and debris. It also has anti-inflammatory properties and high levels of vitamin C. Papaya contains papain, a natural enzyme that can help to remove and exfoliate dead skin cells, as well as high levels of beta-carotene and vitamin C.

You can try applying this mask to cellulite-affected areas. As the enzymes, beta-carotene, and vitamin C support the collagen in those areas, they may help minimize the appearance of the cellulite over time. This mask is also great for your complexion. Please note that the enzymes in fresh pineapple are "tingly" and pretty potent, so if you have sensitive skin, be sure to test a tiny area first to see if this mask irritates your skin.

$3^1/_2$ oz (100 g) freshly cut pineapple*
$1^1/_2$ oz (40 g) freshly cut papaya*
1 teaspoon cold-pressed olive oil

1 teaspoon ground arrowroot, or a little more, as needed

*Note: The pineapple and papaya must be freshly sliced from a whole fruit for this mask to be effective. Precut or canned fruit will not work, as the enzymes will be denatured and some or all of the vitamin C might have oxidized.

Blend the pineapple, papaya, and olive oil in a blender until nearly smooth (but do not overblend or potentially overheat the mixture); because it's a small amount, you can also mash the ingredients in a mortar and pestle. Mix with the arrowroot starch until a thicker paste is achieved. Apply the mixture immediately to your face and leave on for 15 to 20 minutes before rinsing off.

Dry Skin

Dry skin is a common issue that is often the result of imbalances in your diet or environment. Here are a few of the best ways to keep your skin moisturized and glowing.

- Practice *abhyanga* regularly (see page 121) using cold-pressed, unrefined oils. Be sure to rinse off in the shower afterward before applying any additional moisturizer.
- Avoid eating too many dry, crispy foods such as crackers, pretzels, and so on.
- Make sure you are taking a plant-based omega-3 DHA and EPA supplement.
- Incorporate easily digested beauty fats such as avocados, coconut oil, and chia seeds. Make sure you aren't avoiding fat altogether!
- Eat lots of sweet, juicy fruits to hydrate your skin.
- Drink lots of room temperature water.
- If your home environment is very dry, consider getting a humidifier.
- Avoid very hot showers and limit time in hot baths, which can dry out your skin.
- Avoid drying cleansers that can strip your skin of its natural moisture balance, such as ones that contain alcohol.

Here are a few skin-care ingredients to incorporate for dry skin:

HYALURONIC ACID

This is produced naturally in your body and is also found in topical products. It helps attract moisture and keeps your skin moisturized and hydrated.

SHEA AND COCONUT BUTTERS

These are two examples of natural, plant-based occlusives that create a thin film over the skin, lock in moisture, and slow the evaporation of water loss from your skin's surface, helping to create a barrier against water loss.

GRAPE-SEED OIL

This is a great natural moisturizer that helps strengthen cell membranes. It contains antioxidants, vitamins, minerals, and other nutrients. There are many other great natural plant oils, including black cumin seed, hemp seed, tamanu, almond, and so on.

RADICAL BEAUTY SKIN TEXTURE SMOOTHING MASK

Coconut yogurt is a great source of amino acids and probiotics, carrot is high in skin-brightening beta-carotene and antioxidants, and avocado is a rich source of nourishing beauty fats, vitamins, and lecithin to nourish dry skin, leaving it feeling soft and smooth. Try applying this mask on a regular basis (ideally once a week) to see your skin become smoother with diminished age spots.

4 oz (125 g) coconut yogurt (found at local health markets and some supermarkets)
1 avocado, peeled and pitted

3 tablespoons raw, organic honey
1 organic carrot

In a food processor or blender, combine the ingredients and process until you reach a smooth consistency. Spread over your face and neck and relax for 15 to 20 minutes before rinsing.

Red Patchiness

According to Ayurveda, red patches are caused by too much *Pitta* fire present, which may be generated from within by foods that are allergenic or inflammatory.

Try eliminating common allergens, such as dairy and gluten, for two weeks and see if symptoms subside. Here are some additional tips for cutting down on this common skin ailment:

- Avoid spicy and pungent foods and spices such as chilies and chili powder to cut down on internal "fire."
- Take probiotics and eat probiotic-rich foods, such as raw sauerkraut (known in the Beauty Detox community as Probiotic & Enzyme Salad).
- To ensure your digestion is efficient and regular, try adding a magnesium-oxygen supplement in the evenings.
- Try adding some turmeric, which has cleansing properties, to your soups and when cooking veggies.
- Sip warm herbal teas during the day to help keep the microcirculatory channels flowing and free of toxins.
- Drink coconut water, which is cooling.
- Incorporate lots of raw greens into your diet, since raw greens are considered cooling.
- Eat sweet, watery fruits such as pineapples and mangoes to help balance the internal "fire."
- Avoid full body saunas and spa treatments that saturate your face in heat. The half infrared sauna is a great option (see Kimberly's website for recommendations at kimberlysnyder.com).
- Avoid fragrances, dyes, and acids, which can all be irritating to the skin.

Here are a few great skin-care ingredients to incorporate for red, patchy skin:

- Chamomile and aloe are soothing ingredients for your skin.
- Green tea acts as a natural anti-inflammatory and helps neutralize aging and irritating free radicals.

Cucumber, green tea, and chamomile are all cooling, anti-inflammatory ingredients that are fantastic for soothing inflamed skin. You do not necessarily have to peel an organic cuke, as there is lots of zinc and other minerals in the skin. As with all recipes in this book and in general, use organic products as much as possible.

2 tablespoons cucumber, peeled and seeded

1 teaspoon brewed and cooled green tea (preferably loose leaf)

1 teaspoon brewed and cooled chamomile tea (preferably loose leaf)

1 tablespoon aloe vera gel

1 tablespoon ground arrowroot

Blend the cucumber, green tea, and chamomile tea together (if you have trouble blending such a small amount, just mash the cucumber in a mortar and pestle with the teas). Mix in the aloe vera gel and arrowroot until the mixture starts to thicken. Place in the refrigerator for about 30 minutes to cool. Spread over face and neck in an even layer and relax for about 20 minutes before rinsing it off.

Spider Veins

You can blame your grandmother for these beauties. Poor Granny is sweet and innocent, and you sure do love that great lady, but the fact is that vein issues are largely linked to heredity. Most of us never think about our veins and take them completely for granted. That is, until they start rearing their bluish, unwanted heads up to the surface! There are two main types of cosmetically unfortunate vein issues. The first is varicose veins, which can be a more serious form of venous insufficiency. These can lead to pain and soreness, as well as restless legs. If these issues have become a problem for you, get them checked out by your doctor.

On the other hand, telangiectasia, commonly known as spider veins, can indicate a much more mild form of venous insufficiency. They are cosmetically a doozy, but are not health- or life-threatening. So what causes these unfortunate blue malfunctions? Broken-down valves in the veins cause venous insufficiency.

These malfunctioning valves prevent blood flow back to the arteries, which can cause blood to accumulate and pool up. Such vein issues can become more pronounced if one is sedentary or has reduced circulation, and they can even be aggravated by hormonal issues like hormone replacement therapy, pregnancy, or birth control.[4] Here are some things you can do about them:

- Walk around often to keep circulation flowing.
- If you stand still often, look into compression hose to help with support. Some are more visually appealing than others, and you might not want to wear some of them on your bare legs (at least out in public), but you can certainly wear them under a long skirt or pants.
- When showering, massage the area around the broken veins first in a gentle circular motion and then in an upward motion to help improve circulation. (Avoid this with painful varicose veins.)
- Dry brush your skin, as discussed earlier on page 124, which helps stimulate the growth and repair of the tissues and underlying veins by increasing blood flow to the area. It also helps remove the blood that has leaked out of the capillaries by diffusing it into the interstitial fluids for removal. Brushing the spider veins very gently in a circular motion then upward toward the heart several times per day can improve their appearance.
- Vitamins A, B complex, C, D, and E are all great nutrients to help with tissue repair, optimal circulation, and strong veins. Great sources include carrots, nutritional yeast, mushrooms, almonds, lemons, and peppers.
- Avoid inflammatory vegetable oils, especially when cooked, which can become rancid in your body and increase free radicals and cellular damage.
- Make sure you eat the right beauty fats, such as avocados, coconut oil, and olive oil (best taken raw and lightly on certain dishes such as salads). This can help you build nice strong cell walls.
- Eat pineapple! It contains a dietary enzyme called bromelain, which can improve overall circulation by reducing the buildup of fibrin along the walls of the blood vessels.

- Spider veins are often associated with the use of hormone replacement therapy (HRT) and birth control pills. High levels of estrogen from these medications seem to aggravate venous insufficiency. If you are using birth control pills, you may want to ask your doctor for a lower-estrogen-dose formula. If you are on HRT, you may want to consider switching to a lower dose, adding progesterone, or using a weaker formula, such as an estrone cream.

- Try to elevate your legs to hip level for a few minutes several times a day. Frequency is more important than the amount of time in this case. Get out of the habit of crossing your legs, knees, and ankles when seated. If you have a desk job, try to spend a few minutes walking around every hour. If you have a job that requires standing for hours on end, try to sit and elevate your feet to hip level once every hour.

CIRCULATION AND REJUVENATION MASK

Chickpea flour has been used in some Ayurvedic recipe preparations for the skin and is believed to help exfoliate and soften it as well as stimulate circulation and rejuvenate tissues. Bananas are a rich, incredible beauty food high in B vitamins, vitamin A, and minerals such as potassium. Try this simple mask on your face—or even on the spider-vein areas of your legs—when you want to give your skin a revitalization and glow boost.

3 oz (75 g) mashed ripe banana	2 teaspoons sesame oil (or a
1 tablespoon organic chickpea	little more or less, depending
flour	on the size of the banana)

Stir the banana into the chickpea flour and mix in the sesame oil. Apply an even layer to your face and neck, leaving it on for 15 to 20 minutes while you relax, before rinsing off.

Nourish Strong, Healthy Hair and Nails

All of the changes you've made so far to your diet and self-care routine will result in stronger, more naturally beautiful hair and nails. Like your skin, the strength and vitality of your hair and nails is a reflection of all that is happening inside your body, and there are many ways to nourish them both internally and externally.

How to Grow Healthy Hair from the Outside In

If you want strong, healthy hair, it's essential to nourish the hair follicles that grow your actual hair strands. Go ahead right now and touch your scalp with your fingers. Give yourself a little head massage. It feels good, right? Your scalp is rich in nerves and blood vessels. Get familiar with touching your scalp more than just when you are shampooing. It likes it and will respond! Every part of your body needs love and attention to flourish, and that includes your scalp. If you want lovely hair, you have to give some love to your hair. This includes attention from your hands, not just from products you buy. In all areas of life, love can't just be bought.

Fluctuations in hormones and nutrition, as well as your good old genes, can influence the quality and thickness of your hair. The dietary advice in Pillar 1, Internal Nourishment, will help you grow more beautiful hair over time. However, there are also manual, external methods that you can combine with your dietary shifts to help create beautifully healthy, shiny hair. Incorporating these methods from the outside and the inside will help you grow the beautiful hair that is your birthright.

Here are some of the most effective ways to externally nourish your hair.

WASH LESS OFTEN

Unless your hair is incredibly oily, it doesn't need to be washed every day. Washing a few times a week will keep your hair clean but prevent overdrying, allowing more time for the natural oils in your hair to moisturize down to the tips of your strands.

SCALP MASSAGE

This is a fantastic and highly effective way to stimulate your hair follicles and foster healthy new growth. This can be incorporated easily into your daily routine as part of your *abhyanga* practice (see page 121). When you are doing your daily oil massage, be sure to take a few minutes to massage the coconut oil, sesame oil, or specialized herbal formula oil into all areas of your scalp to help stimulate circulation to your hair follicles. If you want to add a few drops of essential oil specifically for the scalp-massage part of your treatment, a few that are extra stimulating to your hair follicles include lemon, peppermint, lavender, basil, and rosemary pure essential oils. Just adding a few drops into the oil will suffice. (If you are new to these oils, and especially if you have sensitive skin, be sure to check with your dermatologist or test a tiny area to see if they irritate your skin.)

SOFTENING HAIR SCALP TREATMENT

This is a great treatment to do once a week to help heal and nourish your hair. It's easy to make and use as part of your hair-care routine. Lavender is healing and nourishing and has been known to relieve tension and headaches when massaged directly into your scalp. Olive oil makes your hair incredibly soft and will improve the elasticity of your hair shaft and protect against breakage.

2 1/2 fl oz (75 ml) cold-pressed olive oil   10 to 12 drops lavender
essential oil

Warm the olive oil in a pan over the lowest setting possible. Turn off and remove from heat and then add the lavender oil. Combine well and massage the warm mixture into your scalp. Twist your hair into a bun, cover with a shower cap, and relax for 20 to 30 minutes before shampooing.

Use Natural Bristles

Brushing your hair with a natural bristle brush can help stimulate your hair follicles and produce more natural oils that lubricate your entire head and all your beautiful hair strands. Start from the top of your head and work systematically down the length of your hair. Gently work out tangles rather than being aggressive; you're not plowing through an overgrown hiking trail. Avoid breakage by being patient and using even strokes.

Deep Clean

It's important to occasionally deep clean your scalp from any dirt and oils that can build up and block your hair follicles. Try periodically using a cleansing shampoo made from natural ingredients or applying an apple cider vinegar rinse. Apple cider vinegar is an excellent rinse to use occasionally to remove impurities from hard water, accumulated sebum, and waxy buildup from products. Pour the apple cider vinegar over your moistened scalp in the shower, massage it in for a couple of minutes, and rinse very well. Then proceed to shampooing and conditioning. You *are* rinsing it out fairly quickly, but as your scalp can absorb so much, it's a great idea to try to source organic vinegar.

Vinegar can also help balance the pH of your hair, which affects the appearance and overall health of your hair. The strands of your hair are made up of keratin protein. When the pH of your hair is properly balanced, your hair will be a sealed, flat cuticle layer on the outside of the strand, which makes your hair more shiny and bouncy. If your hair's pH is imbalanced from lots of heat or chemical treatments, your hair will look dull and frizzy and become brittle and susceptible to more breakage. Try the following pH-Balancing Hair Rinse once every six to eight weeks or so (depending on your hair type), or whenever you feel excessive buildup in your hair. Don't do it too often, however, or it will dry out your hair.

Apple cider vinegar is fantastic for restoring your hair's pH balance as well as helping remove any product residue. Rosemary helps stimulate the scalp and promote hair growth.

8 fl oz (250 ml) organic apple cider vinegar

15 drops rosemary oil
6 fl oz (175 ml) warm water

Combine the ingredients and pour over damp hair, being careful not to get the rinse into your eyes or on your face. Massage for a few moments and rinse out.

Top Ingredients for Hair Care

To pinpoint the best possible ingredients in shampoos and conditioners to help nourish your hair, it's important to look beyond the slogans and pretty packaging devised by marketing companies. Of course, the products you choose must match your individual hair type, but there are some ingredients that are known to work universally well for different types of hair. Products including these ingredients can be sourced at health stores, but they also are increasingly common and easy to find at your local grocery store or pharmacy.

SHEA BUTTER

This is a great natural emollient. It coats the surface of your hair strands with oil, reducing the amount of water that is lost so that your hair stays hydrated and luscious.

COCONUT OIL

This is a perfect fatty emollient to seal moisture into your hair. Coconut oil helps make your hair shiny and healthier.

PURE ALOE VERA GEL

Great for soothing your scalp and hair follicles, aloe vera is said to also contain an enzyme that stimulates hair follicles, helping to promote healthy hair growth.

VEGETABLE GLYCERIN

This acts as a natural humectant, meaning it attracts water and acts as a protective moisture layer, which will help your hair stay moisturized while avoiding frizziness.

JOJOBA

This is a great natural hair oil, which can soothe damaged ends and make your hair look shiny but not greasy by balancing your hair's oil production.

CASTOR OIL

This is a humectant and an antifungal that helps prepare the hair for better growth.

CERAMIDES

Ceramides mend damaged and broken hair fibers by "gluing" them back together and reinforcing your hair's structure. They also help to smooth out frizzy or unmanageable hair.

ANTIOXIDANTS

Antioxidants work great inside your body and also help to nourish your hair from the outside. Applied topically, antioxidants can help protect your hair from free radicals and even protect the integrity of your hair's vital color.

HYALURONIC ACID

Popularly used in skin care (see page 111), hyaluronic acid is also useful for beautiful hair, as it helps to lock hydration into your hair strands.

ACIDIC INGREDIENTS

In this case, acidity can be a good thing! Just as applying apple cider vinegar can cleanse your hair follicles of debris and balance your hair's natural pH, other natural acids in shampoo, such as sodium citrate or citric acid, perform the same functions on a milder, more regular basis.

PANTHENOL

Panthenol is a form of vitamin B that treats and prevents damage to your hair from pollution, free radicals, and sun exposure. It's water soluble, penetrating the hair and acting as a great moisturizer that locks moisture into your hair after cleansing.

ZINC

You can ingest the essential trace element zinc from eating nuts and seeds, such as pumpkin seeds. In shampoo, zinc can soothe the scalp, fight chronic dandruff, and regulate excess sebum, thereby preventing excessively oily hair and even hair loss that results from clogged hair follicles.

RADICAL BEAUTY TIP: KEEP YOUR TRESSES SHINY

Everyone loves hot showers. That's all good, but be sure to end your shower with a cool rinse. (See page 127 to read why alternating temperatures in the shower is a great beauty practice in general.) The cool water will tighten up your hair follicles and cuticle, keeping your hair shinier. Plus, you will feel refreshed!

Hair Ingredients to Avoid

Your hair follicles are very vacuolated, meaning they are rich in blood vessels that are close to the surface of your scalp. Therefore, whatever is in your hair products is quickly absorbed into your bloodstream and into your system. Being aware of the toxic additives in many common hair products and avoiding them goes hand in hand with eating organic foods. It's important to avoid toxins from entering and circulating around your precious body from any source so they do not in any way, shape, or form detract from your natural beauty. Unfortunately, there are thousands of chemicals used in different hair-care products, so it's up to you to scan ingredient labels and be on the lookout. Here are some of the most common harmful ingredients that are important to avoid.

SULFATES

Ugh. These nasty, cheaply produced chemicals, which include sodium lauryl sulfate (SLS), sodium laureth sulfate (SLES), and other forms of sulfate, are used in shampoos (as well as floor cleaners, engine degreasers, and kitchen degreasers like dishwasher soaps) to create foam. It's easy to love a foamy shampoo and feel like you're really cleaning your hair, right? But sulfates can be considered a toxin that creates irritation and itching, as well as more serious issues. A report from the *Journal of the American College of Toxicology* notes that this ingredient has a "degenerative effect on the cell membranes because of its protein denaturing properties,"[1] and that "high levels of skin penetration may occur at even low use concentration."[2] Some studies have noted that sulfates can enter and maintain residual levels in the heart, liver, lungs, and brain from skin contact, and by depositing on the skin surface and in the hair follicles, they can cause damage to the hair follicle.[3,4] Other research has shown that sulfates can create irritation to and impair your immune system.[5]

ETHYL AND ISOPROPYL ALCOHOLS

These petroleum-based alcohols can be very dehydrating to your hair, leaving it dry and eventually leading to breakage. Certain nonvolatile or fatty alcohols, however, such as cetyl alcohol, are okay, as they have a higher carbon count so they are oily and actually condition hair. Be sure to check labels for specific names.

FORMALDEHYDE

Commonly used as a preservative (you might recall the lab rat you dissected in high school biology was embalmed in this), it irritates the skin and can cause inflammation, joint pain, allergies, chronic fatigue, and dizziness.[6] It is also considered a potential carcinogen. Stay away! (Be sure to avoid nail polishes that contain formaldehyde, too.)

RADICAL BEAUTY TIP: HAIR CARE IN THE SUN

Just like your skin, your hair needs adequate sun protection to prevent it from drying out and becoming brittle, damaged, and discolored from overexposure to the sun. There are some sunscreens made for the hair, but the easiest and most effective way to prevent sun damage to your hair is to wear hats! This is especially important when you are out in the sun for extended periods of time. From sun hats to boleros and beyond, you'll be able to express your personal style *and* protect your precious hair, all at the same time.

IMIDAZOLIDINYL UREA AND DMDM HYDANTOIN

On that note, these two ingredients are preservatives that release formaldehyde, so look for them as well on ingredient lists.

PROPYLENE GLYCOL (PG)

PG is a form of mineral oil. This is a controversial ingredient that some believe has some immunotoxicity concerns.[7] It comes in different grades, including an industrial grade that is part of commercial products such as engine coolants, antifreeze, and various enamels and varnishes. For beauty products, it helps to drive ingredients down into the hair (or skin) for deeper penetration. It may break down the proteins that make up your hair in the process (obviously the opposite of what you want!), and also may create allergic reactions or irritations.[8]

POLYETHYLENE GLYCOL (PEG)

PEG is included in shampoos to help dissolve oils, but it can overstrip your hair, leaving it vulnerable and weak.

DIETHANOLAMINE (DEA), MONOETHANOLAMINE (MEA), AND TRIETHANOLAMINE (TEA)

Does this remind you of the song "Do-Re-Mi" from *The Sound of Music*? These rhyming ingredients are not happy like the song. They are, in fact, potential hormone disruptors and irritants[9] and can be absorbed into your hair follicles and enter your body. These ingredients are "foamers," so they're not necessarily even great for your hair, per se, but are included solely for the experience of using them. But really, you should never have to choose between foaming shampoo and your health. Got a shampoo with any of these three-letter acronyms? Into the trash it goes!

FRAGRANCE

This is a tough one because we understand that you want your hair to smell awesome. But fragrance is a generic term for up to 3,100 stock chemical ingredients,[10] many of which are synthetic and toxic. You really don't know exactly what is in your shampoo or conditioner with just "fragrance" on the ingredient list, so you risk getting headaches, dizziness, rashes, and a number of allergic reactions. Tests of fragrance ingredients have found an average of fourteen hidden compounds per formulation, including ingredients linked to hormone disruption and sperm damage.[11] Exposure to these types of chemicals can adversely affect your central nervous system and even affect your mood, making you more irritable. No good-smelling shampoo is worth being moody! Check out products with essential oils, which smell great and are nontoxic.

NATURALLY BEAUTIFUL TEETH AND GUMS

A beautiful smile stemming from authentic joy is one of the most compelling features you can possess. Feeling confident about your teeth can help you smile more naturally. Oil pulling, or swishing sesame or another oil around your mouth for a few minutes in the morning before spitting it out, is something you can incorporate into your morning routine to help keep your mouth beautiful. It is another increasingly popular ancient Ayurvedic practice that benefits your mouth, teeth, and gum health.

Oil pulling is believed to encourage detoxification by attracting, binding, and removing bacteria, toxins, and parasites from your mouth (where a lot of bacteria tend to accumulate) and lymph system, while helping to clear out mucus and congestion from your throat and sinuses. Some even believe that oil pulling can help activate the vagus nerve, which sends information between your brain and the enteric nervous system in your gut, which controls digestion. Stimulating the vagus nerve is said to activate anti-inflammatory pathways in the digestive tract.[12]

Directions for oil pulling are simple:

1. Warm 1 to 2 teaspoons (or a bit less, if you have a tiny mouth!) of pure, cold-pressed sesame oil. (You can do this by parceling the sesame oil you are using into a small vial, and then holding the vial under hot water for a few seconds.)

2. Swish the warmed oil vigorously around all parts of your mouth and back and forth across your gums for 2 to 6 minutes. Don't move it into your throat, and resist the temptation to gargle! Although sometimes you hear recommendations to swish the oil for far longer, traditional Ayurvedic teachings believe that is unnecessary. When you are done, spit out the oil into the garbage.

In addition to oil pulling, another component of the Ayurvedic morning routine is chewing 2 or 3 teaspoons of black sesame seeds, moving them around the entire span of your teeth, for 1 to 3 minutes before spitting them out. This is believed to help polish, strengthen, and mineralize the teeth; remove stains; and also keep your gums healthy. The black sesame seeds are extremely high in calcium, as well as phosphorus, iron, and magnesium.

Radical Beauty Nail Care

It's important to take care of your hands and nails, which are an extension of your beauty. They undergo a great deal of daily wear and tear, from relentless exposure to heat and cold to abrasive soaps and excessive water from hand washing and detergents.

RADICAL BEAUTY NAIL WHITENING TIP

To brighten yellowed nails, try scrubbing them with white vinegar.

Your nails are largely made of a tough protective coating called keratin. A proper diet and excellent circulation are of utmost importance for growing healthy, strong nails. There are also great external ways to support nail health:

- Rather than cutting cuticles, soak your nails in warm water to soften cuticles and then gently push them back. Only trim off hanging, dead skin when necessary.

- Look for polishes free of the "toxic trio": dibutyl phthalate (DBP), toluene, and formaldehyde, which have been associated with development and reproductive issues and dizziness and are potential hormone disruptors and carcinogens.[13] Look for brands labeled "DBP-, toluene-, and formaldehyde-free" or, specifically, "three-free." There are even vegan polishes free of solvents and other toxins, including some that are "ten-free," and some that are water-based. (You may need to reapply these more often due to chipping.)

- Avoid frequent use of nail polish removers, which can dry your nail bed, leading to potential splits. Also look for nail polish removers that are free of acetone.

- Avoid quick-dry nail polishes that contain a great deal of acetone, which can dry out your nails.

- Use gloves when washing the dishes, and otherwise try to keep your hands out of hot water as much as possible.
- Before going out into the cold, always moisturize your hands and protect them with gloves. Avoid direct exposure to cold air.
- Massage and moisturize your nails and cuticles with almond, jojoba, or coconut oil often.

NAIL STRENGTHENING SCRUB

The combination of castor and avocado oils enhances nails' flexibility and renders them more pliable and less prone to chips and breakage. Ground walnuts are high in nourishing omega-3 fatty acids, while the walnuts themselves help to slough off dead surface cells, allowing more moisture and nutrients to be absorbed. Honey is nourishing and softening, and it also contains antibacterial and antiseptic properties.

1 oz (25 g) raw, shelled walnuts
1 tablespoon castor oil

1 tablespoon first cold-pressed avocado oil
1 teaspoon raw, organic honey

Grind walnuts to form a coarse powder. Mix in the oils and the honey to make a thick paste. Rub your entire nails, hands, and cuticles vigorously (but not in an overly abrasive way) for a few moments before rinsing with warm water. Try this treatment once or twice weekly for best results.

Peak Beauty Sleep

Beauty sleep is most certainly a term you've come across before, but you may not have a clear sense of why sleep is so essential to reach your beauty potential or what steps you can take to start sleeping better. This pillar will go into great detail about how sleep specifically affects your natural beauty and how to harness its power to look and feel radically beautiful. The word *peak* is often used in reference to the highest level of athletic performance, or "peak performance." As we are referring to it here in reference to beauty, *peak* means experiencing the optimal level and quality of sleep to fully support your beauty.

While you already know that excellent sleep is important, you may still unknowingly employ tactics that keep you from getting your best sleep. Many of us whittle into our sleeping hours by going to bed later than we should. In part, this is because we tend to prioritize cramming more activity and tasks into the day: cleaning up the kitchen or e-mail box, catching up on work, watching an extra television show, surfing the Internet, online shopping, or whatever else it may be. This often pushes bedtime later and later. At the same time, we shave our sleep away on the other end by rising earlier and earlier in the morning to tend to small children, fit in a workout, or simply get to work.

No matter how much sleep you've been getting up until now, going forward you must shift your priorities in order to start getting peak beauty sleep. In this pillar you'll learn how creating peak beauty sleep can help you lose weight or maintain your ideal weight, improve your metabolism and your immunity, better repair damaged tissues or cells (including in your skin), and delay disease and aging, all around working to increase your beauty. You'll also learn the most effective tips and tools to optimize your beauty sleep, which is key in allowing your most beautiful self to shine through. Hopefully, by the end of this pillar, your perspective on sleep will have radically shifted.

Understand the Sleep-Beauty-Wellness Connection

How Much Sleep Do You Really Need?

No matter how you slice it, most of us aren't getting enough sleep. The National Sleep Foundation suggests that on average adults need about 7 to 9 hours of sleep per night.[1] This is a general recommendation, and you may need more than that depending on your individual constitution, but unfortunately most of us don't get that much. (Contrary to popular belief, only a small fraction of the population can get by for extended periods on less than 7 hours of sleep at night.) Healthy sleep is also uninterrupted, not the kind where you wake up several times a night. Data from the National Health Interview Survey concluded that at least 30 percent of American adults don't get enough sleep. This 30 percent reported only 6 or fewer hours of sleep per night.[2]

Ironically, there's been a lot of talk lately that *oversleeping* can be harmful. In 2002, a study resurfaced that found that people who slept 6.5 to 7.4 hours had lower rates of mortality compared with people who slept either fewer than 4 hours or greater than 8.[3] But before assuming that getting more than 8 hours is "bad," it is important to know that this study was conducted on cancer patients. This might have shifted the results, as those with cancer likely have different sleep needs than the general public. In those with high mortality rates, the lack of sleep or excessive amount of sleep might have been a symptom of the patients' illness and not the cause. This shows how important it is to look at studies very carefully before making broad assumptions, especially as they relate to lifestyle shifts.

Meanwhile, a growing number of researchers don't believe there is such a thing as oversleeping. Dr. Sigrid Veasey of the University of Pennsylvania's

Center for Sleep and Circadian Neurobiology puts it bluntly: "*You can never get 'too much' sleep. When you have had enough sleep, you will wake up.*"

There are other interesting findings as well. Researchers at Stanford University studied the impact of playing sports while involved in academics. The result is that players often get little sleep. They conducted an experiment in which the players slept 10 hours a night for a five- to seven-week period instead of their usual 6 hours. The results showed that their speed and accuracy, as well as their physical, mental, and emotional well-being, all grew measurably better.[4] It's no surprise, then, that many top athletes, including Usain Bolt, Michael Phelps, LeBron James, and Roger Federer, report getting upward of 10 to 12 hours of sleep a night.

You may be asking yourself, What does this have to do with beauty? Well, athletes need to allow their bodies to rest and rejuvenate to reach peak condition for their athletic competitions. Likewise, rest and rejuvenation is key for all of your body's functions to perform at their peak. This has a direct impact on your beauty. An article published on Harvard Medical School's website explains that major restorative functions, "like muscle growth, tissue repair, protein synthesis, and growth hormone release occur mostly, or in some cases only, during sleep."[5]

Ultimately, you must listen to your body to see how much sleep you personally need. It might be 8 hours or possibly even 9 or 10. It is completely individual. You may wonder where you could possibly find more time to get additional sleep, but it is often possible to cut out unnecessary evening activities and simply go to bed earlier. Television is one thing that takes up so much time for most people but is completely unproductive. It may sound radical to suggest giving up TV entirely, but it might be easier than you think and could profoundly improve your life.

Once you have a deeper understanding of how strongly sleep can impact your beauty and overall wellness, you will likely feel compelled to really prioritize your sleep.

The Effects of Too Little Sleep

If you consistently get fewer than the ideal number of hours of sleep for you, here's what you are most likely dealing with.

ACCELERATED AGING

If you've ever wanted actual scientific documentation for the phenomenon of beauty sleep, here it is: A study published in 2015 assessed actual skin aging, and the subjects whose sleep was deemed "good" were found to have lower skin aging scores. This included a 30 percent higher barrier of recovery when compared with poor sleepers.[6]

In another fascinating clinical trial from the University Hospitals Case Medical Center in Cleveland, Ohio, a direct connection was found between poor sleep and accelerating aging, especially of the skin.[7] Researchers examined sixty premenopausal women between the ages of thirty and forty-nine[8] who fell into either a "poor" or "quality" sleep group, based on sleep length and overall excellence. They discovered that the poor sleepers showed twice as many signs of aging as those in the quality sleep group. These measurements included fine lines, uneven pigmentation, slackening of skin, and reduced elasticity.[9] They also found that those in the quality sleep group recovered more efficiently from damage and other stressors like exposure to the sun.[10] This shows that sun is not the *only* big issue with skin aging. Other factors, such as the quality of your sleep, may reduce your skin's ability to recover from sunlight exposure.

Need more proof? A study at Sweden's University of Stockholm found that sleep deprivation produced visible signs of aging, including increased hanging eyelids, darker circles under the eyes, more wrinkles and fine lines, swollen eyes, and more pronounced droopy corners of the mouth.[11] Anything that promotes the use of the word *droopy* to describe your face must obviously be avoided as much as possible!

WEIGHT GAIN

In general, those who do not sleep well tend to weigh more than those who get good levels of sleep.[12] A University Hospitals Case Medical Center clinical trial found that poor sleepers were nearly twice as likely to be overweight than those who slept well. In their study, 23 percent of the "good quality" sleepers were obese, versus 44 percent in the group that reported poor sleep quality.[13] A Wisconsin Sleep Cohort study found that as hours of sleep per night went down, body mass index (BMI) went up proportionally.[14] This further disputes the vastly oversimplified approach that what is on your plate and how much you work out are the only factors that determine your weight.

In another study published in the *American Journal of Epidemiology*, women who slept 5 hours or less a night had a 15 percent higher risk of becoming obese than women who slept 7 hours a night. Over the course of the sixteen-year study, the women who got less sleep also had a 30 percent higher risk of gaining 30 pounds than the women who got 7 hours of sleep per night.[15]

You may be wondering exactly *how* sleep affects your weight. It turns out that a lack of proper sleep can disrupt the key hormones that control appetite, making those who sleep poorly more hungry than those who sleep well through the night.[16] A study published in the *Journal of Clinical Endocrinology and Metabolism* looked at the connection between sleep and the hormone leptin, which controls appetite, and found that circulating levels of leptin in your body are influenced by the quality of your sleep.[17] This means that the more sleep you get, the better your body becomes at sensing when it is full.

The connection between sleep duration, body weight, metabolism, and specific hormones was backed up by a team of researchers from the Stanford University School of Medicine, who found that getting less sleep can lead to higher levels of ghrelin, a hormone that triggers appetite, and lower levels of leptin, which tells your body it's full, as well as an increased BMI.[18] In other words, the less you sleep, the hungrier you will be and the more food it will take to make you feel full!

The Harvard School of Public Health suggests that not getting enough sleep leads to other factors that contribute to weight gain. For example, people who don't sleep enough may be too exhausted to exercise, leading to weight gain. Or perhaps these people simply have more opportunities to eat since they spend more hours of the day awake. And we've all experienced pesky food cravings. When sleep deprived, you may feel more emotional, fatigued, and susceptible to cravings. One study showed that the amygdala, a set of neurons in the brain responsible for emotional reactions in the decision-making process, was more active when subjects did not get adequate sleep.[19]

Interestingly, the ease with which you gain weight or maintain a healthy weight may be related to childhood sleep patterns. A recent study in the *Archives of Pediatrics and Adolescent Medicine* found that not getting enough sleep in early life (through preschool) can be a long-term risk factor for obesity throughout life.[20] The study also found that napping was not a viable substitute for nighttime sleep as it relates to obesity prevention.[21] If you are a parent, you can rest assured that your perhaps frequent bedtime battles are well worth it for the sake of your child's long-term health.

HORMONAL IMBALANCE

Hormones are chemicals that are produced by different organs and glands and send important signals to different parts of the body. As hormones largely regulate repairs that take place in the body, impacting how you look and feel, it is essential to balance your hormones in order to express your Radical Beauty. Hormones can be compared to keys that "unlock" certain cells but not others. Like keys, different cells fit with specific hormones. When the "key" is turned and the cell is "unlocked," it receives a signal to multiply, make proteins or enzymes, or perform other vital tasks, including releasing other hormones. There is a high level of intelligence with hormones. Some may fit with many types of cells but have different effects on each type of cell. For example, a hormone may stimulate one type of cell to perform a task, while the same hormone turns off a different type of cell. To complicate this even more, the way a cell responds to a specific hormone may change over time.

While, thankfully, our bodies and all their intrinsic parts perform their duties without us having to direct them, it's important that we create an ideal environment for our hormones to function properly. The National Institute on Aging teaches us that hormone production fluctuates during the day and also during different points in your life.[22] While some natural fluctuations are normal, we want to avoid the *unnatural* variations that occur if you don't get enough sleep on a consistent basis. Restoration is key to your all-around well-being and for your natural beauty to express itself.

It's been well documented that inadequate sleep can negatively affect certain hormone levels in the body.[23,24] In addition to its effects on the hormones that control appetite, a lack of sleep causes your body to produce excess amounts of the hormone cortisol, which can break down your skin cells and contribute to various skin issues.[25] Cortisol is a stress hormone that tends to accumulate around the stomach, unfortunately leading to weight gain specifically in the belly area, as stomach fat cells are sensitive to cortisol and store excess energy there.[26]

Another hormone affected by sleep is called HGH, or human growth hormone. This is an important hormone for beauty because it helps your skin grow thicker, healthier, and more elastic or pliable in texture, which further helps to protect against wrinkling. Natural production of HGH also helps with muscle building and tissue repair. Unfortunately, disturbed sleep can inhibit your natural production of HGH.[27] This can make it more difficult for your body to build lean muscle and resilient, youthful skin.

WEAKENED IMMUNE SYSTEM

A growing body of research is finding a strong relationship between sleep and immunity.[28] Increasing evidence shows that inadequate sleep leads to a weakened immune response.[29] Sleep may help facilitate the redistribution of T-cells to lymph nodes.[30] T-cells are a vital part of our immune system that help maintain our wellness and vitality, and the more efficiently they travel through the lymphatic system, the better. Since our entire population appears to be suffering from a sleep deficit, our immunity must be reduced across the population as a whole. Can you imagine the health implications for our entire society if we all slept better? The entire health of the community would be bolstered, and health-care costs might be dramatically reduced! But this very much has to start with you.

Getting sick isn't just inconvenient or annoying; it can also be aging. Some theorize that diseases and routine illnesses like the common cold can actually create free radicals in your body.[31] When these sicknesses occur, your immune system creates free radicals on purpose to help neutralize harmful viruses and bacteria. But those free radicals also create cellular damage and contribute to the visible effects of aging. In other words, minimizing and avoiding getting sick isn't just to benefit your health; it can be another powerful tool in your anti-aging arsenal.

SLUGGISH DETOXIFICATION

Sleep gives your body the rest it needs to perform its vital functions, such as detoxification. It is therefore critical to help promote optimal detoxification and clear metabolic waste from your system.[32] As you know, the more detoxed and cleansed your internal body is, the more beautiful you will become.

POOR PERFORMANCE

It's well established that sleep improves your performance and alertness.[33] When you sleep more, you'll drive more safely, and your memory will improve, too.[34] Reduced sleep means you aren't able to perform at your highest potential for all tasks in life. If you aren't able to feel as present and alert at work, when working on your creative pursuits, while playing with your children, or during your workouts, it's very frustrating and reflects a diminishing quality of your life.

ANXIETY AND DEPRESSION

Poor sleep can also contribute to worsening anxiety.[35] In a parallel fashion, insomnia, the extreme end of bad sleep, may be a risk factor for full-blown anxiety disorders.[36] On the opposite end of the spectrum, when you feel fully rested and consistently get enough sleep, it's easier to feel calm and present. Calmness helps you deal better with stressors in life, and as we discussed earlier, dealing with stress better helps delay aging all around.

For someone suffering from depression, bad and irregular sleep is often part of the disorder. In fact, some recent therapies focus on loss of good sleep as the first sign that a bout of depression may soon occur. This onset can be averted by paying close attention to good sleep before the depression actually hits. Is good sleep a preventive for depression? That's not agreed upon, but it's definitely worth trying to incorporate.

PERMANENT BRAIN DAMAGE

An aging brain leads to less vitality overall, and vitality is a big component of being your most Radically Beautiful. Researchers at Duke-NUS Graduate Medical School Singapore (Duke–National University of Singapore) found a relationship between the fewer hours of sleep adults get and accelerated aging in the brain.[37]

Most of us presume that a few nights of missed sleep are not a big deal. We think we can recover by getting more sleep in the future. But a study from researchers at the University of Pennsylvania found otherwise.[38] The lead researcher, Sigrid Veasey, MD, notes, "This is the first report that sleep loss can actually result in a loss of neurons."[39] She continues, "No one really thought that the brain could be irreversibly injured from sleep loss. In general, we've always assumed full recovery of cognition following short- and long-term sleep loss. But some of the research in humans has shown that attention span and several other aspects of cognition may not normalize even with three days of recovery sleep, raising the question of lasting injury in the brain."[40] Whoa . . . now this is a pretty strong reason not to put off sleep!

Sleep deprivation is considered a constant stressor to your system and has been shown in some research to reduce the capacity for learning and memory. Reducing sleep deprivation is even hypothesized to help prevent or slow the progression of Alzheimer's disease.[41] Of course, the sharper and more alert your brain is, the more powerful and confident in your beauty you will be.

All of these findings help us to understand how the most basic of nature's rhythms contributes to every aspect of life. But please don't be alarmed. This shift was not meant to frighten you with the disastrous effects of getting too little sleep, but rather to open your eyes to all of the benefits you'll soon see from getting more, better quality sleep. In the next shift, you'll learn how to tune in to your body's natural rhythms in order to achieve Peak Beauty Sleep.

Tune In to Your Body's Natural Rhythms

Nature's Timetable

Being more in tune with our natural rhythms aligns us to nature's power and beauty. It's easy to think of nature's power in a dramatic flash of lightning or in the heat of the sun, but equal to this power is the strength of rejuvenation. We need to harness this power to retract and go inward in order to have the most effective, deep sleep that fuels our creative power and allows our natural beauty to fully shine through.

Radical Beauty is about living in harmony with nature's inherent wisdom. From a sleep perspective, this means that the more in tune you are with natural light, the better. This shifts every season with the influence and timing of the sun and the larger bodies of energy beyond our planet. The sun coordinates the movement of the Earth around its axis, which influences the larger seasonal shifts as well as the daily shifts that create longer and shorter days. Even though these planetary bodies may seem unfathomably far away from the average person, they actually exert their influence on our bodies. Since we possess all of the main elements found in nature, Ayurveda believes we are miniature representations of the whole universe, the entire cosmos.

Circadian rhythms are physical, mental, and behavioral changes in living beings (including not only animals but also plants and microbes) that follow a roughly 24-hour cycle. These are produced by natural factors in the body and respond to signals from the environment. The main external signal affecting circadian rhythms is light, which influences the turning on and off of an organism's internal clock. Circadian rhythms influence sleep patterns, hormone release, body temperature, and other important bodily functions, while abnormal circadian rhythms have been associated with sleep disorders, obesity, diabetes, depression, bipolar disorder, and seasonal affective disorder.[1]

Circadian rhythms are important for us to consider in promoting Peak Beauty Sleep. If we live in tune with our natural body clocks and circadian rhythms, we will naturally be more active in the morning and wind down in the evening. An ideal time to work out, for instance, is in the morning, around the rising light and rising energy, or in the middle of the day, in the peak of sunlight, as opposed to late in the evening, when the sun is naturally descending, indicating a return inward toward relaxation. Late workouts can be overly stimulating and wake you up rather than bring you closer to sleep.

The brain's electrical response to rhythmic sensory stimulation, such as pulses of sound or light,[2] synchronizes with the natural, rhythmic changes in our environment. Our health, down to the minute cellular level, depends on the degree to which we are in harmony with the natural cycles of daytime and nighttime. Even basic functions in our body that we often take for granted, such as our blood pressure, immune system functions, and cellular growth, all depend on our rhythmic melatonin cycle. This in turn depends on syncing up properly with nature's rhythms. We are, after all, inseparably one with nature.

Artificial Light: Friend or Foe?

When you consider the fact that Thomas Edison successfully tested the first electric lamp in 1879,[3] you might be a little jolted (pun intended) to realize that artificial lights haven't been around very long in the broad scope of human evolution. While the benefits of electricity are enormous and obvious, it has also introduced a set of health and beauty issues. This is due to the fact that artificial lighting allows us to experience daytime around the clock if we wish, making us completely out of tune with the natural rhythms of the planet.

The body's master clock is made up of about 20,000 neurons, with sleep signals traveling from the pons, an area at the base of the brain, to the thalamus and then on to the thinking part of the brain, the cortex.[4] The pineal gland produces melatonin, a hormone that communicates to the body information about light levels in the outside world. The light seen by your eyes influences how your brain interprets this information. When your body clock senses a decrease in light, ideally in the evenings, it signals your brain to produce more melatonin to induce drowsiness and sleep.

But now we are in an age where we are exposed to numerous new assailants on our inner sleep mechanism, including illuminated smartphones, tablets, e-readers, and laptops. We use these devices often right in our beds and directly before bedtime with increasing frequency. The eye is registering daytime levels of light later and later at night. A National Sleep Foundation survey found that nine out of ten Americans reported using a technological device in the hours before bed.[5] With the increased light stimulation to our brains, hormones, and entire being, how can we expect the body to maintain normal sleep patterns?

The result is that we've lost the connection to our natural rhythms and the cycles of the environment around us. It's important to refoster that connection. While your life might be extremely busy and hectic, shifting your schedule as much as possible toward going to bed closer to sunset and waking up closer to sunrise will help you align and synergize with the higher power of universal nature. *Closer* is the key word here, as it might seem impossible in modern life to go to bed at sunset and rise right at sunrise. But start with the baby step of going to bed half an hour earlier and waking up half an hour earlier. Also try at least eating dinner earlier, closer to sunset, which is also helpful for syncing closer to natural rhythms.

Yin and Yang: How the Day Affects the Night

Exposure to natural light during the day is important as a contrast to the dark cycles of the night. This helps promote overall healthy sleep and waking cycles. If you want to have a peaceful nightly rhythm of sleeping, you have to also balance the opposite, the daylight. It's important to have exposure to natural light on a regular basis. Just as our sleep rhythms have become corrupted by artificial light exposure long after daylight has naturally reduced, so our daily rhythms have been worn away by minimized exposure to natural light. Most of us spend the vast majority of our days indoors under artificial lights.

The neurotransmitter in our brain called serotonin increases with the light of each day. Serotonin influences daily and nightly rhythms, memory, appetite, and so on—in essence, all the factors that play a part in our internal rhythms. The amount of melatonin made available to the body in response to the darkness of the night actually depends on the concentration of serotonin secreted in response to the natural light we are exposed to during the day. Serotonin is broken down into melatonin, so there is a beautifully coordinated, natural rhythm present between the cycles of serotonin and melatonin, which depend on each other and are controlled by a changing environment.

The Importance of Color

Clearly, avoiding artificial light around bedtime is important for Peak Beauty Sleep, but interestingly, it turns out that not all light is created equal. In fact, using light color strategically might be helpful in smoothing out nervous-system activity.[6] Research on the "color temperature" of light and its effects on the brain suggests that the "temperature" of the light is more important than its brightness. This means that on a color spectrum, yellow-white through red lights (which are considered low-color-temperature lights) have a far less detrimental effect on our systems than the blue lights on the other end of the spectrum.

Research has now pinpointed that electronics emanate blue light, which affects the brain more strongly than other colors and, in particular, disturbs our sleep. In other words, reducing light all around can be very helpful, but it's critical to reduce blue light specifically. Unfortunately, blue light is emitted strongly and consistently from many different electronic devices. Using these devices near bedtime can have a detrimental effect on your sleep patterns and consequently your natural beauty expression.

A photoreceptor in the eye called melanopsin plays a role in establishing our day/night cycles and is particularly sensitive to a narrow band of blue light in the 460–480 nanometers (nm) range.[7] Researchers at the University of Pennsylvania School of Medicine and School of Arts and Sciences studied the biological effects of blue light[8] and found that melanopsin is very sensitive to blue light, which is emitted by digital devices, including smartphones, tablets, and computers.[9]

This means that if you work on a tablet or laptop, or look at your smartphone before bed, you might find your sleep is delayed. This results in all of the adverse beauty and wellness implications we mentioned earlier, including accelerated aging, reduced performance in all your tasks,[10] and suppression of natural human growth hormone, which you need to increase muscle mass and induce tissue repair.

Electronics and Sleep Don't Mix

An alarming 51 percent of people who text specifically in the hour before going to bed reported they were less likely to get a good night's sleep, "every/almost every weeknight."[11] In a similar fashion, up to 77 percent use their computers or laptops in the hour before bed. Of those, 50 percent reported they were less likely to get a good night's sleep, "every/almost every weeknight."[12]

According to more than thirty years of studies conducted at the Division of Sleep Medicine at Boston's Brigham and Women's Hospital and Harvard Medical School, the light from electronics has a significant effect on circadian (i.e., daily) rhythms of waking and sleeping. Throwing off your circadian rhythm affects how quickly you fall asleep as well as the quality of sleep you get.[13] According to Dr. Charles A. Czeisler of Harvard Medical School, "Artificial light exposure between dusk and the time we go to bed at night suppresses release of the sleep-promoting hormone melatonin, enhances alertness and shifts circadian rhythms to a later hour—making it more difficult to fall asleep."[14]

Answering work e-mails late at night, whether from your boss or regarding pending stressful deadlines, might also stir up anxiety that is not so conducive to sleep. You may be wondering, what about e-readers? These are one of the newest electronic phenomena to have an effect on our brains and biorhythms. A report from the *Proceedings of the National Academy of Sciences* found that using such devices near bedtime caused users to take longer to fall asleep and led to disturbances in their circadian rhythm, suppression of the sleep-inducing hormone melatonin, delays in the timing of REM sleep, and decreased alertness the next morning.[15]

In short, the bright light from these devices stimulates your brain and, unfortunately, makes it think it's daytime. This keeps your brain alert instead of allowing it to wind down when it senses that it is night. While there are some apps you can download onto devices to help reduce the emission of blue light, there is still some remaining stimulation from your electronic devices. You'd be better served turning them off earlier every evening.

Action Steps to Align Yourself to Nature's Rhythms

Here are some of the most important steps you can take to cut down on sleep disturbances from artificial lights—especially electronic devices—to promote Peak Beauty Sleep.

FOLLOW THE ONE-HOUR RULE

It's critical to put down your devices, including tablets, cell phones, and e-readers, at least an hour before bed if you want to get that profound beauty sleep that is critical to how you feel and look.

USE AIRPLANE MODE

While you're at it, be sure to fully turn off your cell phone when you go to bed—or at least put it in airplane mode. That way you won't be disturbed by the sounds or lights from nighttime calls, texts, and e-mails. Plus, by cutting off the signal, you'll have fewer electromagnetic frequencies, or invisible electric and magnetic fields radiating away from appliances that may have potentially harmful health effects, targeted at you during the night. You certainly don't need that signal beaming at you all night long.

FLASHLIGHT IT TO THE BATHROOM

We all have to get up in the middle of the night for a bathroom break sometimes. If you turn on the bathroom light, however, the brightness can interrupt your circadian rhythms, making it difficult for you to go back to sleep. Instead, try using a night-light in the bathroom that isn't visible from your bedroom, or keep a dim flashlight next to the bed. Avoid drinking large quantities of fluids before bedtime as well, in order to avoid this problem altogether.

CHANGE YOUR ALARM

Unfortunately, LED alarm clocks pose the same problems as other electronic devices: they introduce a source of light into your room that disrupts your circadian rhythm. Your alarm clock also gives off an electromagnetic frequency (EMF). Some studies link EMF exposure to melatonin interruption and depletion in rodents and humans,[16] which is not good since melatonin is a hormone necessary for sound sleep. Switch to a battery-operated alarm clock or use your phone's alarm, which should be in airplane mode at bedtime and throughout the night. Avoid placing other electronic devices such as radios or MP3 players on your bedside table as well.

CAN'T SLEEP? CHILL OUT

If you simply can't fall asleep for more than half an hour or so and are finding yourself getting increasingly agitated, get up and go into the other room and read a book or magazine, listen to some relaxing music, or meditate. Whatever you do, *don't* do anything stimulating, such as go on your computer or watch television. The other thing to avoid is staring at the clock or constantly checking the time on your phone. (There goes that blue light again!) Focusing on the time can stress you out and make it even harder to fall asleep. So just try to let it go, and keep your phone (in airplane mode of course!) far enough away that it takes some real effort to reach over and pick it up.

PICK PRINT

While e-readers may be convenient for your commute or when traveling, opt for printed books at night. Reading from a printed book at night is actually relaxing and can help promote Peak Beauty Sleep.

BALANCE LIGHT DAYS AND DARK NIGHTS

To sleep better at night, get more natural light into your days. Wake up to the light by opening your curtains and letting it shine in. If you have to be indoors for much of your day because of your job, make an effort to go for a walk during the day, even if it's just briefly to run errands or walk around your local park. Try to eat lunch outside when the weather permits. Even in the winter, get outside and into the light as much as possible. Bundle up when it's cold. The more natural light exposure your eyes receive, the more in balance you will be, in rhythm between the alternating beauty sleeping and waking hours.

Establish Healthy Sleep Routines

The Importance of a Regular Schedule

We humans are natural creatures of habit, and our daily routines establish our bodily rhythms. One of the best ways to regulate and normalize your sleeping schedule is to regulate and normalize all the other rhythms in your life, including when you eat and exercise. Your body will better be able to feel settled and ready for bed if everything else in your life is on a regular schedule, too. The more you can stick to as regular a schedule as possible (even when traveling), the better your body will "know" its expected routines. You will naturally settle into sleep at the same time night after night, and thus enhance your beauty.

Here are some general guidelines:

- Exercise at the same time every day, ideally in the morning or at lunchtime, and avoid heavy physical stimulation later in the day. Late workouts can be overly stimulating and keep your mind and body alert. Try to end workouts at least 3 to 4 hours before bed. But do make regular workouts a part of your routine. A study from Northwestern Medicine found that exercise in general was helpful in relieving insomnia.[1] In the study, adults who were previously sedentary and then started doing aerobic exercise four times a week reported an increase in sleep quality and vitality, along with less sleepiness during the day and fewer depressive symptoms.[2]

- Keep regular mealtimes for breakfast, lunch, and dinner (though the particular foods that make up those meals may vary with the seasons).

- Always strive to eat dinner at least a few hours before bed. Digestion slows at night because your body is meant to be rejuvenating, not digesting! Plus, feeling heaviness in your stomach as you are drifting off is not a recipe for deep or peaceful sleep. Ideally, try to eat dinner 3 to 4 hours before bed. (It's really not *that* crazy; if you go to bed at 11 p.m., aim to finish dinner at least by 8 p.m., for instance).
- Complete your *abhyanga* (see page 121) and other skin-care routines at the same time every day.
- Establish a regular morning routine that includes drinking hot water with lemon and allowing enough time for elimination.
- Establish a regular evening routine (see below) and stick to it to signal to your body that it's time to wind down and prepare for sleep.
- Keep your sleeping hours consistent. This is perhaps most important of all! It will set your internal clock so your body is better able to get drowsy naturally and sleep more deeply once you climb into bed. Even on the weekends, try not to get too thrown off your regular weekday schedule. This will make it easier for you to maintain optimal sleep patterns overall.
- Avoiding napping. Ayurvedic teachings frown on daytime sleeping for adults, believing that it can contribute to illness. Napping may be tempting or even a habit that you love, but if you find yourself engaged in irregular sleep patterns, it's better to avoid napping in general, especially after 4 or 5 p.m.

Establish an Evening Routine

While your overall daily routine is important to promote Peak Beauty Sleep, the most important piece of this routine takes place in the evening before bed. This was discussed in *The Beauty Detox Power,* but because it is so important to help you achieve Radical Beauty, we are going to discuss it here again.

Followed daily, a regular evening routine will help you prepare mentally and physically for sleep by giving cues to your internal clock. This will help you get the best possible beauty sleep every day and in the long-term, which is where the real benefits are to be had. What you choose to do for your evening routine is completely up to you. Every person will respond differently to each activity. You can choose one of these suggestions, a combination of them, or come up with your own ideas for how to wind down in the evening before bed. The most important thing is that you pick something that makes you feel relaxed and that you do it at the same time every day as often as you can. Here are some suggestions for your evening routine.

SIP SOMETHING SOOTHING

After dinner, sip some herbal tea or hot almond or hemp milk while relaxing or getting ready for bed. (See the Evening Replenishing Elixir on page 180.)

GET DIM

After 6 p.m. in the winter or 7 p.m. in the summer, start dimming the lights in your home. Try using candles at dinner and in whatever room of the house you are in to start reducing your exposure to artificial lights. You don't have to go full precolonial style, but any time you can reduce artificial lighting, the better.

PRACTICE *ABHYANGA*

If you are too rushed in the mornings, you can perform your *abhyanga* routine (see page 121) in the evening. Or practice a shorter variation of *abhyanga* followed by a relaxing hot bath or shower. If you completed your *abhyanga* in the morning, a nice warm bath or shower might be relaxing by itself.

RELAX TO MUSIC

Try a routine of listening to some music you find truly relaxing. Music can help to powerfully relax your mind. Find some music you connect to with a slower vibration that leaves you feeling soothed and chilled out. No stimulating hip-hop or hard rock at this time!

HONOR THE SACRED HOUR

Treat the last hour before bed as sacred time for you. Try reading something relaxing or spiritually uplifting, or meditating. There are excellent ways to set the energetic tone as you drift into sleep. (See Pillar 6 for more specifics about meditation.) Your nighttime reading should be done with real books instead of an electronic reader that can disrupt your internal cues and sleep patterns.

During the sacred hour, what you avoid is just as crucial as what you engage in. Avoid stressful or stimulating activities. Late at night is not the ideal time to complete last-minute work on a presentation, hit the gym, or engage in a dynamic Vinyasa yoga flow. It's also not the best time to get into a big emotional discussion with your partner or a friend. You'll be better off saving that for morning tea or a Saturday hike, if you can put it off until then. Stressful activities just have no place before bedtime. They can induce your body to secrete the stress hormone cortisol, which can make you feel more alert. Chill out and steer clear of anything non–chilled out.

SECURE THE BEST BEAUTY SLEEP POSE

Research has shown that exactly how you sleep on your pillow can influence wrinkle formation. One study from the journal of *Clinical and Experimental Dermatology* studied mechanical forces on the face and how they influenced wrinkles and superficial facial changes, including the formation of crow's-feet and lines around the mouth. They found that redistributing pressure could help reduce wrinkles.[3]

So what can you do? First, ensure that you have the right kind of pillow (see page 178) and avoid sleeping on your stomach, which may create pressure and enhance wrinkles to an even greater degree. Also avoid crossing your legs when you sleep. It's not only bad for circulation, but can also twist your spine, leaving you feeling unbalanced in the morning. Try sleeping with a pillow between your legs, which will keep your legs and hips more balanced.

Create a Personal Bedroom Cave

One of the most important routines you can create is the habit of sleeping in an ideal environment. If you look at the sleeping habits of other animals, regardless of whether they sleep during the day or the night, you will find bears and bats burrowed deep in cool, dark, quiet caves. Let's take this cue from nature as a guide to create an ideal sleep environment. There are three factors that are essential for creating your own personal beauty sleep "cave" right in your own home.

COOL

Warm temperatures might feel great during the day when you're outside, especially if you like to hike, bike, or go to the beach. But high temperatures are not great for sleep. In fact, some research has shown a connection between insomnia and elevated body temperatures.[4] You've perhaps already experienced how much easier it is to sleep soundly when you can snuggle under the covers. When you sleep, your body's temperature drops mildly, which actually helps prepare you to sleep through the night.

While the National Sleep Foundation recommends a cool 65 degrees Fahrenheit (18 degrees Celsius)[5] for sleep, somewhere between 65 and 75 degrees Fahrenheit (18 to 24 degrees Celsius), depending on your particular body constitution, is a good range to help you drop off to sleep faster and more deeply. Some researchers believe that keeping temperatures steady throughout the night is important, and that if there is a rise or fall in temperature you might experience less quality REM sleep. If possible, set your home thermometer to hold steady at a certain temperature. From a beauty perspective, excessive heat can cause you to lose even more fluids throughout the night, and sleep is already dehydrating. Chronic, excessive nighttime dehydration over time can contribute to drying out and taxing your skin.

DARK

Your whole bedroom needs to be as dark as possible. Move as much electronic equipment out of your bedroom as possible (surely the printer can fit somewhere in the living room) and get rid of digital alarm clocks that are plugged in and introduce their own lights and electromagnetic frequencies. Then go through and use black tape to cover any little blinking lights that can't be avoided. Light tells your brain that it's time to wake up, and even a small amount of ambient light from your cell phone or computer can disrupt the production of melatonin,[6] which regulates sleep cycles.

It's also very helpful to equip your room with heavy blackout shades that completely block out the sunlight along with outside streetlights or car lights. This is especially important if you live on a busy road or in a city. An eye mask is also a great tool to help block out light. If you don't like the feel of a mask, which can feel constricting to some, simply drape a dark T-shirt over your eyes. Strive for the complete darkness of a deeply burrowed cave, trying to re-create that natural environment of peace and relaxation.

SACRED BEDROOM ACTIVITIES

There are (probably) multiple rooms in your house or apartment for all the functions you perform daily as a human being. While it's not a bad idea to work on your computer at the kitchen table or sometimes eat dinner on your couch in the living room if you feel like it, it's important to keep your bedroom activities to the bare minimum: sleep, relaxation, and sex. *That's it*. Ban laptops, TVs, and work materials from your bedroom. Keeping your bed only for relaxing or lovemaking will help strengthen your mental association between your bedroom and sleep—or lovemaking and then sleep, on those occasions!

Some light reading in bed, especially of inspiring or spiritual material, is highly recommended. This content can seep into and positively influence your mind as you are drifting off to sleep. But TV, with its stimulating lights and images, should be avoided. Keep your TV in your living room, not your bedroom.

Depending on where you live, you may not be able to control the noise in your external environment, which may include barking dogs, chattering teenagers, noisy car engines, and the like. As much as we would like to, we can't make all the outside signs of life go away when it's time for bed. But you *can* control the noise inside your cave. Creating white noise by using a fan, an excellent air filter, or even a specific white-noise maker can help you sleep more soundly. Another option is to block out the noise as much as possible with earplugs. The more disruptive outer noises you can avoid, the more peaceful your inner sleeping cave will be.

Bonus Cave Factor: Comfort

Caves in nature are not necessarily "comfortable" per se, as they are made mostly of rocks; slippery, damp surfaces; and even pools of water. But your home cave can deviate from the strict natural variety to include all the tools to help you get comfortable for sleep. These include soft sheets that don't irritate your skin, calming scents, an excellent mattress, and the right pillows.

What's the best kind of mattress? There isn't a lot of scientific evidence to conclusively show that one type of mattress is better than another kind.[7] Plus the right mattress for your neighbor or brother may not necessarily be the best one for you. It's best to lie down on different mattresses and see which one feels best for you, especially if you have neck or back pain. Howard Levy, MD, an Emory University assistant professor of orthopedics, physical medicine, and rehabilitation, comments, "If you're on too soft [of] a mattress, you'll start to sink down to the bottom. But on too hard of a mattress you have too much pressure on the sacrum, and on the shoulders, and on the back of the head."[8] In other words, a mattress of medium firmness might work the best for your spine and give you enough balance and support.

If you have medical conditions such as chronic obstructive pulmonary disorder (COPD) or frequent heartburn from gastroesophageal reflux disease (GERD), you may want to utilize an adjustable bed that can help you elevate your head at night when you sleep to help you breathe easier and experience fewer symptoms. If you have allergies to dust mites, try getting a washable mattress cover that you can slip on and off and wash easily.

The Better Sleep Council recommends spending at least 15 minutes on the bed in the store before buying it, as it may take that much time to relax and really feel out your new mattress.[9] So don't be embarrassed to march right into the store and plop down on the mattresses for a little while on each one. It's *your* beauty sleep. Set aside a few hours on a Sunday afternoon, roll into the local mattress stores, and prepare to spend some time curled up on the various beds you find. Toting a good read along is totally optional (but recommended!).

Pillows are also pretty important when it comes to sleep comfort. They can greatly contribute to your beauty sleep or diminish it. If you have headaches or aches and pains through your neck, shoulder, or upper back, your pillow can either help provide relief or exacerbate these pesky issues.

The position you sleep in also has some influence over the type of pillow you should choose. If you sleep on your back, look for a thinner pillow so your head and neck are not positioned too far forward, which can consistently throw you out of alignment. You can also seek out a pillow that has a more structured shape in the lower part to help cradle your neck and provide more support. If you sleep on your side, look for a firmer pillow that can stabilize your neck and head and keep them from dropping down too far. This will help fill in the space between your ear and shoulder and give you enough support to avoid tension or cramps that keep you from falling asleep or wake you up with an aching neck. Stomach sleeping is not recommended for skin beauty reasons (see page 174), but if you do choose to sleep on your stomach, try looking for a flat pillow or using one underneath your stomach to help support your lower back and spine.

The right scents can also bolster your sleep on a nightly basis. The keys to enhance all the moods in the universe, including drowsiness and relaxation, are found in nature. Certain essential oils distilled from nature's bounty, especially lavender, neroli, vetiver, valerian, chamomile, and clary sage, activate alpha wave activity in the back of your brain, which leads to relaxation and helps you sleep more soundly. Lavender is believed anecdotally to stimulate the pineal gland and the secretion of melatonin, perhaps promoting sleep.

You can try making your own room or pillow spray by mixing a few drops of these essential oils (alone or a combo that suits you) and some distilled water into a spray bottle. Another option is to buy an essential oil ring for the lightbulb in the lamp at your bedside table.

PET LOVE

Do your furry friends belong in your cave? Dogs and cats may be unconditional sources of love and comfort, but some research has found that having your cats and dogs sleep in the bed with you can wake you up during the night and interfere with your best sleep.[10] While you love your four-legged friends, it might be best to have them sleep in their own space away from yours.

The Best Foods for Sleep

Many people don't realize that what they do (and don't) eat can have a dramatic impact on the quality of their sleep. Certain foods have different properties and qualities that can help promote Peak Beauty Sleep. Try incorporating these foods into your dietary routine in the afternoons and evenings to enhance your sleep at night.

HEMP MILK

Hemp milk is high in the amino acid tryptophan, which is a precursor to serotonin and helps to promote sleep. It also contains all the essential amino acids and lots of minerals. Try the Evening Replenishing Elixir on page 180, which is made from a hemp milk base.

WHOLE, UNREFINED CARBOHYDRATES

Try some quinoa, brown rice, amaranth, gluten-free teff- or brown rice–based wraps, or buckwheat (soba) noodles. Carbohydrates increase the level of tryptophan in your blood, helping to promote sleep.

BANANAS

Bananas help promote sleep because they contain the natural muscle relaxants magnesium and potassium. They also have carbohydrates that will make you sleepy. They are a low-water, starchy fruit that digests slowly, so you can have one ideally a few hours before bed if you find yourself getting hungry but want to eat something that is sleep inducing rather than stimulating.

SWEET POTATOES

These hearty root vegetables contain muscle-relaxing potassium and are a whole, complex carbohydrate. Try baking some sweet potatoes and eating them at dinner with a big salad.

EVENING REPLENISHING ELIXIR

This elixir contains nourishing essential beauty fats and spices known to help soothe inflammation and your nervous system.

Mugful of hemp milk
$^1/_2$ teaspoon powdered turmeric
$^1/_2$ teaspoon ground
    cardamom

$^1/_4$ teaspoon ground cloves
Raw, organic honey or raw coconut nectar, to taste

Heat the hemp milk to just under a boil, and stir in the turmeric, cardamom, and cloves. Remove from the heat, add the raw honey, and enjoy hot.

CHERRIES

This bright, beautiful summer fruit is one of the few foods that naturally contain melatonin. A study found that drinking tart cherry juice offers some slight improvements to the duration and quality of sleep in those with chronic insomnia.[11]

CHIA PUDDING

This snack, made by soaking chia seeds in a liquid base, has a great mix of complex carbs, omega-3 fatty acids, and amino acids to help you feel satiated but not overly stuffed and enjoy a great night's sleep.

The Worst Foods for Sleep

Just as there are excellent foods for sleep, there are foods that are not so great for promoting sleep. Review this list and avoid these foods in the evening to best support your Peak Beauty Sleep.

HEAVY PROTEIN MEALS

Meals that are high in concentrated proteins should be avoided late at night. They take a great deal of digestive energy to break down and can keep you up by overactivating digestion. If you are going to have a heavy dinner, try to eat it early. If circumstances force a late dinner, choose a lighter, plant-based meal.

HIGH FAT MEALS

Fat stimulates the production of acid in the stomach while encouraging the loosening of the esophageal sphincter. This can cause food to spill up into your esophagus, creating heartburn. Lying down to go to sleep after eating heavy, fatty foods makes it even easier for acid to get in all the wrong places. This is a super uncomfortable beauty sleep no-no.

CHOCOLATE

While a little piece of dark chocolate might quell your sweet craving, do not overindulge in chocolate late in night. Remember that it does contain caffeine as well as theobromine, another stimulating compound that can adversely affect your beauty sleep.

SPICY FOODS

These can be overstimulating and actually keep you up at night. A study out of Australia found that on nights the subjects ate spicy meals, there were adverse changes in their sleep patterns.[12] The researchers also found that subjects had elevated body temperatures during their first sleep cycles, which has been shown in other studies to be linked to poor sleep quality.[13]

CAFFEINE

Even if you feel you are used to caffeine, it still keeps your body working. Research published in the *Journal of Clinical Sleep Medicine* found that caffeine ingested as early as 6 hours before bedtime could negatively affect sleep patterns.[14] In a practical sense, this means you should stop drinking coffee (if you drink it at all), green tea, or yerba maté by the afternoon. By the way, the tradition of drinking coffee after dinner is one you should abandon. Make your own tradition with herbal tea if you'd like to sip on something hot, and your beauty will surely benefit.

NICOTINE

If you smoke, you should stop for many health and beauty reasons! We are sure you know this, and hopefully you are working on eliminating that habit long-term. But in the very short-term while transitioning completely, be sure to refrain from indulging in any nicotine products too close to bedtime. Nicotine can be stimulating, which is not conducive to your beauty sleep.

ALCOHOL

This is a tough one, because if you do want to have some drinks, you likely won't have them in the middle of the day or in the morning unless it's a very rare special occasion, such as a tailgate or a celebratory brunch. The problem is that even though the alcohol (especially wine) may feel as if it's inducing sleep, alcohol actually interferes with the restorative functions of sleep.[15] This means that although it may feel relaxing, after a few hours it may encourage you to wake up during the night, decreasing the quality of your overall sleep.

SUPPLEMENT YOUR SLEEP WITH VITAMIN B$_{12}$

This important water-soluble vitamin is used for many functions of the body, including maintaining energy and preventing fatigue. Vitamin B$_{12}$ promotes healthy brain and cardiac function and helps us sleep better, as it has a critical role in the formation of melatonin. It also supports the optimal metabolism of fats and carbohydrates, promotes healthy cell growth and repair, and activates the vitamin folate in the body. While it can be stored in your liver for some time, you can get a blood test to see if your body currently has the proper amount.

Vegans and vegetarians are definitely encouraged to supplement with B$_{12}$ because it is found mostly in animal products, but if you do eat meat, that does not necessarily mean that you have optimal levels of Vitamin B$_{12}$. Absorption and utilization of B$_{12}$ might still be compromised even if you consume foods that contain it (such as animal protein, fortified cereals, and nutritional yeast). For instance, if you are low in hydrochloric acid, which releases B$_{12}$ from food, your body may have issues absorbing B$_{12}$. Your stomach lining could also be lacking in its ability to produce intrinsic factor, a protein that must bind to B$_{12}$ in the small intestine so the body can absorb it.

Check with your doctor if you are unsure of how much Vitamin B$_{12}$ your body needs, but 500 to 1,000 micrograms (mcg) is generally considered a good daily amount. You can take a B-complex supplement to get a balance of all the B vitamins.

If you really value your sleep, you may have to make some serious lifestyle changes around your alcohol habits. This may seem difficult at first, but once you experience more daytime bliss and start feeling great in so many other areas of your life (including having increasingly beautiful skin), you may naturally taper off your imbibing. When you do, you may find that your "cleaner" system needs far less alcohol in general to feel relaxed or to enjoy the taste of your favorite Cabernet or Pinot. In an ideal world, you should avoid drinking within 3 hours of bedtime. But if you are going out for a night with friends, this obviously won't be realistic. Just be aware, drink responsibly and moderately (ideally keeping it to one or two drinks maximum), and perhaps find other ways to spend time with friends and relaxing that don't involve alcohol.

Hopefully by now it is clear to you just how important Peak Beauty Sleep is for your overall health, vitality, and beauty. It's so important, in fact, that achieving your full potential of Radical Beauty would be hard to realize without working to optimize your sleep. Be sure to make the necessary shifts to prioritize your sleep so you can enjoy your best beauty for the long-term.

Primal Beauty

If you want to see true beauty personified, all you need do is gaze at a sunrise or sunset, the mighty rivers or wide oceans, or the harmonious synergy in any forest. We can stand in awe of nature's perfect beauty while recognizing that we are a part of it. Each of us is a part of the natural world, and living in accordance with natural principles and rhythms aligns us with Mother Nature. This powerfully supports our natural beauty to flow through.

Shakti is the Sanskrit word for the creative power of nature that we are all a part of. Living in accordance with nature is as essential to our being as breathing or sleeping, but it's easy with a modern lifestyle to stray further and further away from our attunement with nature. When we superimpose synthetic or unnatural rhythms over the fabric of our lives, our natural beauty suffers.

Nature is our teacher. We can learn a lot from watching the cycles of the sun and moon, listening to the sounds of nature, and tuning in to the effects they have on our energy. The more you are in harmony with nature and her rhythms and energies, the more positive effect you'll see on your well-being and beauty.

Harness the Beauty of the Seasons

One of the most important ways to allow the power of nature to support your health and beauty is to tune in to the changing seasons of the year. Every part of the year has a different collective energy, which in turn affects your personal energy. Riding this wave and adjusting your dietary and lifestyle patterns to be in sync with the flow of the seasons will help you achieve Radical Beauty. The more in sync you are with the universal energies taking place on a larger scale beyond you, the better your skin, hair, and nails will look, and the more power you'll feel supporting you in everything you do.

For instance, by eating according to the seasons and largely focusing your diet on the produce that is being grown locally during the current season, you will be eating food that is at its peak of freshness. Not only will it taste its best, but it will also have the most beauty nutrition because it was picked close to when and where you consume it. Seasonal foods also tend to be more affordable since crops for each season are naturally in abundance and sellers don't have to account for shipping costs.

If you focus on eating seasonally and shopping often at the local farmer's markets, you may find that you end up eating a far wider variety of what happens to be growing around you at the moment instead of reaching for your favorite staple veggies. This will help you naturally get a greater variety of beauty nutrients into your diet, as different foods contain different compositions of minerals and phytonutrients to help support your Radical Beauty. You will also feel more integrated into your surrounding environment if you can eat what is grown there. Besides your personal benefits, eating this way reduces your carbon footprint and allows you to support Mother Nature. It requires less fuel (from trucks, trains, planes, and so on) to transport food from local farms to your table than from overseas growers.

From a beauty standpoint, you may notice that each season has a different effect on your skin, and it is important to adjust accordingly. The seasons will influence your exercise and activity levels, as well, and you must honor that flow. In a larger sense, as the overall environment is shifting, you can tune in to that collective energy and work with it in each season, not against it. For example, during the peak light of the summer you may feel a tremendous drive to work on creative projects that you previously decided to "plant" in the spring. Being authentic to those natural urges will make you more beautifully powerful.

Let's explore all the seasons and how to best shift your dietary and skin-care routines as well as your energy goals to maintain your natural beauty in alignment with the larger picture of nature all around you.

Winter Lifestyle Beauty Practices

Winter is the season with the least amount of light. Your skin might need more moisture at this time, and you might naturally want to eat meals that are more hearty and hot, temperature-wise. With the deepening darkness, you may sense a natural tendency to go inward and take stock of your goals and what you are creating in your life. Here are the best practices to attain Radical Beauty in the winter:

- Eat more freshly made hot meals. Your body will naturally crave hot soups and stews, baked vegetable dishes, and the like, so be in tune with those needs and supply yourself with hot, comforting foods. Though you may, of course, keep some raw foods in your diet, be sure to balance them with warming foods.

- Incorporate a lot of root vegetables such as acorn, butternut and coquina squash; yams, sweet potatoes, and pumpkins, which you will find in the local farmer's markets at this time of year. These vegetables are particularly high in beta-carotene, which converts into vitamin A in the body and is an excellent nutrient to keep your skin healthy and bright in these dimmer months.

- Add warming spices such as ginger, cloves, and cinnamon to your teas and recipes.

- Switch to organic, cold-pressed sesame oil to moisturize your skin for your *abhyanga* practice. Sesame oil is said to have warming properties.

- Due to the dryness of winter, you might need a heavier facial moisturizer. Switch accordingly and look for one that is oil based rather than water based, as the oil will provide a protective layer on your skin and hold in moisture longer. Products containing pure plant oils like coconut, almond, avocado, and primrose oil should not make your skin break out. On the other hand, shea butter may clog your pores; especially if you are acne-prone, avoid products on the face that contain shea butter (though it's great to use on your body). Avoid products that contain synthetic, petroleum-based oils, such as mineral oil.

- Your skin will likely be dry and dehydrated not only from the wind and cold elements, but also from indoor heat, so make sure your moisturizer contains hyaluronic acid and other humectants to attract more moisture to your face and keep it supple.

- Increase your fat intake slightly—but not dramatically—with whole plant foods such as chia seeds, walnuts, and avocados. These essential fats will nourish supple skin. Just an extra few tablespoons of chia seed pudding (see kimberlysnyder.com for the easy recipe) or another half of an avocado will keep your skin moisturized from the inside out. Extra fat in the winter may also feel grounding during this dark period.

- Use a creamy cleanser rather than a gel one. The cream will have fewer stripping surfactants and help keep the natural oils on your skin intact during these times when you want to hold on to all of the moisture you can.

- Do a weekly at-home oil treatment to keep your hair protected from the drying weather. At least once a week, massage coconut oil into the tips of your hair and throughout the strands, pile it into a bun or tuck it into a shower cap, leave it in for at least 30 minutes to 1 hour, and then rinse out and shampoo as usual.

- Slough off dry skin cells with an at-home sugar scrub. Combine equal parts coconut oil and organic sugar and then add 15 to 20 drops or so of your favorite essential oil. Keep the mixture in a glass or BPA-free container. In the shower, gently rub off dead skin cells from your entire body, including your elbows and heels. Shaving is also a great exfoliator for the large surface area of your legs.

- Stay active. It's tempting to just curl up during winter, but the diminished light and the cold weather can contribute to depression, stagnation, a weakened immune system, and sluggish feelings. It's a great time of year to begin or deepen a home yoga practice, whether on your own or with a yoga DVD. You don't have to expose yourself to the elements to stay active and move every part of your body.

- Honor the natural tendency for more "darkness" and allow yourself to rejuvenate and rest by staying at home more. Don't push yourself to go out more than you naturally like out of obligation. You might feel that evenings at home with herbal tea, a warm bath, and a good book simply serve you more.

- If you live in a place that has limited sunlight for extended periods of time throughout the winter months, you might want to consider supplementing with vitamin D^3, or getting a special light designed to help stimulate vitamin D in your body. Vitamin D plays a vital role in maintaining healthy, beautiful bones, strong immunity, balanced moods, and all-around health and wellness.

- With the very slowly burgeoning light of the winter solstice near the end of the year, complete an honest and deep assessment of where you would like to put your energy in the upcoming year and what is nurturing and authentic for your beautiful spirit at this time. In nature, new seeds are growing at the root level now, and a lot is taking place beneath the surface. This is a great time for you, too, to evaluate where you want to plant your "seeds," which projects you want to pursue, and where you want to put your energy, which will bloom later in the year. You can determine this only by being honest and listening to your heart.

Spring Lifestyle Beauty Practices

In spring, life emerges again. No matter how long the cold winter months may seem some years, spring always follows. You can see the burgeoning beauty of fresh flower buds, leaves, and shoots and feel the urge to express your natural beauty outwardly with sundresses, skirts, and perhaps brighter makeup colors. As the light increases, you naturally feel like shedding the stagnation and heaviness of winter. This includes a tendency to start eating lighter and perhaps lightening up on your skin-care products, too. You may also feel a natural rise in energy, a newfound spark of powerful inspiration that can now be directed toward whatever goals you decided to pursue when taking stock in the darkness of winter. Here are the best ways to harness the beauty of spring:

- Spring is the very best time of the year to complete a cleanse or engage in some detoxing. If you're interested in a liquid cleanse, check out the organic, strategically designed ones offered from Glow Bio (myglowbio .com) or do your own version by making fresh green smoothies or juices and abstaining from heavier foods for a few days.

- Lighten up your diet. This is a great time of year to shift into eating more raw foods (though you don't have to eat 100 percent raw, by any means). Reduce your ratio of fats so you feel less weighed down. You might want to eat lighter, broth-based soups and favor smaller amounts of avocado and nuts. Use all oils sparingly.

- If you indulged over the winter, it's a great time to reset bad habits and patterns and renew your resolve to improve your eating habits. Feel in tune with the bursting energy of spring by letting go of heavier, dense, or clogging foods. Ditch the dairy, refined sugars, gluten, and excess animal protein, and eat more light, plant-centric meals.

- Increase your consumption of raw apple cider vinegar by adding it into salad dressings or hot water that you sip, as it has antiseptic qualities to help you cleanse for spring while building healthy bacteria in your gut. It also offers the beauty-balancing electrolyte potassium.

- Sprouts and microgreens very much capture the emerging energy of the spring and are bursting with living enzymes, vitamins, minerals, and phytonutrients. Wash them well and sprinkle them liberally into salads, on top of soups, and on just about any dish you eat. Even though they are so pretty to look at, you can also throw a handful into a smoothie!

- Add some natural diuretics to your smoothies and other dishes to help flush out some spring water weight. Some good options include coriander, parsley, asparagus, cranberry, and pineapple; as it gets closer to summer, try aubergine and watermelon.

- Take full advantage of your farmer's market, which will have a much wider array of foods than it did during the winter. Lettuces, fennel, broccoli, asparagus, watercress, and spring greens are just a few of the farmer's market spring treasures you will discover.

- Sweat any way you can! This is a great time of year to hit the infrared sauna or get out into the light of day for some vigorous hiking, walking, or jogging. Sweat is a great way to purge out toxicity and excess stagnation that built up during the winter.

- If you have a home yoga practice, this is a great time to increase the Surya Namaskars, or sun salutations, and other standing flow sequences, as you'll naturally feel like moving more vigorously this season.

- Take advantage of the growing light. Get up earlier to enjoy the mornings, and perhaps take an afternoon or post-early-dinner stroll to enjoy the evening light and watch the sunset. This is a beautiful way to sync with the changing rhythm of the environment.

- Gently exfoliate dead skin cells that may have accumulated from winter with a cleanser that contains alpha or beta hydroxy acids.

- Try sloughing off excessive dead skin cells on your body with a salt scrub rather than the sugar scrub you might have used for winter. Salt scrubs are considered slightly more exfoliating, and salt is said to have a negative ionic charge, helping purify negative energies and impurities that you may have picked up from the environment.[1] This is the theory behind the rock salt lamps sold at local health markets, which are said to help neutralize home environments from electronic devices that are believed to give off a positive ionic charge. Combine equal parts coconut oil and salt with 15 to 20 drops of your favorite essential oil (such as lavender or neroli). Keep the mixture in a glass or BPA-free container, and gently scrub your entire body in the shower.

- Pay extra attention to moving stagnation through your lymphatic system, as this is the season to detox. Refer back to page 120 for more tips on this.

- Ayurveda encourages *Panchakarma* methods to help cleanse the body and renew digestion. These are detoxification methods that include colon cleansing. If you're up for it, try getting an at-home enema kit or a gravity colonic from a recommended therapist.

- Increase your water intake to flush out impurities. Also try incorporating hot water with lemon in the afternoons and/or evenings. This is a fantastic cleansing, flushing drink.

- With the growing light, be sure to properly protect yourself from the sun with wide-brimmed hats, large sunglasses, and nontoxic sunscreen (see page 115).

- Synchronize with the creative power flowing through nature and the universe. Take the time to put energy into your creative ventures and longings, and cultivate them. Be selective with your time, cutting out excessive television watching and other more passive activities you might have engaged in over the cold winter. Spend more time going for what you want. You have all the power of the universe supporting you now to go for it!

Summer Lifestyle Beauty Practices

Summer brings the most intense sunlight, which is activating and exciting. Depending on where you live, it might be extremely humid or extremely dry at this time. You might also be contending with a vacillation between hot outdoor weather and freezing indoor air-conditioning. It's important to protect and nourish your immunity and energy during these vital summer months. Here are some of the most effective Radical Beauty summer practices:

- Eat lots of cooling, juicy in-season fruits, including apricots, grapes, blueberries, blackberries, cherries, plums, raspberries, strawberries, figs, nectarines, and melons.

These are among the bounty of summer

- Enjoy beetroot, cucumbers, peppers, radishes, courgettes, endives, and beans. These are among the bounty of summer foods you'll find fresh and available at your local farmer's market.

- It's easier to get more agitated, impatient, and annoyed during this "fiery" season of *Pitta,* which governs our internal fire. It's a good idea to avoid overactive foods that might enhance those qualities, including chilies, spicy tomatillos, and excessive garlic and onion.

- Drink cooling, herbal teas such as fresh mint tea or chamomile. It's easy to grow a little mint plant at your kitchen windowsill and have fresh mint tea all summer.

- Honor your body's natural inclination to eat lighter during the heat of summer. Listen to your body and never force it to eat. It's important to recognize that you shouldn't necessarily eat the same meals or foods during every month of the year. This is a great time to eat lots of raw foods such as fresh salads and fruit.

- Drink coconut water, which is hydrating and helps to replenish electrolytes and minerals that you lose from sweating.

- Enjoy lots of raw greens this season, which are by nature *yin,* or cooling. Be creative with the range of lettuces and greens you see at your farmer's market, and rotate them to create some new, tasty salads.

- Since you may already feel puffy or somewhat swollen from the heat, it's a good idea to cut back on salty foods. Try using more fresh herbs for flavor rather than lots of salt. Your taste for salt will naturally reduce over time.

- As your skin increases in oiliness, try the Radically Clear Skin Mask (page 129) or other clay-based masks to help ward off breakouts and congestion in your complexion.

- Unless you have very dry skin, try switching your cleanser from a creamy one to a gel-based one, which is lighter and can help clear out excess sweat, dirt, and grime.

- If oil-based creams are starting to feel too heavy, switch to a highly absorbable, lighter, water-based moisturizer for the summer.

- Aloe is a fairly sturdy plant to try growing in a pot indoors or outdoors (depending on where you live). You'll have a fresh source to use on any burns from excessive sunlight. (Let's really hope that doesn't happen, but just in case, be prepared!)

- Since coconut oil is said to have cooling properties, switch to coconut oil for your *abhyanga* practice (see page 121).

- Wear light-colored, natural fabrics such as linen and cotton, which allow your skin to breathe.

- Fill a spritzer bottle with rose water, and spray it across your face and décolleté whenever you need a soothing refresher.

- Honor changes in movement this time of year. You might be drawn to yoga (especially a self-practice) rather than super intense aerobic activities (unless they involve beach or water sports!), which might feel depleting. This is not necessarily the best time for hot yoga in an enclosed, artificially heated room.

- You might feel activated and excited not only by your creative or professional pursuits but also to explore and revel in being outside in nature's raw elements. This might mean beach time or more time to lounge in a park. Allow yourself to have this outdoor time and to explore feeling stimulated from nature as well as your personal interests. Your energy will naturally be high, so get outside and enjoy. At the very end of summer, however, depending on your environment, you might feel overheated and the need to chill out more, and it's important to honor that as well.

Fall Lifestyle Beauty Practices

The beauty of fall is seen in the full range of colors among Mother Nature's changing leaves. The air gets crisper, and the wind can pick up, making it important to protect your skin and body. You may find yourself craving less coconut water and more hot teas and elixirs to feel balanced, as well as hot, nourishing meals you may have largely avoided in the summer. From an energetic standpoint, it's important to take measures to feel grounded, as *Vata*, the air-based element, dominates the fall season. When imbalanced, this can exacerbate stress and anxiety, which is particularly true if activities dramatically increase after a leisurely summer. Here are the best fall beauty practices:

- It's the natural time of year to start eating more grounding, warm cooked meals again, so be sure to adjust your dietary rotation accordingly.

- Brussels sprouts, turnips, daikon radish, cauliflower, and mushrooms are some of the vegetables you'll find in season in the fall, so be sure to take advantage and find creative and simple ways to cook and enjoy these fortifying foods.

- Quinoa, brown rice, and amaranth are great gluten-free grains to incorporate this time of year, especially if eaten with lots of vegetables.

- Sip on lemon balm, chamomile, valerian root, ashwagandha or holy basil/tulsi teas, which are fantastic for helping you destress and unwind. You can source these teas, which can often be found combined in "anti-anxiety" formulations, at health stores.

- The drying wind and drop in humidity may make your skin feel rougher. Be sure to spend a little more time with your *abhyanga* practice (see page 121), which is also good for pacifying excess *Vata,* which can lead to feeling overwhelmed and anxious when imbalanced. *Abhyanga* is a great practice to help alleviate stress.

- Since *Vata,* or the air element, is so prevalent in the fall, you may experience some constipation. This is a symptom of *Vata* being out of balance. Be sure to eat lots of fibrous foods, take some magnesium-oxygen supplements as needed to help keep things moving, and eat mindfully and slowly, always chewing well.

- Be sure to protect your skin from the quickening changes of the weather, including dry wind. Use scarves and gloves to protect your hands, neck, and face during walks or periods outside, keeping out drafts that can lead to chapping and excessive dryness.

- Your skin may need extra nourishment with the change of seasons, and it might start to feel drier. The Radically Timeless Beauty Mask (page 115) is particularly excellent at this time of year.

- Be sure to protect your delicate lips, which may become increasingly chapped. Apply lip balms regularly that contain natural ingredients such as shea butter, olive oil, and vitamin E. Avoid lip balms that contain petroleum-based, synthetic ingredients (which you don't want to continually ingest, an inevitable occurrence with anything you put on your lips).

- Since you might have gotten your fair share (or more!) of sun, salt water, and chlorine over the summer, your skin might feel a bit taxed. Try going back to a gentle sugar scrub (see Winter tips on page 189) and adding more coconut oil if you feel that your skin needs extra lubrication.

- Avoid using stripping soaps on your skin in the shower. Choose all-natural, mild, and simple cleansers with essential oils instead of potentially irritating artificial fragrances.

- With the cooler temperatures and chilly wind, it's time to switch back to thicker moisturizers with an oil base, which can feel more hydrating and protective.

- Pay extra attention to your hands. They have the long winter ahead of them with lots of potential cold and wind exposure. Be sure to keep your hands moisturized with a good hand cream (shea butter or other natural ingredient based), and reapply often, especially after washing your hands.

- After the leisure of summer, you may feel an increased swirl of activities in the fall: kids going back to school, increased work projects, or new-found intensity in hitting goals by the end of the year. Be sure to balance the stress. Make it a priority to create downtime for yourself as the holidays gear up so you don't feel overwhelmed and resort to stress eating or other unhealthy outlets. Take time to cultivate nurturing, grounding activities such as meditation, massages, spending time at home reading, or whatever makes you feel soothed.

Making an effort to gracefully acknowledge the energy shifts as the earth makes her yearly progression around the sun and to shift your daily lifestyle routines in accordance with the different seasons is an important way to maximize your health, energy, and expression of beauty. Whether we are aware of it or not, we are impacted by the larger energy influences of our environment. Why not recognize, embrace, and align with them to your advantage? You only have heightened beauty and a greater sense of energy to attain. Start applying these modifications for the season you are in right now to feel more in tune with the collective universal energy of which you are intrinsically part.

Balance Solar and Lunar Energy and All the Earth's Elements

Solar Beauty

Of course, no one would claim that going out and baking in the sun is good for your skin. By now, it's well established that overexposure to the sun can lead to skin cancer and seriously accelerated skin aging. But that's not to say that we should shun the sun completely. The sun is a vital component of nature that provides life and vitality to the entire planet, including us. Even in the dawn of increased modernism, we cannot divorce ourselves from Mother Nature; our connection to her is indivisible.

While you have to be very careful about how and where you engage in sun exposure (which we will discuss further below), we don't want to completely eschew the sun. Robyn Lucas, an epidemiologist at Australian National University who led a study published in the *International Journal of Epidemiology*, concluded that far more lives are lost to diseases caused by a *lack* of sunlight than to those caused by too much.[1] There are many health and beauty benefits to limited sun exposure, including the following.

ENDORPHIN AND HORMONE PRODUCTION

Just being around sunlight—even if you're not directly exposed to it—can help improve your mood by causing your body to synthesize "feel good" endorphins and hormones such as serotonin. This can be as simple as gazing out of a window into the natural light while eating lunch or working on a laptop (though you won't absorb vitamin D through glass). A lack of sun exposure can cause a melatonin imbalance and lead to seasonal affective disorder (SAD), a form of depression caused by a deficiency of natural sunlight during the winter months. This is a very real issue for those in certain environments that don't have enough sunlight, and it demonstrates how important natural elements such as the sun are to our beauty and well-being. As we mentioned in Pillar 3, Peak Beauty Sleep, it's critical to have a healthy amount of daylight to balance the night. Your pineal gland produces melatonin based on the contrast of bright sun exposure in the day and complete darkness at night.[2] If you don't have enough exposure to daylight during the day, your body can't appreciate the difference and will not optimize your melatonin production, which is important to regulate healthy beauty sleep cycles.[3]

VITAMIN D SYNTHESIS AND IMMUNE BOOST

Sunlight helps your skin synthesize vitamin D, which makes it possible to absorb calcium. Vitamin D also helps with skin issues like psoriasis, and boosts your immunity so you can better fight infections such as colds and the flu. Some researchers believe it may even help protect against the development of some cancer cells.[4] Vitamin D is really a hormone and not a vitamin, and it has been shown in some research to help increase testosterone levels in men[5] and regulate estrogen and progesterone levels in women.[6] This assistance in balancing hormones is another huge benefit of sun exposure. Though you can supplement with vitamin D, it's preferable and more reliable to get vitamin D through moderate sunlight exposure whenever possible.

IMPROVED CIRCULATION AND METABOLISM

The sun is good for blood circulation, which, as we discussed earlier, is important to ensure the optimal distribution of beauty nutrients throughout your entire body, and some research is even linking sunlight exposure to a boost in metabolism.[7]

POSSIBLE PREVENTION OF HEART DISEASE AND CANCER

New research out of the *Journal of Investigative Dermatology* has found that when sunlight touches the skin, a compound called nitric oxide, which helps lower blood pressure, is released into the blood vessels.[8] Head researcher Richard Weller and his colleagues state, "We are concerned that well-meaning advice to reduce the comparatively low numbers of deaths from skin cancer may inadvertently increase the risk of death from far higher prevalent cardiovascular disease and stroke, and goes against epidemiological data[9,10] showing that sunlight exposure reduces all-cause and cardiovascular mortality."[11] The researchers noted that for every person who succumbed to skin cancer, about sixty to one hundred people succumb to stroke and heart disease linked to high blood pressure. This translates to eighty times more people dying of cardiovascular disease than skin cancer.

A study published in the journal *Cancer,* as well as a systematic review published in the *European Journal of Cancer,* found that insufficient exposure to sunlight can be a risk factor for cancer in western Europe and North America, and the malignancies that showed the greatest increase with inadequate exposure to sunlight were reproductive and digestive cancers, namely breast, colon, and ovarian cancers.[12,13]

Sun Exposure vs. Sun Damage

You may be wondering, what about sun damage and aging? Again, we are definitely *not* suggesting that you bake out in the sun 1960s-style, when it was the thing to reflect the sunlight back onto your skin with aluminum foil. What we're talking about is much more strategic and controlled. When managed this way, limited sun exposure might actually reverse sun damage! Research out of Stanford University found that by triggering the synthesis of vitamin D within the body, limited sun exposure may cause immune cells to travel to the outer layers of the skin, where they are available to protect and help repair damage caused by excessive sun exposure.[14]

So how much sun is the right balance for your beauty? Well, first of all, we don't recommend exposing your delicate facial skin to the sun. It's too precious, and it's obviously the first place you want to protect against visible signs of aging. Always wear a hat when you are exposed to sunlight, and be sure to use nontoxic sunscreen protection.

To get healthy sunlight, focus on your limbs. Michael F. Holick, MD, PhD, who heads up the Vitamin D, Skin, and Bone Research Laboratory at Boston

University and is the author of the book *The UV Advantage,* agrees. He recommends sensible sun exposure of 5 to 10 minutes of direct sunlight on bare legs and arms two or three times a week.[15] Applying sunscreen is definitely recommended for any sun exposure beyond that. The sun will feel great on your arms and legs during short walks in the sunlight. Try parking your car a little farther away from the mall or grocery store the next time you go shopping and enjoy some extra time in the sun. Take 5 minutes to read outside, to sip your favorite tea, or just to look at the beauty around you, whether you are in the suburbs or in the city. Even in most industrial areas you can usually find something beautiful. This will naturally feel fantastic and delicious for your whole body, which loves getting some light, even for a very short time! Holick also recommends supplementing with 1,000 IUs of vitamin D,[16] especially in the winter, when you may not get adequate sunlight.

You can also balance the beauty of natural sunlight with foods that are rich in vitamins C and E as well as selenium. These are great skin beauty foods that protect against sun damage. Karen E. Burke, MD, PhD, of the Mount Sinai School of Medicine says, "These antioxidants work by speeding up the skin's natural repair systems and by directly inhibiting further damage."[17] Some great natural sources of these Radical Beauty nutrients include acai, blueberries, Brazil nuts, almonds, oranges, and peppers.

Capturing Energy Directly from the Light

We all know that plants convert sunlight into energy. But in 2014 a groundbreaking study published in the *Journal of Cell Science* suggested that animals that consume a chlorophyll-rich diet are also able to derive energy directly from the sunlight.[18] Previously, we believed that green plants were the only organisms that were able to convert sunlight into biological energy in the form of adenosine triphosphate (ATP). This study showed that the mitochondria in animal cells "can also capture light and synthesize ATP when mixed with a light-capturing metabolite of chlorophyll."[19]

In other words, this study implies that animals—including humans—can borrow the light-harvesting capabilities of chlorophyll when consuming a diet rich in plant food and use it for energy (ATP) production. Some of the animals researched that were fed such a diet and exposed to light also saw an increased life span. Furthermore, the energy coming from the chlorophyll-induced diet and light exposure was believed to help animal mitochondria function in a healthier way.[20] This is super exciting from a beauty standpoint, because healthier mitochondria function means a reduction in the aging caused by free radicals and thus a reduction in cellular damage.[21]

This is a whole new way to think about our diet and the role green vegetables play when it comes to our beauty. Besides providing us with an abundance of vitamins, minerals, and thousands of beauty-building compounds, according to this research consuming green vegetables may also help us generate energy directly from the sunlight! This further shows our timeless and infinite connection, an unbroken continuum, with nature. Greens are grown in nature and make up a large part of the diets of our close genetic relatives. The big takeaway here is the reinforcement of what we've been saying all along: eat close to nature and become more naturally beautiful and have more beautiful, natural energy.

Lunar (Moon) Energy

Like the sun, the moon and her cycles have an impact on our energy, albeit in more subtle ways. While it's not as obvious as the sunlight that grows plants and has a visible impact on our skin, the moon, another larger energetic body in our macrocosmic orbit, also impacts our beauty. Our ancestors were more in tune with the moon's waning and waxing rhythms and observed and noted them to create timetables for tending and harvesting crops and organizing community life. The planting calendar of biodynamic farming, a type of sustainable organic farming practiced globally from France to India and beyond, considers soil fertility, plant growth, and livestock care as a set of ecologically interrelated tasks,[22] and is synced with the lunar phases of the moon.[23]

There's been some documented influence of the moon on certain animals, such as the body weight of honeybees that peaks during a new moon.[24] Different ancient cultures, verified in some writings from Babylonia and Assyria, have connected a lunar influence on humans. It's recognized that the tides are caused by the gravitational relationship between the moon and the earth, known as the tidal force. On a micro level, we are made up of around 72 percent water and might experience some of the lunar influence from this larger body of energy, such as periods of feeling more expansive and energized or more retracted and inward.

The female menstrual cycle and the complete cycle of the moon, which is approximately the same number of days, has caused much intrigue over the years. Ayurveda believes that the cycles of the moon and the tides of the ocean are mysterious and powerful ways to display the deep connection a woman has to nature.

Just as it is important to keep your waking hours closely tied to the sunrises and sunsets, traditional systems worldwide believe that there is power in syncing up your activities to the cycles of nature such as the moon cycle. Attuning the collective natural force between certain activities and efforts helps us live more in harmony with nature.

The new moon is like a mini New Year's every month. Think of it as a wonderful way to refresh each month and create new goals or refocus on your goals with new vigor. It's a good day for cleansing and a great time to start implementing positive new habits to benefit your beauty, such as a commitment to drinking hot water with lemon each morning, drinking more fresh water and giving up soda, or making more time to prepare and benefit from some at-home beauty masks. Why wait for New Year's? You can experience a personal, renewed commitment to improving your beauty every single month.

The full moon is when you may feel the strong influence of completeness in your projects. You can time your creative projects or goals to reach their peak in sync with the full moon. Beauty-wise, this is a great time to prepare and enjoy a very nourishing beauty meal that may take a little more effort than usual for you and your loved ones. Try to enjoy even a few minutes' "moon bathing" out in the fullness of the moon's natural light, which has a cooling, soothing energy that balances the activating sunlight energy in your being.

Ancient mystics believe that the waxing, or growing energy, of the moon is a great time for fertility, taking in nourishment, and building on your intentions from the new moon, while the waning energy that comes after the full moon is a good time for taking stock and cleaning up any old business. This might be a great time to clean out your fridge, kitchen cupboards, and bathroom cabinets of any old beauty products or toxic ingredients that don't serve you anymore. Reclaim only what is fresh and supportive of your life force.

Balancing the Elements in Your Body

According to Ayurveda's *panchamahaboota* theory, everything in the universe—including you—is composed of five main elements: earth, water, fire, air, and space (or ether). This theory holds that the elemental constitution that makes up your body is not unique, but it is shared with all things throughout nature. In the Chinese medical system there are also five elements: earth, water, fire, wood, and metal. Without going into too much detail about these complex ancient systems, we can use some understanding of them to benefit our beauty by creating more balance. According to Ayurveda, an imbalance of these elements can lead to beauty disorders such as acne, brittle hair, and skin that ages faster than it should.

The Ayurvedic *dosha* theory holds that we all possess each of the five elements, but certain elements are dominant in our bodies. Building on what we said earlier about the *dosha* system, we have three dominant elements: *Vata,* or air constitution, is represented by the wind in nature; *Pitta,* or fire constitution, is a representation of the sun; and *Kapha,* or earth/water constitution, is represented by the rocks and solid elements on earth as well as bodies of water. When we are out of balance, the elements within our bodies are also imbalanced. On the other hand, balancing our elemental constitution promotes health and delays or reduces visible signs of aging. Radical Beauty requires balance and avoiding extremes so you can fully express your natural beauty.

Again, this whole concept goes into much more depth, but there are some general principles that you can use for introspection to survey potential areas of imbalance within yourself while using tangible tools to work on creating a beautiful balance within your body, mind, and spirit. Here are some of the symptoms of balanced and imbalanced elements and a sampling of the most effective tools to get back in balance.

VATA (AIR/WIND)

Like the wind, this represents the force behind all movements, including internal movements such as digestion, elimination, breathing, and circulation.

Symptoms of balanced *Vata*: creative thinking, inspired, enthusiastic, supple skin

Symptoms of imbalanced *Vata*: constipation, excessive worry and anxiety, insomnia, and dry skin

Some basic tips for balancing *Vata* include the following:

- Incorporate *abhyanga* into your regular daily practice with a real commitment, as it is especially important for helping to ground and destress the mind.
- Get to bed earlier and establish a regular schedule to get more rest.
- Protect yourself with proper measures in cold, windy weather since air-based *Vata* types may be more susceptible to chills and imbalances from chilly weather.
- Prioritize regular, proper elimination (with diet, oxygen-magnesium products, probiotics, etc.).
- Establish a regular daily routine, which is especially important for *Vata*.
- Avoid caffeine and stimulants.
- Favor fresh, light, and easy-to-digest foods. Heavy proteins (red meat, dairy, and the like) are especially hard to digest, so limit or avoid them.
- Avoid foods that are extremely light and dry, such as crackers, cold cereals, and packaged snacks.
- Incorporate cardamom, cumin, ginger, cinnamon, salt, cloves, mustard seed, and black pepper in your diet.

PITTA (FIRE/SUN)

Fire is the transformative element in nature that can enable change, so it has an important role in digestion and metabolism, governing the digestive *agni* in your body.

Symptoms of balanced *Pitta*: being confident, expressing charisma and intelligence, and taking action with a clear sense of vision, direction, and purpose

Symptoms of imbalanced *Pitta*: inflammation, diarrhea, indigestion, heartburn, hives, skin rashes, chronic irritation, premature graying of hair, acne

*Note: Excessive internal overheating/*Pitta *is considered very aging.*

Some basic tips for balancing *Pitta* include the following:

- Avoid spicy food, such as chilies, and "heating" foods and spices, including tomatoes, radishes, aubergine, beetroot, garlic, onions, peppers, and mustard seed.
- Avoid the tendency to overwork; take more time to rest and rejuvenate.
- Incorporate more cooling foods, such as green leafy vegetables, courgettes, green beans, and cucumber. The Glowing Green Smoothie (see recipe, page 27) is particularly excellent.
- Drink "cooling" beverages, such as coconut water, or lemon balm or tulsi tea.

KAPHA (EARTH/WATER)

Like the tangible elements of earth, such as rivers and rocks, *Kapha* is what gives structure to our body and mind and lubrication for our joints and tissues, and helps to form healthy structures (*dhatus*) of the body.

Symptoms of balanced *Kapha*: stamina; strength; healthy lubrication and moistness in skin, hair and joints; devotion; good at following through; even-tempered; patient; compassionate

Symptoms of imbalanced *Kapha*: easily gaining weight (and having a hard time losing or maintaining ideal weight), slow metabolism, lethargy, excessive sleep, problems feeling motivated, congestion, stagnation in the lymphatic system, oily skin

Some basic tips for balancing *Kapha* include the following:

- Incorporate some cardio to help ward off stagnation and lethargy. Hiking and biking are some great examples.
- Favor light, dry foods and decrease all oils and excess fats. Try cooking with water or preparing soups and steaming or baking vegetables with little (or even no) oil. (Good fats can be consumed in moderate amounts from avocados and other whole plant foods.)
- Reduce consumption of large amounts of nuts, which are dense.
- In warmer months, enjoy a diet made up largely of raw foods, including vegetables, fruits, some seeds, and small amounts of nuts.
- Reduce sodium levels.
- Try avoiding gluten and wheat-based products.

As micro expressions of the greater macrocosmic universe, we have an inherent connection to the greater bodies of the sun, the moon, and all the elements of nature, which also reside within us. Working to optimize their influence on us and balance the universal elements within our own bodies is an important way to align to your highest expression of Radical Beauty.

Get Closer to Nature Indoors and Out

Healing by "Grounding"

Most of us intuitively feel good being in nature. You may not realize that there is actually a word for making direct contact with the earth, but actually there are two: *grounding* and *earthing*. Both terms refer to the healing that takes place from making direct contact with the earth.

There are now studies that show that grounding has major benefits for health as well as beauty. For instance, a study published in the *Journal of Cosmetics, Dermatological Sciences and Applications* found that even an hour session of making direct contact with the earth restored the regulation of blood flow to the face, helping to enhance skin tissue repair and improve facial appearance.[1] Our intrinsic connection with nature is so great that just by making direct contact with it, our skin beauty measurably benefits! Mother Nature indeed can be a powerful supporter of our skin and overall health.

How does touching the earth actually improve our health and beauty beyond just feeling "good"? Just touching the earth, which is electrically conductive,[2] neutralizes free radicals and brings you back in sync with the earth's energy field. Upon contact, the negative ions from the earth's surface rush into our bodies to discharge the many unpaired positive ions (or free radicals) we've picked up from modern living. These free radicals stem from regular exposure to environmental pollutants, heavy metals, radiation, toxicity, and chemicals in the food supply. Those free radicals are associated with disease, aging, and inflammation, but when you expose your bare skin to the soil, sand, or grass, the healing powers of the earth neutralize them to keep inflammation and aging in check.

Think about how soothing it feels to dig your heels into the sand during a day at the beach. Now there is science to prove what we've intuitively felt all along: contact with the earth really is healing and necessary to achieve Radical Beauty. A paper by Dr. James Oschman in the *Journal of Alternative and Complementary Medicine*[3] explains how "electron deficiency" from not making enough contact with the earth's surface causes the immune system to suffer and inflammation to spiral out of control.

Free radicals are some of the biggest offenders when it comes to aging, and neutralizing them with negative electrons from the earth quells inflammation and slows or prevents many chronic diseases. A study published in 2013 found that grounding has some beneficial effects on cardiovascular risk factors.[4] It was surmised that this is because contact with the earth naturally thins the blood. Other research, from 2011, showed that grounding improves heart rate variability, which is not only beneficial for the heart but for reducing stress.[5] Lowered stress levels can help allay aging.[6] Grounding also helped alleviate muscle soreness in some research,[7] possibly due to better circulation, blood pressure, and blood flow. This is important from a beauty standpoint, as better circulation of nutrients and oxygen will ensure beautiful, healthy skin and hair.

HELP FOR BONE HEALTH RIGHT FROM THE EARTH

The *Journal of Alternative and Complementary Medicine* discussed a possible reduction in the likelihood of developing osteoporosis due to less loss of calcium and phosphorus through urinary excretion[8] when subjects spent time earthing. The loss of these minerals over time is tied to the development of osteoporosis, so finding out how to reduce the loss could do wonders for bone health and to help us maintain a beautiful, upright, and graceful structure.

How to Get Grounded

Grounding couldn't be easier—and it's free! All you have to do is touch the earth whenever you can and as much as you can. Here are some general tips:

- Make as much contact as possible directly through your bare feet, whether it means popping your shoes off at the local park or just walking around in your backyard.

- Even a few minutes spent in contact with the earth is beneficial. Try to work it into your life regularly. You can read with your feet on the earth, or have a conversation with friends while strolling barefoot through the park. If they need extra motivation, share with them how it's been proved to be good for skin health and reducing aging and inflammation.

- If you have access to a grassy backyard, a nice park, or just a field of grass, lie down sometimes so your spine has full contact with the earth. You can even try taking a nap on your back in the grass; you'll wake up feeling radically recharged.

It seems so simple, but remember that some of the most beautiful things in life are truly simple. Pets and children intuitively love to frolic in the grass, and it's time for all of us to focus on reestablishing that sacred connection. Nature is so healing to us; all we have to do is reach out and make contact with her, and she will help us heal from the inside out, while your beauty benefits as well. You will be able to feel how authentically good earthing is for you because the more you participate in earthing, the more reconnected and recharged you will feel in the most Radically Beautiful way.

Making Our Indoors Closer to Nature

Though it would be ideal to be outside in nature more, the fact is that most of us spend the vast majority of our time indoors. We certainly can't change that, and we also can't control everything in our environments, such as when you're walking down the street and a passing bus blows a spray of nasty exhaust on you, or when you step into a restaurant and get a whiff or two of nasty cigarette smoke from the smokers lined up outside. You also can't help it if the soap in public restrooms contains chemicals like sulfates that you wouldn't want to use at home, or you step into a taxi saturated with a sickeningly sweet air freshener dangling from the rearview mirror.

Studies on human exposure to air pollutants by the Environmental Protection Agency (EPA) indicate that indoor levels of pollutants may be two to five times—and even upwards of over one hundred times—higher than outdoor pollutant levels.[9] While this may seem shocking if concerns about indoor pollution have never really crossed your mind, further consider the fact that indoor air pollutants have been ranked among the top five environmental risks to public health.

The problem is that with air-conditioning, heating, and modern office buildings and hotels, many windows are permanently sealed, and very little circulating air enters indoor spaces. This allows indoor pollutants to accumulate to levels that can affect your health and, yes, your beauty. Taking measures to reduce indoor pollution is especially important for those who are pregnant, nursing, or have children, as these pollutants may even disrupt normal brain and organ development.[10] Anything toxic is not in alignment with the natural biorhythms of your body and is going to create free radicals, disrupt your system, and diminish your natural beauty.

But we are not completely helpless to external factors. We *can* control our personal environments to a great extent, and there is much you can do to transform your personal environment into one that nourishes rather than hinders your beauty. It's empowering when you realize all you can do to make these important shifts. There are a lot of them.

Here are some measures you can take to reduce toxicity in your home and in any indoor spaces you spend time in.

DITCH AIR FRESHENERS

Nobody likes a smelly bathroom, but spraying air fresheners into the air regularly is far worse for you than enduring temporary unpleasant bathroom smells. A study from the University of Washington found that eight unnamed, widely used US air fresheners released an average of eighteen chemicals into the air,[11] including some volatile organic chemicals (VOCs) that are considered toxic or hazardous.

If you want to make your home or office smell fresh (as we all do), just open a window, burn a nontoxic soya candle, fill an essential oil diffuser, or crack open a box of good ol' bicarbonate of soda, which naturally helps to fight odors. Also work to get rid of the source of the smell in the first place; it might mean replacing something that's old or past its prime (like an old carpet), which would end up being a positive change all around.

USE NATURAL CLEANING METHODS

It's absolutely critical to reduce toxic cleaning products in your home across the board—from dish soaps to carpet cleaners, all surface and cleaning sprays, and so on. Go green all the way! Your health and beauty are worth it. Get a big trash can and clean house (pun intended), ridding your whole space of toxic chemicals. You can find some nontoxic DIY natural cleaning products to get your space spic-and-span without any toxic petroleum-based chemicals (see page 216). Lemons, bicarbonate of soda, and vinegar are fantastic natural cleaning ingredients, and you might be surprised at how well they work compared with their toxic, chemical-filled counterparts.

VACUUM REGULARLY

Regularly vacuum all indoor spaces using an appliance with a HEPA filter, which stands for "high-efficiency particulate air." A HEPA filter is a type of mechanical air filter that works by forcing air through a fine mesh filter that traps harmful particles and ensures they don't get blown back out into your space (which obviously would defeat the purpose of your hard work!). These particles include pollutants, allergens, dust, and brominated fire-retardant chemicals (known as PBDEs). Be sure to wash out your filter regularly.

MOP IT

According to the Environmental Working Group, ordinary house dust is a complex mixture of pet dander, fungal spores, particulates from indoor aerosols, soil tracked in by foot traffic, volatile organic compounds (VOCs) that evaporate at room temperature, and traces of metals, and these contaminants may degrade more slowly in dust.[12] Regular mopping, especially with the use of microfiber mops, captures dust and dirt from surfaces that vacuuming tends to leave behind. You can mop with plain water (after vacuuming), a nontoxic soap, or some diluted white vinegar.

KEEP A STRICT SHOE-FREE POLICY

If you've ever traveled to Asia, you know that in many countries it's customary to remove your shoes upon entering a home or traditional restaurant. This is an excellent policy to greatly reduce pesticides, pollutants, and toxins that can be tracked into your home from the bottoms of shoes and then absorbed through bare feet (yuck!). This is especially true if you practice yoga at home and place your face near the floor, or if you have toddlers and children whose hands often make contact with the floor.

Think about it... what is on the bottom of your shoes? If you've ever been to New York City or any other large city and seen the sidewalks there, it might feel pretty nasty to want to have any skin contact with the bottoms of your shoes. It's like walking barefoot on the sidewalk, which is something you would probably never want to do! It is coated with visible and invisible amounts of garbage (including a range of hazardous products to simply nasty decaying food), chemicals, human spit, dog feces and urine (probably human also mixed in there), and who knows what else. But no matter where you live, you might be unknowingly tracking in a whole host of toxins into your home with just your shoes. It might be an adjustment to kick off your shoes as soon as you walk into your home and encourage everyone else to do the same, but your home will feel so much cleaner, and you will soon be happy you made the switch to shoes-free. You won't want to go back!

TEST FOR RADON

Radon is a radioactive gas that is linked to lung cancer. It stems from the natural decay of uranium found in soil that potentially moves into homes through cracks and holes in the foundation. Even if your home is new, it could still have a radon issue. Granite countertops are also linked to radon. You can test for radon and even get a do-it-yourself radon kit. If the results show that something needs to be shifted, call a qualified radon mitigation specialist to help.

USE NATURAL LAUNDRY DETERGENT

While it's tempting to buy the jumbo-sized detergents that are inexpensively priced at the local drugstore, unfortunately the synthetic fragrances in laundry products are often a source of petroleum-derived chemicals—not to mention the other chemicals in the detergents themselves, which not only can be irritants but also emit toxins into the air that can also be absorbed through your skin. All these chemicals may have negative health effects when inhaled, just as phthalates are known to disrupt hormones. There are great, highly effective, and nontoxic laundry detergents available now, some even coming in jumbo sizes also, so make sure to seek them out.

GIVE UP AEROSOL

Anything that spews out micro particles you can inhale is something you want to eliminate from your space. These include deodorants (see a clean DIY version on page 119), hair sprays, furniture and carpet cleaners, and definitely air fresheners and sprays. Just use natural and nonspray versions of the items you want to use.

OPEN YOUR WINDOWS

It's important to let fresh air regularly flush out your space to keep pollutants and chemicals from building up. Cross-ventilation is especially great if you can open opposing windows and let the breeze flow through. Bathroom and kitchen fans that exhaust to the outdoors also increase ventilation and help remove pollutants.

DIY HOME CLEANING PRODUCTS

One of the most powerful ways you can take charge of your personal space and make it one that supports your Radical Beauty is to ban chemicals whenever and wherever you can. These natural cleaning solutions are effective at keeping your space clean but won't add beauty-diminishing chemicals to your space.

RADICAL BEAUTY NON-STREAK, NONTOXIC GLASS CLEANER

All you have to do is peer at the bright blue color of most commercial glass cleaners or check out the warnings on the back of such products to know that these cleaners are not a beautiful thing to have around your space. This recipe works. It does contain rubbing alcohol, which you, of course, do not want to ingest or even make contact with your hands, but for the intended cleaning purposes, it is a great alternative!

2 fl oz (50 ml) white vinegar (apple cider vinegar will work as well)

2 fl oz (50 ml) rubbing (isopropyl) alcohol

8 to 10 drops grapefruit or orange essential oil

Mix all ingredients together and pour into a BPA-free spray bottle. Spray onto glass surfaces and wipe clean with a microfiber cloth.

ALL-GOOD OVEN CLEANER SCRUB

One of the last places you want to spray nasty chemicals that circulate in a contained space is in your oven, where your food actually bakes. This is a reliable scrub to use instead.

1 1/2 oz (45 g) bicarbonate of soda

2 teaspoons salt

2 1/2 fl oz (75 ml) water

Combine all the ingredients thoroughly to make a paste. Set to the side for at least 5 minutes. Dip your scrubbing tools into the paste and clean the inside of your oven.

Surfaces are meant to be touched, and they are—some of them very often! You never want to spray chemicals on such places, where they come into contact with your skin and then can be absorbed into your body. This is a great cleaner recipe, and the combination of all the citrus does well to hide the vinegar smell.

8 fl oz (250 ml) apple cider vinegar
8 fl oz (250 ml) water
2 fl oz (50 ml) lemon juice

30 (or so) drops orange or grapefruit essential oil, or a combination

Combine all the ingredients and mix well before transferring to a BPA-free spray bottle. Spray onto surfaces and wipe down.

STOCK UP ON HOUSEPLANTS

Houseplants not only bring beauty into your home, but they can also clean the air in your home. A two-year research project conducted by NASA found that plants—even the microorganisms in the soil—can reduce indoor air pollutants substantially.[13] The plants help purify your home, absorbing chemical pollutants given off by synthetic materials. According to NASA, some of the best plants to promote indoor air quality are spider plant, peace lily, bamboo, snake plant, heartleaf philodendron, elephant ear philodendron, and different varieties of dracaena.

MAKE YOUR HOME A NO-SMOKING ZONE

Okay, this is an obvious one, but it's a biggie when it comes to air pollution. Secondhand cigarette smoke is rife with contaminants, and exposure is linked to issues like bronchitis, asthma, and ear infections. Have smoker relatives or friends? Besides encouraging them to quit, politely let them know that they have to smoke outside (and far, far away from doors and open windows).

CHANGE FILTERS

Just because your air conditioner hasn't broken down yet doesn't mean you don't have to pay any attention to it! Most air conditioners and heaters have replaceable filters, so it's a good idea to replace them often (well before they bite the dust) to keep debris and pollutants out of your beauty space.

WASH UP

Once a week, wash your sheets, pillowcases, mattress pads, duvet covers, and blankets with hot water to clean out any compiling dust, mold, and the like.

ADJUST THE HUMIDITY

Humidity can have an effect on the concentrations of some indoor air pollutants. The ideal range is between 30 and 50 percent. If it's too humid in your home, try opening the windows or using a dehumidifier.

CHOOSE MORE BEAUTIFUL DRY CLEANING

Most of us drop off our dry cleaning and don't give it another thought until it's time to pick it up. But most dry cleaners—around 85 percent, in fact—use a solvent called perchloroethylene, or "perc," a chemical the Environmental Protection Agency (EPA) considers both a health and environmental hazard that has been identified as a possible human carcinogen and been linked to neurological effects, kidney and liver damage,[14] and possibly birth defects and reproductive issues.[15]

There are, however, dry-cleaning methods that do not use perc; seek these out to alleviate the concern of this toxin leaching into your beautiful body. Look for dry cleaners advertised as being "green," which can use several alternatives. One of these is wet cleaning, which the EPA considers one of the safest professional cleansing methods, as there is no hazardous chemical use. Carbon dioxide cleaning is nontoxic and is also considered environmentally friendly.

CHECK APPLIANCES

Inspect fuel-burning appliances regularly for leaks, and make repairs when necessary.

SET BOUNDARIES WITH PETS

Pets are indeed wonderful, but the truth is that dogs and other outdoor pets can track in a lot of environmental pollutants on their paws. Ideally, it would be a good idea to keep furry friends out of your bedroom and certainly off your bed, as well as off couches and fabric-covered furniture. Think about it: paws are like your pets' shoes, and you wouldn't want *anyone's* shoes tramping around directly all over your bed and couch!

Electromagnetic Field Pollution

In the modern world we live in, we are constantly being assailed by an invisible form of pollution from electromagnetic fields, also known as EMFs. Electric and magnetic fields are invisible force lines that surround any electrical device. Even smaller devices, such as a radio alarm clock near your head on your nightstand table, can emit EMFs. Today, there are many various sources of EMF pollution, including cell phones, computers and laptops, TVs, wireless baby monitors, wireless gaming consoles, microwave ovens, high- and low-voltage power lines, cell phone towers, and other types of electronic equipment.

EMF pollution can affect every organ and every cell of your body. In a simplified sense, when an electromagnetic wave passes through your body, it induces an electric current inside you that can interfere with many of your body's natural biological processes.

There is controversy about the extent and specificity to which EMFs can affect human health. But most researchers would agree that taking reasonable steps to help reduce your EMF exposure is warranted. Some research has concluded that magnetic fields are potentially carcinogenic,[16] and the World Health Organization stated in a 2011 press release that cell phones could be a carcinogen with excessive use.[17] The BioInitiative Working Group, made up of an international group of scientists, researchers, and public health professionals, put out a report in 2012 with their conclusion that magnetic fields can be linked to various health issues, including impaired stress responses, childhood cancers such as leukemia and compromised immune function, neurology, and behavior.[18]

What can you do?

- Switch off electronic devices when possible. This includes turning your cell phone off (or at least to airplane mode) at bedtime to prevent the signal from coming in.
- Avoid electronic alarm clocks in your bedroom and switch to battery-operated ones.
- Replace wireless devices with wired alternatives, such as swapping out a wireless headset for a wired one. Use corded baby monitors, or if that is not possible, keep your baby monitor at least 6 feet away from your baby.
- Try to reduce cell phone use as much as possible (seemingly hard but not impossible) by talking on landlines and using wired headsets as much as possible.
- Avoid microwaves. In addition to their EMF output, microwaves may potentially alter or even destroy your food's nutrition. For instance, research published in the journal *Pediatrics* found that microwaving breast milk cuts down on lysozyme activity, reduces key antibodies, promotes potentially dangerous bacteria, and destroys immunoglobulin A antibodies, which fight invading microbes.[19]

Beautiful Movement

Nature designed the body to move, and when it moves correctly, the body maintains itself exquisitely. Stasis is the enemy, which doesn't come as good news in a society where sedentary lifestyles are on the rise. How you choose to move your body has an effect on your entire being, including your health and your mental and emotional states, as well as the more obvious physical results like the tone of your muscles and your external beauty.

The first and greatest single benefit you can receive comes the moment you decide to get up out of your chair to stand, move, and be active. Gravity itself creates healthy movement in the lymphatic system, which is well understood, but there seem to be hidden reasons why standing up and letting gravity do its work is important. A key study of college varsity athletes put them in bed for two weeks without getting up—once considered the best regimen for patients recovering from serious injury, surgery, and even childbirth.

But total rest does the opposite of what it was intended to do. At the end of the two weeks, the athletes had lost the equivalent of two years of muscle building. Most of this so-called disuse atrophy is prevented by having patients stand up and move around as soon as possible in their recovery. On the other end of the spectrum, popular fitness maxims like "No pain, no gain" inspire us to believe that in order to see results, we have to virtually torture ourselves at the gym, pushing ourselves to the point of gasping for air or dripping with sweat. While these methods will certainly get you some results, overdoing it can be aging. There are other types of movements that more effectively support your overall energy and beauty while delaying the aging process.

There are other benefits to strategic movements. In a study of people who wanted to lose weight, one group was put on a running program, another on a jogging program, and a third group was simply asked to walk. The walking group lost the most weight. They demonstrated the fact that muscles stop burning oxygen during heavy activity, and therefore the metabolism that burns fat is shut down. Some studies show markedly improved health and longevity among people who stand more than 13 hours a day, compared with workers who stand less than 2 hours. We recommend, as do many experts, that you stand up and move around briefly at least once an hour.

If you move in a strategic way, you will not only see the tangible results of a sculpted, lithe, strong body, but you will also optimize the flow of energy throughout your joints, spine, and entire being. This stimulates your endocrine and other glands and keeps your body more energetically open so it can function at its peak.

When you stop moving, energy stagnates, and illness and sickness can build up.[1] Body tension is created by the resistance to the flow of energy and a lack of oxygen. As your body stiffens, so can your mind, and you can become resistant to change. There is an uninterrupted flow of energy between the emotional, mental, and physical aspects of your being, and properly moving your body affects each part equally. In this pillar you'll learn which types of movements age you and which ones are the most beneficial in terms of making you Radically Beautiful.

Incorporate Fluid Movement Throughout Your Day

Your Movement Affects Your Entire Life Experience

The foods you eat cannot adequately be reduced down to a series of numbers, and the same is true for how you move. The sole utility of your workouts isn't the number of calories or the amount of fat you burn. Moving affects your overall life. Here are just some of the many ways that moving benefits you:

- Increases energy
- Makes you feel strong and powerful in your body
- Helps you create and maintain a healthy weight
- Lowers cholesterol, triglycerides, and the risk of high blood pressure
- Builds healthy bones
- Reduces inflammation[1]
- Promotes better sleep
- Releases "feel good" chemicals called endorphins to improve mood and combat depression[2]
- Increases focus, memory, and sharper thinking and learning[3]
- Improves circulation
- Increases longevity
- Works on a cellular level to decrease the toll of stress on your aging process[4]

- Improves self-esteem and body image (critical to being beautiful is *feeling* beautiful!)

And while it's been well documented that moving and exercising in general improve your mood, the *types* of movements that flow through your body affect your overall mentality, your emotions, and your state of being. Try to recall the last time you were at a party or a wedding and danced in a free-form way, just feeling the music and having fun. Afterward you probably felt free, alive, and exhilarated. This feeling of freedom is magnetic and beautiful, and translates to an outwardly joyful energy that is very attractive. This is a perfect example of how your bodily movements have a profound impact on the state of your mind and your overall beauty.

If you only move in a linear, straightforward, and rigid fashion, such as on a treadmill or stair climber, you may start to become more linear in the way you think and feel in your body. In contrast, incorporating flowing movements, such as dance or yoga, can help inspire creative thinking. But it's not just the actual movements your body makes that have an impact—the environment in which you move your body also makes an enormous difference.

Surfing the dynamic waves of the ocean can make you feel connected to the natural world around you in a way that's impossible when slugging it out on weight machines or even on a simulated surfing machine. Hiking on uneven terrain in the fresh air can help you feel more vigorous and free in your body than doing the same incline level on a treadmill. If you live in an urban environment, trekking up some local hills in neighborhoods with sidewalks or nearby parks would also allow you to gain the benefits from much-needed time outside and away from indoor buildings.

Your mind and body are fused together, and one closely affects the other. It's not that any particular forms of movement are necessarily "bad" and should be avoided altogether, and factors like the weather, convenience, and your schedule might mean that the gym is your only option on certain days. That's fine. But we encourage you to balance the movements in your life and incorporate free-form, natural movements outside in the elements whenever possible. This will help keep your energy circulating in the most dynamic and free way, which is a key component to Radical Beauty.

RADICAL BEAUTY EXERCISE GUIDELINES

- Weave activity and movement into your daily life.

- Strive for around an hour of movement at least five days a week.

- According to the Physical Guidelines for Activity for Americans put out by the US government, at least 2.5 hours a week of moderate-intensity aerobic activity is recommended for adults. For more extensive health benefits, increase aerobic activity to 5 hours of moderate intensity weekly, and include two days or more a week of muscle-strengthening activities.[5]

- Make an effort to get out in the fresh air and nature as much as possible—ideally weekly.

- Remember that smaller, shorter activities throughout the day add up!

- Find forms of movement that you enjoy and will stick with.

- Mix circular and nonlinear forms of movement into your weekly routine. Try Vinyasa yoga, dance classes or free-form dance, rock climbing, various kinds of team sports (like volleyball), or other outdoor activities you can try in your area.

- Another option if you are crunched for time is high-interval training, which is a short, intense workout for a few minutes that requires recovery time.[6] These types of exercise may compact the time for working out due to their more vigorous nature, but they may feel too depleting for some, so listen to your body and stick to the type of movement that feels good to you. If you always dread something, you likely won't stick with it long-term.

Every component of the Radical Beauty lifestyle is tied together. Earlier we talked about grounding (see page 209) and the profound benefits of making contact with nature. Even if you aren't literally grounding by walking barefoot while you walk, jog, or hike, you'll reap a lot of the same benefits from being around trees, including fresh, oxygen-rich air and the inexplicable joy of connecting with nature. We are part of nature, and it inherently feels wonderful for us to reconnect with the bigger whole of which we are part.

Sitting and Lack of Movement Diminish Your Beauty

Failing to move your body has an extremely adverse effect on your overall beauty. But even if you regularly engage in intense exercise, you might still be accruing body fat and harmful health effects from sitting for long periods during the day. In other words, an hour of exercise does not necessarily balance the negative effects of a nonstop hour of sitting.[7] If you want to feel and look your most beautiful, it's critical to break up your periods of sitting during the day.

If you take a moment to tally the amount of time you spend in your car, at your desk, and perhaps in front of a television set, you might be shocked to see how much it all adds up. Dr. James Levine, director of the Mayo Clinic–Arizona State University Obesity Solutions Initiative, promotes the phrase "Sitting is the new smoking."[8] Studying the adverse effects of the increasingly sedentary Western lifestyle for years has led Levine and others to believe that sitting and being inactive for long periods is extremely dangerous to your health. For example, researchers have found evidence that prolonged sitting affects the blood sugar levels and insulin in the body, and that sitting too much can actually increase the risk of developing several serious illnesses, such as heart disease, type 2 diabetes, and colon and endometrial cancer.[9] An article published in *Diabetologia* examined the results of eighteen studies with nearly 800,000 participants and determined that those who sat the most were twice as likely to develop type 2 diabetes compared with those who sat the least.[10]

Sitting too much can also keep you from feeling beautifully joyful. If you sit for longer periods, your circulation can be reduced, and it may be harder for your "feel-good" brain chemicals (neurotransmitters, endorphins, and endocannabinoids) to make their way to receptors.[11] A study published in the *American Journal of Preventive Medicine* that looked at over 9,000 middle-aged women found that women who sat more than 7 hours a day were 47 percent more likely to suffer from depression than those who sat 4 hours or fewer.[12] Our natural state is to be dynamic and moving, and if we don't live in alignment with our authentic nature, we simply won't feel as genuinely happy.

The negative impact of sitting nearly all day is a relatively new problem. Our ancestors spent most of their days upright and moving, first while seeking out and gathering their own food, and in later generations while working in the fields, building structures, and getting around by foot or horseback. Technology and modern farming have put us in a position where we hardly need to move at all in order to get everything done. This may be a luxury in some ways, but as a result, we as a society move around on average 90 percent less than our ancestors did just one hundred years ago.[13]

WALKING FOR DIGESTION

A central belief in Ayurveda is that energy has to stay in motion within us and in our lives in order to continually nourish us and create harmony. On the opposite end of the spectrum is stagnation, which leads to *ama*, or toxicity buildup. It is a highly recommended practice in Ayurveda to go for a 15-minute walk after dinner. This practice is believed to help promote digestion, as well as the assimilation and circulation of nutrients all around your body.

This easy practice of walking after dinner could be coupled with gazing upon the sunset, particularly in the summer, or doing some errands like taking out the trash, dropping off dry cleaning, or picking up pet food. Strolling around the neighborhood can be a great bonding experience to share with your family or roommates as you do something great for your health and promote your Radical Beauty. Try it for yourself.

Movement shouldn't be an all-or-nothing proposition. Just because you can't get to the gym doesn't mean you have to sit and be completely inactive, forgoing all movement for the whole day. Remember, it's all about balance. Research has shown that whether or not you exercise regularly, taking breaks from long periods of sitting can stave off some of the negative effects of inactivity such as high cholesterol, triglycerides, and inflammation.[14] Even very short breaks can be beneficial.[15] Whether or not you set aside time each day to exercise, incorporating micro movements and mini routines into your daily life can be great for your health.

A study from *The Journal of Physiology* tested levels of an enzyme that breaks down fat in three groups of mice: mice that lay down for most of the day, stood for most of the day, or exercised.[16] Not surprisingly, the enzyme activity in the lying mice was very low, while the levels rose more than ten times when the mice simply stood. However, a surprising finding was that exercise had no additional effects on the enzyme levels in the mice's legs. The researchers surmised that even if you don't exercise rigorously, simply spending much of the day standing over sitting would lead to big benefits.

SUPPORT FOR THE STANDING DESK

Since many of us have jobs that require us to sit for several hours, an option that is growing in popularity is the standing desk. A standing desk is built specifically for you to work at while standing up. Many of them convert into seated desks so you can alternate periods of standing and sitting throughout the day. It may take a bit of getting used to if you're accustomed to sitting all day, but you'll probably soon find that you feel more awake and think more creatively when working standing up. Some companies have even reported an increase in productivity when employees use standing desks. If you spend several hours a day working at a desk, this might be an ideal option for you. If getting a new desk is out of your budget at the moment, you can try creating your own standing desk by stacking books or solid boxes in one corner of your desk to your standing height, and propping your laptop on them to work.

Make sure to get up and stretch or go for a quick walk to the printer, to grab more water, or just to circle around your office or home at least every 20 to 30 minutes. Eventually it will feel like second nature to get up more often, even if it feels like a lot of moving around at first. Whether or not you exercise, you can't sit the rest of the day and expect your body to respond by reflecting its maximum health and beauty potential.

Radical Beauty Daily Movement Solutions

It's clear by now that your life shouldn't be drastically divided into two opposing states: exercise and inactivity. Movement needs to be broken up during the entire day in order for you to glean optimal health and beauty benefits. Here are some of the top ways you can incorporate movement throughout your day.

TAKE FREQUENT BREAKS

At least every 30 minutes or so, stand up and stretch, walk around for a few minutes, or run an errand. You can even do a few exercises like push-ups or with free weights next to your desk if you work from home, or if it doesn't feel too weird in your office. If you sit in an open space, just walking around might be a more feasible (and less awkward) option.

TAKE THE STAIRS

This is an oldie but goodie recommendation that you may have been hearing for years but never followed. Taking a deep breath and bypassing the elevator in favor of the stairwell is an easy way to incorporate more activity in your everyday life. You can start with two floors and build from there, using the elevator to fill in the rest.

SOCIALIZE WHILE MOVING

Instead of meeting friends for coffee, tea, lunch, or dinner, meet up for a hike or a walk through your neighborhood. You'll be able to chat and catch up while being active together.

MAXIMIZE YOUR LUNCH HOUR

Use this time to walk around the neighborhood near your office. You can get in at least a good mile if you walk for a brisk 15 to 18 minutes. Keep some sneakers at your desk and pop them on before heading out at lunchtime.

WALK AND TALK

Walk around while talking on the phone. Thanks to cell phones, no longer do you have to be rooted in a seated position to talk. This practice alone could create a lot of movement during your day.

TALK FACE TO FACE

Walk down the hallway to see a colleague rather than e-mailing them. This encourages more social interaction as well as movement—two diminishing yet healthy aspects of our society. After all, we were meant to have *some* regular social interactions as human beings.

TRADE YOUR CHAIR FOR A STABILITY BALL

This will encourage you to use your core muscles during the day to remain stabilized. Don't worry if your colleagues chuckle at your "chair ball" at first. Eventually they will probably want to get one also, and you can feel smug that you were the office trendsetter who started it all.

PARK FARTHER

Get in the habit of choosing a spot in the back of the parking lot so you can get a longer walk into the store. This is especially great while you're out running errands during lunchtime to break up all of that sitting you do.

DITCH THE CAR

If possible, walk or bike to work or to do any errands you can. If you take the bus or the subway, get off at an earlier stop so you can walk some distance to get home or to work.

PLAY WITH YOUR KIDS

Get outside and try kicking or throwing a ball around. This is a great way to establish regular movement practices for the whole family and help your children set healthy habits for an active life.

MULTITASK DURING TV TIME

If you do watch TV, this is one great time *to* multitask (unlike at mealtimes). Keep a yoga mat near your television set and get in the habit of doing a few yoga poses (see pages 246–55) or stretches while watching your favorite show. And try to avoid "binge watching" whole seasons in one or two sittings, which is now possible with streaming. Try to discipline yourself to old school, prestreaming style: one episode at a time.

The Aging Effects of Overexercising

While there are so many benefits to moving throughout the day, there *is* such a thing as overdoing it. It's well established that moderate amounts of exercise can increase antioxidant defenses and offer innumerable health and beauty benefits such as increased circulation and blood flow. Excessive movement, however, can actually be depleting and create oxidative stress, a form of free-radical creation that leads to accelerated aging.[17] This is when your workout stops working for you and may actually start doing more harm than good.

First, let's define oxidative stress. Free radicals are morphed cells that your body creates as a result of exposure to pollutants and toxicity, as well as natural processes like metabolism. Your body uses different antioxidants to prevent and control damage from these free radicals. When free radicals overwhelm your antioxidant defenses, your cells become damaged. This damage is called *oxidative stress*.[18] There's a lot of data suggesting that oxidative stress contributes to inflammation and aging in different ways,[19,20,21] including aging of the skin[22] and the hair,[23] and numerous studies, including research from *Advances in Clinical Chemistry,* show that acute bouts of exercise can induce a state of oxidative stress.[24]

You don't have to be fearful of any amount of oxidative stress. It would be nearly impossible to live without having *some* in your body, and even newer research is finding that oxidative stress is beneficial in small amounts by prompting your body to increase its antioxidants.[25] Over time, this can help your body recover more quickly. In other words, you can become slightly more immune to the effects of oxidative stress. Research on serious athletes with the highest training volumes, experience, and levels of fitness shows that they handle oxidative stress well.[26]

So how much is too much oxidative stress? Your body only has so many antioxidants to combat free radicals before inflammation and the effects of aging weigh down the beauty of your skin, hair, and body. Too much oxidative stress could deplete your antioxidant reserves. It is generally believed that long, intense exercise such as running marathons and endurance training causes more oxidative stress than humans can handle.[27] During extreme and prolonged exercise, your body runs out of antioxidants, allowing free radicals to overwhelm your cells and oxidative stress to rise far beyond healthy levels.

Dr. James O'Keefe, a cardiologist who authored a review for the Mayo Clinic on the adverse cardiovascular effects of excessive exercise,[28] stated in a TED talk that "if we went out for a run right now and you ran hard . . . by 60 minutes something starts happening. . . . The free radicals blossom, and it starts *burning* the heart. It starts *searing* and inflaming the inside of your coronary arteries."[29]

Hearing the words *burning, searing,* and *inflaming* to describe what excessive exercise can do to your cardiovascular function probably makes you want to cringe. It sounds horrifying! It's easy to paint visual images around these visceral words. But just as excessive oxidative stress can "sear" your heart, it can also "sear" your beauty, showing up as weathered and wrinkled skin. Remember that everything in your body affects everything else. Earlier we talked about how cardiovascular function has an impact on the distribution of beauty nutrients, so the harmful effects described by Dr. O'Keefe extend beyond your heart and include your beauty.

If you are a competitive athlete, you'll want to be sure to eat a superior, antioxidant-rich, high-plant-food diet every single day to compensate for your intense training. However, being a "weekend warrior," or someone who doesn't have as much time to work out consistently during the week and slaves away for long hours on the weekend, may cause a disruption to your body's overall balance, or homeostasis.[30] As we discussed extensively earlier, breaking up your movement over not only the week but throughout the day is the healthiest and most beautifying way to approach your exercise routine.

BEAUTIFUL SWEAT

While you don't want to overexert and deplete yourself in order to break a sweat, sweat in and of itself is a beautiful thing. You may not feel so beautiful while you are drenched and sticky, but after a shower and perhaps a drink of coconut water, you'll likely feel more energized and beautiful than you did before your sweating session.

Sweat, a by-product of the circulatory process to cool down your body, is a fantastic way to promote detoxification. The increased blood flow that comes with sweating increases your circulation, which improves your skin's elasticity and tone, making it more beautiful over time. Because sweating is a great way to promote more overall movement throughout your system, it can even enhance digestion and help eliminate constipation, thereby removing waste products and promoting youthful energy and beauty.

Through the skin, we can detoxify heavy metals (including mercury and lead),[31] pesticides, herbicides, and other toxins from our system and keep them from circulating within our bodies, where they can contribute to inflammation and free radicals,[32] diminishing our health and beauty. Sweating is also a great way to boost your endorphins,[33] which can improve your mood and make you feel happier.

Some of the most beneficial ways to break a sweat are by moving outside in the fresh air. This includes hiking, biking, walking, and playing outdoor sports like tennis. Some indoor activities such as yoga (which can also be practiced outside when the weather permits) and dance or dance-fitness classes can also be highly beneficial. There are different forms of heated yoga that use an artificial heat source in a closed room with stagnant air. While this is certainly a way to promote sweat, it's more natural to pursue yoga where the heat builds from your own breath and movement rather than from an artificial source.

Infrared and regular saunas are also great sweating resources. Try breaking a sweat ideally twice or more on a weekly basis throughout the year, hydrating well before and afterward, to get maximum beauty benefits.

Everyone has a different capacity for exercise, but working out at a moderate to high intensity for more than 1 to 2 hours a day can generally be considered extreme (unless you happen to be an Olympic or otherwise very competitive athlete). That being said, overdoing it is different for each individual and can shift over time. If you naturally build up your fitness levels over the long-term, your body can begin to handle oxidative stress levels better than if you don't work out for months and then jump right into a killer workout. Make sure to progress at a reasonable pace and allow for adequate recovery time between training sessions.

Listen to your body, and be on the lookout for signs of overtraining, such as feeling sick, moody, anxious, or irritated. If you experience changes to your sleep, appetite, performance, or libido, or feel chronically sore or achy,[34] you just might be exercising past your optimal limit. If you listen to your body, you can feel when you are overwhelming yourself with oxidative stress instead of getting the healthy amount of exercise that produces a toned, lean body and glowing skin.

Properly Timing Your Exercise and Food

Unless you are an endurance athlete who needs to fuel up in extreme amounts, exercising right after eating a meal or consuming heavy snack foods is not recommended. This impairs your *agni*, or digestion, and splits your energy between digesting and nourishing your muscles for your workout. Blood flow is pulled out of your stomach and digestive tract to go into your muscles. It's akin to multitasking for your body. Imagine if you had to have a serious conversation while writing a meaningful e-mail; your communication on both fronts would suffer. It's just not possible to do two things really well at the same time. Focusing your energy and attention on one task at a time is the best way to be really successful at anything, and this also applies to your body's energy. Allow it to be used maximally either for digestion or exercise.

Space your meals and workouts out so you have energy for your beauty-building movement practices. Ideally, heavy foods should be consumed at least 2 hours before exercise to allow for enough energy to break them down, although as discussed previously, a gentle 15-minute walk after eating is highly recommended. Here are some specific tips for workouts at various times of the day.

MORNING WORKOUTS

BEFORE: Depending on how early your workout is, it might feel better on an empty stomach (especially for a yoga practice). Or, if you need something in your stomach, a banana, some berries, or a Glowing Green Smoothie (see recipe on page 27) are light choices that digest well. Fruit, an easy-to-digest carb, consumed prior to exercise could be beneficial and would not limit fat burning.[35]

AVOID: Anything very heavy like a big breakfast of eggs and bacon right before a workout requires a great deal of energy to digest. You'll have a less-than-efficient workout and less-than-efficient digestion. Beauty-wise, you lose out on both sides.

AFTERWARD: If you didn't have it before working out, this is a great time for your Glowing Green Smoothie. If you're still hungry after the GGS, follow it with some porridge oats or a Power Protein Smoothie (see kimberlysnyder.com for recipe). If you did a high-resistance workout and are interested specifically in building lean muscle tone, follow your GGS with a simple mix of coconut water, banana, and spirulina. This is low in fat but provides the carbs and amino acid spectrum needed for recovery. Since spirulina is an algae that breaks down and digests easily, you could also add spirulina to your Glowing Green Smoothie (though concentrated protein powders are not recommended in your GGS; save them for shakes later in the day).

AFTERNOON/EVENING WORKOUTS

BEFORE: Get fuel in the form of carbohydrates and protein during the day. There is research indicating the importance of consuming amino acids and carbohydrates before resistance exercise to help build muscle.[36] Try having some quinoa for the carbs and protein at lunch or some mushrooms or baked veggies, an avocado or sunflower seed kale salad, soup, or a protein shake, or chia seed pudding so you'll be fueled up and ready to go a couple hours later. The Glowing Green Smoothie would also fill this need as a snack, as greens are high in amino acids and the banana and other fruit in the recipe supply some carbs.

AVOID: Eating heavy foods within 2 hours of your workout, whatever time that might be. If you end up getting really hungry and needing something, a banana or another Glowing Green Smoothie are two good ideas.

AFTERWARD: If you are hungry before dinner, a banana can also be good post-workout, as it has complex carbs, potassium, and fiber. Having some protein is important to rebuild your muscles after a strengthening workout, so a Power Protein Smoothie, veggies and hummus, nuts, seeds (chia seeds are especially beneficial), protein-rich veggies such as Brussels sprouts, or some legumes like lentils are good choices, if eaten 3 to 4 hours before bed.

AVOID: Don't eat a late, heavy dinner at all costs. If you do have to exercise in the evening, a light kale salad with some avocado (remember, greens have protein, too) or a smoothie are two great choices.

ALL DAY: Hydrate well before and after exercising to prevent dehydration. Drink adequate liquids between meals so you aren't tempted to drink a lot during meals, which would dilute your digestive enzymes. If you sweat a lot during your workouts, coconut water is a great natural sports drink.

DO YOU NEED MORE PROTEIN TO BUILD MUSCLE?

There's a general belief that if you are an athlete or even someone who wants to increase strength and muscle tone, you need to eat more protein. Is this true? And when exactly should you consume it?

Research from the *Journal of Sports Sciences* shows that even elite athletes in training need only about 0.59 to 0.82 grams of protein per pound (or 1.3 to 1.8 kilograms) of body weight for optimum performance.[37] So a male weighing 180 pounds in training would not need much more than 106 grams of protein a day (remember more protein is *not* necessarily better; see page 72). This amount is easily obtainable with a vegan protein shake, nuts or seeds, and a moderate protein-containing meal, plus a variety of other whole foods during the day—and of course if you are not an elite athlete and weigh less you would need less. If you are a woman and are not an elite athlete in training, 40 to 60 grams of protein a day should be plenty for your daily needs and keeping toned. This can easily be acquired from a plant-based diet that includes some seeds, nuts, legumes, lots of veggies, especially green veggies, and protein shakes.

PROTEIN INTAKE IN A DAY (IN GRAMS)
WITH A PLANT-BASED DIET

With these two sample meal plans, you can see how easy it is to get the average daily protein requirements for women with a plant-based diet. For men, larger portion sizes or some extra nuts and seeds would also easily fulfill protein requirements. (Approximate/estimated grams of protein for foods listed; some variations may occur.)

SAMPLE MEAL DAY #1

MORNING

Hot water with lemon: 0 grams

16 fl oz (500 ml) Glowing Green Smoothie (page 27): 6 grams

Steel-cut porridge oats (1 oz (25 g) dry) made with water: 4 grams

LUNCH

Large kale salad topped with 1½ oz (40 g) sunflower seeds: 13 grams

Spring green wraps with nut pâté (see page 95): 11 grams

SNACK

Chia pudding (page 28): 5 grams

DINNER

6 oz (175 g) of cooked quinoa with 6 oz (175 g) of broccoli; side of green salad: 11 grams

1 oz (25 g) dark chocolate (at least 72% cacao): 1 gram

DAILY TOTAL: 51 GRAMS OF PROTEIN

SAMPLE MEAL PLAN #2

MORNING

Hot water with lemon: 0 grams

16 fl oz (500 ml) Glowing Green Smoothie (page 27): 6 grams

Apple: : 1 gram

Coconut yogurt with 4 oz (125 g) gluten-free granola: 4 grams

LUNCH

Gluten-free veggie and quinoa wrap (wrap made from teff): 6 grams

SNACK

Power Protein Smoothie (see kimberlysnyder.com): 24 grams*

* Could be more or less, depending on protein powder used

DINNER

Lentil and Kale Soup (page 295): 9 grams

Grilled portobello mushrooms with large mixed green salad: 6 grams

Almond milk-based hot chocolate: 2 grams

DAILY TOTAL: 58 GRAMS OF PROTEIN

A study from the *Journal of Applied Physiology* showed that it is best to consume amino acids and carbs up to 3 hours post-workout to increase muscle synthesis.[38] The other macronutrient—fat—was not found to be part of this equation, perhaps because fat can slow the uptake of the key nutrients. If you are engaging in endurance sports or workouts, some research has shown that consuming fat before exercise helps improve results of conserving muscle glycogen levels, or fuel needed to supply your muscles with energy, for these longer exercise periods,[39] but it should be forms of fat that are easy to digest, such as avocados and chia seeds, and consumed with enough time to allow for digestion (ideally at least 2 hours before workouts).

So exactly how much do you need? Though it really depends on your size and the type of workout you do, around 20 grams of protein should suffice post-workout (research has shown that for the average adult, muscle protein synthesis saturates at 20 grams of protein and increasing to 40 grams does not make a difference,[40] which would be at least as much as you get in the Power Protein Smoothie or in a typical shake made from almond milk and vegan protein powder).

WEIGHT/PROTEIN REQUIREMENTS

Weight	World Health Organization (WHO) Requirements for Protein, 0.34g/lb	Higher Activity Levels, Pregnancy, or Other Reasons, 0.5 g/lb
120 lb.	41 g	60 g
140 lb.	48 g	70 g
160 lb.	54 g	80 g
180 lb.	61 g	90 g
200 lb.	68 g	100 g
220 lb.	75 g	110 g
240 lb.	82 g	120 g

Practice Breathing and Yoga Exercises for Beauty

Pranayama: Secrets to Breathing for Beauty

Breath is perhaps the subtlest form of movement that we engage in minute to minute, even while we sleep. Since we all breathe automatically, many of us don't pay attention to our breath and take it for granted. Yet one of the secrets to youthfulness and energy is proper breathing. There are specific breathing techniques that can be used to enhance the efficiency of your exercise and movements and circulate oxygen and vitality-enhancing energy, or *prana,* more efficiently around your body. This increases your Radical Beauty.

Pranayama, which in a very simplified definition translates to "breathing exercises," is really a deeper concept that has to do with consciously controlling your *prana.* It is one of the most beneficial and effective techniques to help dissipate stress and balance your mind.

Prana is the universal life energy that permeates the entire universe. By becoming aware of it and working with it deliberately through *pranayama* techniques, you'll be able to expand your energy beyond any perceived limitations. Your rejuvenation will expand, as will your magnetic energy and true beauty. A grounded, calm, yet tangibly magnetic energy is possible to attain through regularly practicing *pranayama* (and meditation, which we'll talk about in Pillar 6). These are among the most powerful practices available to us.

Pranayama is considered alkalizing and cleansing since it promotes efficient elimination of toxins through the lungs. *Pranayama* practices work best in tandem with a cleansing, alkaline diet (see Pillar 1). This helps open up the channels for more *prana* to enter. Deep inhales and exhales can move toxins through the lymph, acting as a pump for the lymphatic system. Tibetan yogis demonstrate the extreme power of breath and mind control. Using these dynamic practices, they can generate such intense heat that they are comfortable in cold temperatures and can even melt the snow around them.

Breathing techniques can certainly ramp up your beauty potential. Imagine if you breathed improperly day after day, year after year. You wouldn't get the full potential of nourishing oxygen to all of your cells, which can accelerate aging. Deeper, more efficient breathing that results in improved circulation equals better distribution of oxygen and nutrients. This in turn will help create more glowing, youthful skin and help you feel more naturally energized.

The first step to *pranayama* is to become aware of your breath in the first place and start to slow it down. When you slow down your breath, you tend to breathe more fully. This helps you become more efficient at ingesting oxygen and expelling waste. You will also feel calmer and more balanced as you release stress and absorb fewer of its toxic effects.

States of Breathing

There are three states of breathing we all naturally do throughout the day and night.

PURAKA: This is the state of inhalation, when your lungs are filled with air. Work to take deeper inhales, filling your upper and lower lungs to pull in the maximum amount of oxygen possible and allowing your stomach to expand like a balloon. Also take care to breathe in slowly, probably much more slowly than you are used to. You can even try counting to four as you inhale to consciously slow down your breath.

KUMBHATA: This is the state of retention. In normal, everyday breathing, this equates to the very subtle pause between your inhales and exhales. *Prana* and oxygen from the lungs enter the bloodstream to be delivered to all of the cells in your body as gases from the cells enter the lungs and prepare for expulsion out of the body.

RECAKA: This is the state of exhalation of toxic substances from the body. It's important to exhale very deeply, perhaps even more deeply than you inhale, to ensure that you fully expel wastes and by-products of the breath out of your body. Your belly should pull in slightly toward your spine.

Basic *Pranayama* Techniques
That Promote Beauty

These practices are ideally performed at the specific times that are noted for each technique. Practicing these in the open air is ideal. Otherwise, find a peaceful environment where you can sit with your spine straight. It might be more comfortable for you to sit cross-legged on a firm pillow or to sit in a chair with both feet firmly planted on the ground. But do avoid saggy couches and cushions, which can cause you to inadvertently sink down, preventing optimal breath flow and reducing these *pranayama* techniques' strong benefits.

Please check with your doctor before starting if you are new to these or any other *pranayama* breath techniques, or if you are pregnant or have a medical condition.

UJJAYI

This is the primary way of breathing while practicing yoga *asanas,* or poses, but this is also a fantastic form of breath to use anytime you feel stressed. *Ujjayi* helps you bring the maximum amount of oxygen into your body; efficiently distribute nutrients; avoid shallow, chest-based, and inefficient breathing; and give more magnetic beauty energy and a glow to your skin and eyes.

This form of breathing has been used for thousands of years in both Taoist and yogic traditions. It is often referred to as "the ocean breath" because it sounds like gentle ocean waves. *Ujjayi* is a deep, abdominal-based breath that fills your lower belly first, then rises to fill the lower rib cage, then all the way up into the upper lungs, chest, and throat.

To begin, open your mouth wide and let out a vocal exhale. Now, inhale and close your mouth and try to exhale and make the same sound, which will produce a noise somewhat akin to the ocean at the back of your throat. If you're in public, you can just focus on breathing deeply without tensing or raising your shoulders, allowing your entire belly to expand without making the audible sound. You'll still benefit from this slow, deep breathing. In either case, inhale and exhale through your nose for roughly the same length of time. If you are a particularly fast breather or have a hard time knowing how to slow down, try breathing in and out for a count of four. Practice this any time of the day and into the evening.

BHASTRIKA

This is an especially beautifying *pranayama* technique because it is cleansing and raises the metabolism. Breathe in and out through your nose in a quick rhythm. This expels negativity. Think of a sniffing dog. The rhythm is even and fast. You can do one or a few rounds of 20 to 30 seconds each, working your way up to 3 to 5 minutes a day. After finishing, you will feel euphoric and energized in a profound way. Since this is an energizing practice, it's best to practice this in the mornings and daytime rather than the evenings. It can take a while to get the rhythm down, but it's worth the effort.

NADI SHODHANA

This breathing technique creates balance in the body, which is a key component of Radical Beauty. The term *Nadi Shodhana* literally means "clearing the channels of circulation." This technique is also referred to as "alternate nostril breathing" and is effective in helping you deeply relax your body and mind while balancing the energies between the left and right side of your body. Yogis believe the left is the *ida*, the cooling or lunar side of your body, while the right is the *pingala*, or the solar or warming, fiery energy in the body. These contrasting but complementary sides need to be balanced. If you have too much fire you can burn out or get overanxious or overheated, which ancient Indian philosophy warns might speed the aging process. If you are too cool and don't have enough fire, you can become lethargic and depressed.

Try practicing *Nadi Shodhana* in the evenings after work and before bed or before meditating to balance your fire and cooling elements; release anxiety, depression, or stress; and create a deep sense of equilibrium and balance. Start by taking a big exhale and clearing the breath completely out of both nostrils. Then take your index and middle fingers (as if you were going to make a "peace sign"), and curl them into your palm or place them on the bridge of your nose. Now hold your right thumb over your right nostril and inhale deeply through your left nostril. At the top of your inhalation, close off your left (*ida*, or lunar, cooling) nostril with your ring and pinky fingers and exhale fully through your right nostril. After a full exhalation, inhale through the right (*pingala*, or solar, warming) nostril, closing it off with your right thumb at the top of your inhalation. Repeat this over and over, without force, just watching your breath and feeling the power of this practice to balance your entire, beautiful being.

KAPALABHATI

This is also a purifying beauty breath that is sometimes referred to as "skull shining breath." It can help your entire being as well as your complexion radiate with the glow of cleanliness and peace. This toning *pranayama* technique cleanses your respiratory system and encourages the release of toxins. It is made up of short, powerful exhales and passive inhales.

To practice *Kapalabhati,* sit in a comfortable position with a straight spine. Rest your hands on your belly so you can tune in to the sharp exhalations. If you prefer, rest them on your knees with your palms facing down. Bring your attention to your lower abdomen and inhale through both nostrils deeply. Contract your lower belly or use your hands to gently press on this area, forcing out the breath in a short burst. This should feel strong and powerful. As you quickly release the contraction, your inhalation should be automatic and passive. Your focus should be on exhaling.

Begin slowly, aiming for 65 to 70 contractions per minute. Gradually pick up the pace for 95 to 105 exhalation/inhalation cycles per minute. Always go at your own pace and never force yourself. Stop if you feel at all light-headed or dizzy. After one minute of the exercise, inhale deeply through the nostrils and then exhale slowly through your mouth. Depending on your experience level, you can work up to doing multiple repetitions. This is a great exercise to do in the morning to warm up for your morning yoga practice or meditation. As this practice is energizing, it is not recommended for the late evening.

Yoga for Detoxification and Beauty

Of all the types of movement out there, yoga is one of the best for promoting Radical Beauty. The *asana,* or pose part of yoga, incorporates twisted and circular movements of different muscle groups. This includes flexing your spine in all directions. There are many advantages to this over linear movements with a limited range of motion.

YOGA GEAR

To start practicing yoga, you'll want to invest in a decent yoga mat that will prevent you from skidding and sliding during your *asanas* and is thick enough to provide padding for your knees and hips during various poses. There are a lot of great eco-friendly mats available. You may also want to invest in two yoga blocks to help modify poses, especially as a beginner. These are fairly inexpensive but enormously helpful in making sure you don't compromise the integrity of the pose as you naturally increase your flexibility. For some poses, such as *Parsvottonasana*, or Pyramid pose (see page 248), you can use one block on either side of your leg to help you modify the pose. Other gear, such as yoga belts and blankets, are not fully necessary, especially as a beginner. You can think about investing in them later if you find a need. For now, a pillow or any sturdy blanket you already have at home can be used to help elevate hips for seated poses and, while practicing *pranayama*, to increase your comfort and help align your spine.

Yoga is cleansing in many different ways. It allows you to physically stimulate your abdominal organs, including your liver, kidneys, and digestive organs. This makes yoga incredibly beneficial for digestion, which you now know is key to beauty and health. Yoga also stimulates your endocrine glands, including the thyroid gland, which controls your metabolism. It also helps cleanse your liver, your main detoxifying organ. Far beyond simply burning calories or working your limbs and core, when practiced properly yoga can be a very powerful tool in helping to keep your body limber, strong, youthful, and beautifully healthy with an all-around glow and beautiful, healthy skin.

Yoga *asanas* are the ideal physical movements to couple with the other shifts in this book to physically support a clean, beautiful body and mind. The deeper benefits of yoga extend to settling and balancing your mind, preparing you for meditation, and aiding in the meditation practice itself, which we will discuss in Pillar 6. For now, let's focus on the physical, movement-based aspects of yoga so you can begin reaping its many beauty benefits.

Top Radical Beauty Poses for Beauty and Detoxification

Below are among the most effective and beneficial poses to incorporate into your lifestyle. You can try a few of these poses that you feel the most connected to, or try all of them and see which ones your body and mind respond to. You can work them into your daily routine right after rising in the morning, as many of these can easily be practiced in the space next to your bed or even perhaps in bed if you have a firm mattress. Others, such as *Paschimottanasana,* which is a nervous-system-soothing seated forward bend, are excellent to incorporate into your evening routine for added digestive and anxiety-quelling benefits as you get ready for some all-important beauty rest.

If you are new to yoga, are pregnant, or have a medical condition, please talk to your doctor before beginning.

TADASANA (MOUNTAIN POSE)

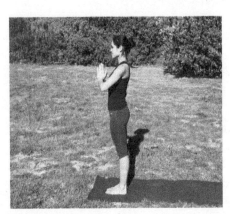

BENEFITS: This pose can bring profound awareness into a seemingly simple stance. It strengthens the legs, firms your abdomen and glutes, and improves your posture.

DESCRIPTION: Stand straight with the insides of your big toes together. Line up your feet parallel, heels a little apart, middle toes pointing forward. Ground your energy evenly through the four corners of your feet, and gently pull up from your spine. Open your chest and shoulders slightly, but keep your chin parallel to the floor. Hands come together in *Anjali* mudra (with palms pressing), or arms drop gently to your sides.

BEST TIME TO PRACTICE: This can be practiced anytime, but it's a fantastic way to start the day while feeling tall, confident, and grounded.

OTHER TIPS: Try doing this pose at first standing sideways in front of a full-length mirror so you can get a visual image of your own posture and consequently learn to feel what is proper posture in your own body.

SUPTA MATSYENDRASANA (SUPINE TWIST)

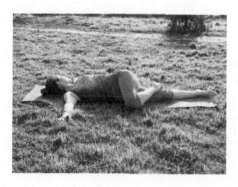

BENEFITS: Twists literally squeeze toxins out of your liver and kidneys, stimulating digestion and cleansing and encouraging a healthy blood flow to energize your entire spine. Practiced regularly, twists will help leave you with a more clean and beautiful body. There are many different variations of yogic twists, including ones practiced while standing, sitting, and lying down. This particular supine twist is great for all levels.

DESCRIPTION: Begin lying on your back. Open your arms out to the side in a T. Bend your left knee, and lift it up, allowing it to start to drop and twist over your right thigh as far as it feels natural and comfortable. Continue to breathe slowly as you let your head turn naturally to the left and root your shoulders down. Let your knee drop open as much as feels natural, allowing the spine and organs to twist and wring out. Stay in the twist for at least five to ten breaths or more. Repeat on the right side.

BEST TIME TO PRACTICE: Any time of the day.

OTHER TIPS: Always twist your left leg over first in order to follow the path of your digestive tract and encourage wastes to exit your system efficiently.

MĀRJĀRYASANA BITILASANA (CAT-COW)

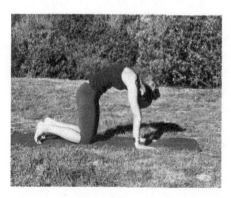

BENEFITS: Regularly flexing your spine as you do in this sequence is one of the best long-term beauty movements. By stimulating all your organs, especially your vitality-enhancing kidneys as well as your colon and digestive tract, *Mārjāryasana* boosts your overall circulation and stimulates your entire spine, relieving stress and revitalizing your energy.

DESCRIPTION: Start by kneeling on your hands and knees, keeping your hands underneath your shoulders and your knees underneath your hips. Exhale deeply through your mouth and contract your abdominal muscles up toward your spine, rounding your spine to the ceiling as you tuck your tailbone under and bring your chin toward your chest. This arch is known as "cat" since it resembles a cat arching its back. Inhale and relax your belly so it drifts toward the ground for the "cow" portion (resembling the bulge of a cow's pronounced udder), lifting your head so you are facing forward, opening your back into a slight backbend, and sliding your shoulder blades down your back. Continue to flow your spine through several rounds of these arching motions, feeling the movement of each vertebra.

BEST TIME TO PRACTICE: Try practicing a few rounds of this right on your bedroom floor upon waking (or near your kitchen while heating up the water to make your hot water with lemon!) to get energized for the entire day ahead.

OTHER TIPS: Be sure to practice this on a yoga mat or a carpet to provide some padding for your tender knee joints.

PARSVOTTONASANA (PYRAMID POSE)

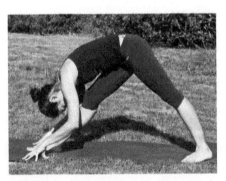

BENEFITS: This pose stimulates and tones your abdominal organs and supports digestion. It also improves your posture and balance.

DESCRIPTION: Start in a wide stance with your right leg forward and pointing straight ahead and your left leg behind and pointed at a 45-degree angle. Square your hips so both are pointing straight forward. On an exhale, fold forward from the hips until your torso is parallel with the floor or, if comfortable, fold in more deeply toward your right leg, placing your fingertips on the floor or on two blocks on either side of your right leg. Breathe deeply for five to ten breaths. Repeat on the other side.

BEST TIME TO PRACTICE: Any time of the day.

OTHER TIPS: This and other forward-bend poses are great to call upon when you feel stressed or overwhelmed.

UTKATASANA (CHAIR POSE)

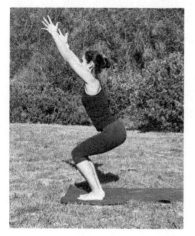

BENEFITS: Not only does this stimulate your abdominal organs and promote cleansing but it is also a powerful pose to tone your thighs and entire legs.

DESCRIPTION: Begin in *Tadasana* (Mountain pose), with your feet touching and your spine erect. Move back and down as if you are going to sit down in a chair; this might only be a few inches back to start if you are a beginner. Then lift your arms in front of you at around ear level with your palms facing each other, your shoulder blades moving down your back, and your chest broad while you root back strongly into your heels. Keep drawing in your abdominal muscles to support your back as you "sit" back. Breathe deeply.

BEST TIME TO PRACTICE: Any time of the day.

OTHER TIPS: For an added bonus, add a round or two of *Kapalabhati* breath (page 244) while in Chair pose.

UTTHITA TRIKONASANA (EXTENDED TRIANGLE POSE)

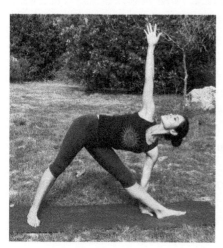

BENEFITS: This excellent pose stimulates digestion and elimination while providing a wonderful stretch all along your leg muscles, back, chest, shoulders, and oblique muscles.

DESCRIPTION: Begin in *Tadasana* (Mountain pose). Step back with your right foot, turning it outward at a 45-degree angle, toward the top corner of your mat. Point your left toes forward so that your hips open to face the side of the mat. Inhale and move your arms out in a T shape, with your palms down and shoulders relaxed. Exhale and push your hips toward your back, right, foot. Lengthen your spine while keeping both legs straight. Keep your left quad muscle engaged and rotated outward. Move your left hand toward your shin, a block, your ankle, or the floor while your right arm moves up toward the ceiling. Keep your spine and torso lengthened as you breathe for at least five breaths. Repeat on the other side.

BEST TIME TO PRACTICE: Any time of the day.

OTHER TIPS: It's easy in this pose to collapse down into your spine as you try to reach your leg while in this sideways position. A block is especially helpful here to help establish the feeling of lifting upward instead of drooping down into your lower leg.

BHUJAṄGASANA (COBRA POSE)

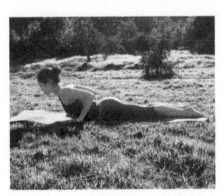

BENEFITS: This is one of the most effective poses to support optimal digestion. It also works well to increase your circulation and stimulate your kidneys while stretching your spine and activating your thyroid. This balances your metabolism and helps you feel revitalized and radiant.

DESCRIPTION: Begin by lying on your belly. Place your palms under your shoulders with your fingertips pointed straight forward and your elbows tucked straight back behind you, close to your rib cage. Lengthen your legs, with the tops of your feet pressing down into your mat and your toes pointing straight back behind you. While you inhale, press your hands or fingertips down into the mat to gently lengthen your arms as you stretch back into a backbend. Do not strain. Only bend as much as feels natural. Lift your chest up and radiate your heart wide open, rolling your shoulder blades down. Breathe in this backbend for at least five breaths. To come out, bend your elbows to gently lower back down to your mat.

BEST TIME TO PRACTICE: In the morning or afternoon; backbends can feel too stimulating in the evening.

OTHER TIPS: Try different variations, such as staying on your hands and coming up to your finger pads, to see which version feels best for you. You can also try carefully turning your head from side to side while in the backbend for a gentle neck stretch.

DHANURASANA (BOW POSE)

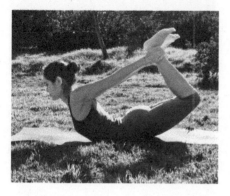

BENEFITS: This pose stretches and stimulates your abdominal organs and is great for enhancing detoxification. It also is a great pose for strengthening your back muscles and thighs.

DESCRIPTION: Lie on your stomach with your arms by your sides and your palms facing upward. Roll your shoulders up and back. Bend both knees, flexing your heels and bringing your feet toward your buttocks. Grasp your outer ankles with your hands if possible, or, if not, energetically press your ankles and feet toward one another. Keep breathing deeply as you press your knees toward each other into the midline and your heels back, gradually increasing the opening of your chest and heart. Rock gently if that feels natural. Breathe for at least five breaths. You can repeat up to three rounds.

BEST TIME TO PRACTICE: Mornings and afternoons are ideal, as backbends can feel too stimulating in the evening.

OTHER TIPS: Be patient and do not overstrain or try to bend too deeply before your spine is ready. Keep your legs really active and strong in this pose and avoid contracting your buttocks.

NĀVASANA (BOAT POSE)

BENEFITS: This core-building pose supports digestion as well as detoxification through the kidneys. It also tones and firms the hips and thighs as well as entire midsection.

DESCRIPTION: Sit on your mat and place your feet and bent knees together. Hold the backs of your knees or thighs. Lean slightly back and strongly engage your core. Keep your spine tall and, depending on what feels comfortable, either leave your feet on the mat, raise your heels to the height of your knees, or slowly stretch your legs out straight. In any case, reach your arms forward so they are straight at the height of your shoulders. Maintain the pose for fifteen to twenty breaths.

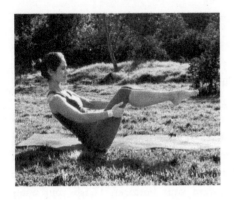
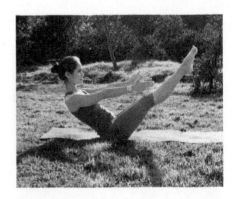

BEST TIME TO PRACTICE: Any time of the day, but as suggested for your entire practice, this pose in particular must be practiced on an empty stomach.

OTHER TIPS: For added detoxifying benefit, try adding *Bhastrika* breath (page 243) while in this pose.

SETU BANDHA SARVANGASANA (BRIDGE POSE)

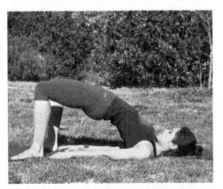

BENEFITS: This highly effective *asana* is both therapeutic and beneficial. It stimulates the thyroid, balancing your metabolism, aiding digestion, and relieving menstrual symptoms. At the same time, it calms the mind and opens the spine, chest, and heart, reversing the forward-bending motion most of us are in all day while at our computers and on our phones.

DESCRIPTION: Lying on the floor, bend your knees and place your feet flat on the ground. Position your heels hip width apart, directly under your knees. Be sure your feet are facing straight forward. Press your palms into the floor and slowly lift your hips and lower back off the floor to a comfortable level, ideally to the height of your knees, as you root your feet down strongly into the ground. Stay in this pose for five breaths or more. To come down, gently lower your hips down to the mat. This can be repeated for one to three rounds.

BEST TIME TO PRACTICE: Any time of the day; as this is a mild backbend, it may not be as stimulating in the evening as other backbend variations.

OTHER TIPS: To enhance the benefits, try slowing down your *Ujjayi* breath (page 242) even more while in this pose.

PASCHIMOTTANASANA (SEATED FORWARD FOLD)

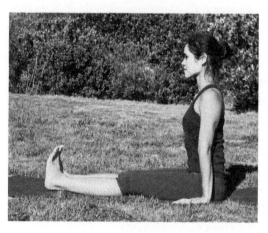

BENEFITS: Besides massaging the internal organs and aiding digestion, this forward-bending pose calms anxiety and soothes your nervous system. Taking action to destress regularly is important to maintain your Radical Beauty.

DESCRIPTION: Start with your legs out in front of you, heels flexed and big toes pointed upward. Inhale and reach your hands up, with your arms at the sides of your ears to create length in your spine. As you exhale, lean forward from your hip joints, creating as much length as possible by stretching your arms forward. You may not come anywhere close to your legs, and that is okay. Do not force this at all! It takes a while to open up your hamstrings and other leg muscles. You can rest your hands, fingertips, or forearms down on the mat for support. You can also grab on to the outside of your calves.

BEST TIME TO PRACTICE: Any time of day; forward-bending poses such as this one are great whenever you feel stressed or overwhelmed.

OTHER TIPS: For a very safe and comfortable version, you can bend your knees deeply so that your chest touches your thighs and then start to wiggle your hips back as long as your chest and thighs keep touching, which will help protect your lower back. Pause at your "edge," never overstraining, and breathe. To exit the pose gently, press back up.

JANU SIRSASANA (HEAD-TO-KNEE FORWARD BEND)

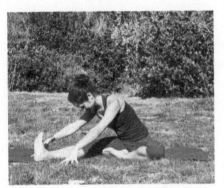

BENEFITS: This is a great pose to stretch and stimulate your internal organs, particularly your liver, kidneys, and intestines. This pose helps calm the mind and relieve anxiety and stress.

DESCRIPTION: Sit on the floor with your legs straight in front of you. Inhale, bend your left knee, and draw your heel back toward your groin, pressing against your inner right thigh. Keep your right leg straight with your right foot flexed. Stretch both arms up overhead, then exhale and twist your torso slightly to the right, lining up your navel with your right big toe. Start to stretch your arms forward, lengthening your spine forward as much as possible and bringing your hands down to the mat on either side of your leg for support. Eventually you may be able to clasp either side of your right foot. To exit, gently bring your torso back up. Straighten your left leg and repeat on the other side.

BEST TIME TO PRACTICE: You can practice this pose on or next to your bed or at the end of any exercise session or yoga practice to increase flexibility, reduce tightness, and return to balance.

OTHER TIPS: If it's really hard to find traction, try wrapping a towel around your flexed foot and gently pulling back with both hands.

HALASANA (PLOW POSE)

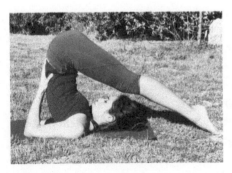

BENEFITS: This is a wonderful pose to increase circulation and proper blood flow for an all-around beautiful glow. It calms the central nervous system and aids with stress and anxiety, while boosting digestion and removing mucus and congestion.

DESCRIPTION: Lie flat on your mat with your arms beside you and your palms facing downward. As you inhale, use your abdominal muscles to lift your feet off the floor and sweep your legs over your head. Your feet *may or may not* touch the floor behind you. Support your hips and back with your hands, palms facing up. To avoid overstretching your neck, the tops of your shoulders should push down into the mat. Maintain the pose for five to ten breaths or more. To exit the pose, lift up into *Nirālamba Sarvāṅgasana* (Shoulder Stand; see below) or gently roll back down to your mat.

BEST TIME TO PRACTICE: Any time of the day.

OTHER TIPS: Be sure to always practice this pose on a yoga mat or carpet and never on a bare floor where your shoulder blades can dig in.

NIRĀLAMBA SARVĀṄGASANA (SHOULDER STAND)

BENEFITS: The great yoga master B. K. S. Iyengar states in *Light on Yoga* that "the benefits of shoulder stand cannot be overstated."[1] By reversing the flow of blood, this inversion stimulates your entire circulatory system, bringing a beautiful glow to your face while also calming the brain and relieving stress. It stimulates the thyroid while increasing your energy and metabolism, which may help promote weight loss.

DESCRIPTION: Lie on your back and gently lift your legs backward into *Halasana* (Plow pose, page 254), with your legs over your head. Bend your elbows and bring your hands onto your back with your palms facing upward for support. Tuck your shoulder blades underneath you. Next, lift your legs up off the floor and toward the ceiling. Point your toes and engage your legs and core. Once you raise your legs, keep your gaze up and neck straight. Lift up through the balls of the feet. Bring the hips toward the front of the room and the feet toward the back to straighten the body, engaging your core and avoiding a bowed-out position. Breathe evenly and deeply. Try to stay up there for at least 30 seconds and build up to a few minutes. To exit the pose, carefully bring your feet back over your head, returning to *Halasana*.

BEST TIME TO PRACTICE: Any time of day.

OTHER TIPS: If you find discomfort in your shoulders in this pose, try folding your mat over a few times or folding a firm blanket into a rectangular shape and placing it right underneath your shoulder blades so that your head is off the mat or blanket but you get a slight elevation in your shoulder blades.

PILLAR 6:

Spiritual Beauty

Inner beauty is the most precious kind of beauty—and also the most mysterious. All of us have heard about "living in the light" and "finding your soul mate," until these phrases have lost their meaning. But spirit and soul are real experiences, and the love of someone who holds you up as a perfect partner in life is not just a dream. Pillar 6 takes Radical Beauty this final step, into the light of spirit, where your daily experience will validate your highest personal values. Your highest potential for beauty will be unfulfilled without spiritual beauty.

Pause for a moment and ask yourself what "living in the light" means to you personally. For one person it might be like waking up to greet the dawn—there is a sense of joyful freshness and renewal. Another person would immediately imagine the gleam of love in a child's eyes—the light is love. No matter how you define it, the light is a source of beauty from within.

Because beauty is natural, so is spiritual beauty. There is no reason to feel that spiritual beauty must be something rare. We were born to live in the light. There's a beautiful expression of this truth in the Indian spiritual tradition, which says the following: To know who you really are, imagine two birds sitting in a tree. One bird eats the fruit of the tree while its mate looks on lovingly—this is your true self, where inner and outer beauty are bonded by love.

The true self is another element of Radical Beauty, one that transcends appearances and calls out to us from some place deeply personal and universal at the same time. While you go through your daily life—working, loving, pursuing all the things you desire—there is a hidden, silent part of you that doesn't engage in action. It merely looks on. This silent aspect of the self lives in the light. From it radiates spiritual beauty.

How to Find Your Personal
Path to Spiritual Beauty

Finding your spiritual beauty isn't a difficult task like climbing a mountain. Let's say that you've had a hard day at work and are driving home in slow traffic. There's nothing delightful about your situation. You are trapped by the daily grind. Suddenly a rain shower passes overhead, and a few minutes later a gorgeous double rainbow appears in the sky. What happens to you inside? Almost everyone would say that they feel a moment of delight, and while it lasts, this moment is all-embracing. You don't want to be distracted because the spell of beauty has captivated you.

In Radical Beauty, we want you to be just as captivated by your own self, the true self that is made of light. You have glimpsed it thousands of times in moments when any of the following experiences happened to you.

> You felt happy and peaceful inside.
>
> You felt inspired by the sight of something beautiful.
>
> You felt safe and protected.
>
> Your mind became quiet and settled.
>
> You felt loved and lovable.
>
> You felt connected to a higher power, whether you labeled it
> as God or not.
>
> You felt refreshed and renewed.
>
> You longed to know the truth about life.
>
> You realized that you belong.

These aren't rare experiences—everyone has had them. They make us feel, even for an instant, that life is beautiful. Our true self was peeking through. As part of Radical Beauty, we want these glimpses to become lasting and permanent. This is actually the most natural way to live. On a cloudy day, you don't think, "Gray is how it should always be. A sunny day is the exception." Everyone takes for granted, even in the gloomiest climates, that the sun represents a permanent force while clouds come and go. It's the same with spirit. No matter how clouded over it becomes—due to negative emotions, distractions, old wounds, or painful conditioning—the true self is steady and ever-present.

There are many reasons why we can't see our own inner beauty, but the most important is that we were never taught how. A rainbow catches your attention automatically, not just because it looks beautiful but because we were all trained from childhood to see with the eyes of the body. Seeing with the eyes of the soul is just as easy and natural—once you have learned how.

There's nothing new here. For thousands of years people have wanted three things very deeply: love, healing, and awakening. In the world's wisdom traditions, a rich storehouse of knowledge has accumulated about the path that leads to these things. The most valuable knowledge can be stated in a few sentences:

> The path must be inspiring.
>
> It must fit with your own personality and tendencies.
>
> It should be without stress and strain.

The challenge is to turn these three principles into a practical plan. Here is where the traditions of wisdom lay down three main approaches. These are blueprints or strategy plans, we might say, that have proven to work time and time again. As we describe them, stop and consider which approach suits you personally.

- The path of love and devotion: On this path the incentive is joy. Seeing the beauty of the world, you seek more of it, and the more you find, the more blissful you feel. Moments of love start to deepen. You are inspired to contemplate a creation permeated by love. This path is very private, because it takes place entirely in the heart. Further along the path you sense that love can be unconditional, and you find yourself offering devotion to the source of such pure love.

  > Qualities of this path: Bliss, joy, love of beauty, desire to give and receive love, hunger for the divine, a sense of heartfelt warmth
  >
  > The goal: To live in the light of divine grace

- The path of action and service: On this path the incentive is spiritual growth. Having glimpsed what is best in yourself, you want to act from your best self always. There is a strong desire to fulfill your inner potential. This is achieved by expanding your awareness, because the more expanded you feel, the more complete you are. This path is dynamic and takes place in the hustle and bustle of the real world. Further along, the most fulfilling action is no longer selfish. You feel more fulfilled by service to others. The more you give of yourself, the more you receive back. This motivates you to surrender all attachment, because you realize that what you desired all along was pure freedom.

> Qualities of this path: Evolution, growth, fulfilled potential, giving, serving, longing for freedom, renewal, sense of expansion, becoming unburdened and free while still acting in the world

> The goal: Liberation

- The path of knowledge and truth: On this path the incentive is a thirst for understanding. You have glimpsed the reality that peeks through the veil of illusion. The physical world isn't enough to satisfy your need to know the truth. You delve into scriptures, poetry, and other writing that speaks to you about a deeper reality. This path is mental. Every day is about seeking a new level of understanding. Wisdom inspires you. Further along the path, the mind realizes that wisdom can't be found in books or by any set system of thought. The ultimate understanding is based on silent awareness, which simply knows. By relying on the silent mind rather than all the fleeting thoughts that fill the mind, you discover that reality is unbounded, pure consciousness. With this understanding, all seeking ceases.

> Qualities of this path: Seeking, being true to yourself, thirst for knowledge, self-reliance, the pull of wisdom, spiritual teachings, inspiration from what the mind discovers

> The goal: Unbounded awareness

The three pathways are equal and have been tested for centuries, wherever people have wanted to find more from life than what is presented on the surface. Once you find the path that matches you personally, it becomes the easiest and most natural one for you to follow. Each path implies a new way of life, but it is important to note that if this way of life imposes stress and strain, you will sooner or later lapse back into your old way of life.

Setting the Stage

Do you see yourself taking one of the three paths? Each one awakens Radical Beauty at the deepest level, yet you must be comfortable finding the way that suits you best. For some people the choice is very clear. For others, there's a degree of uncertainty. They can see a bit of themselves in all three paths, the way of love, the way of action, and the way of knowledge. To help you choose, take a closer look at how your life is being lived today. Even before we think about getting on the path, the stage has been set for taking the first step.

A way of life that's naturally compatible with *love and devotion* is drawn to community and togetherness. It involves taking care of others. Family comes first. A loving household is considered the ideal. Warmth and heartfelt emotions come naturally. There is usually an attraction to church or temple. Feelings of reverence come naturally. You seek communion with nature, the people you love, and all of humanity. You believe in the power of prayer, and you have experienced moments of grace. Your personality is likely to be shy and self-effacing, but this isn't always true. At your best you feel gratitude and devotion for the gifts that fill your life.

A way of life that's naturally compatible with *personal growth* is drawn to new possibilities. This is more than the ordinary life of action, which is dominated by external demands and duties. The spark instead comes from inside, through constant, often restless, seeking. Discovery and curiosity occupy your mind. You like to challenge yourself to find out what you are capable of. Spiritually you are attracted to groups that offer a better way of life and the fulfillment of hidden potential. You have a strong sense of purpose, grounded on a secure sense of self. You measure your self-worth not by visible rewards like money and possessions but by how expanded you are becoming inside. You are impatient with the demands of your ego, which thinks only of itself and the next pleasure it can experience. Your seeking looks beyond the ego to higher states of consciousness. Being the best you can be appeals to you, and this turns into a strong motivation spiritually. Although others may see you only in worldly terms, you can surprise them by being selfless, generous, and willing to serve others.

A way of life that's naturally compatible with *understanding* is drawn to the truth. There is a constant need to know more. A high value is placed on living your own truth, which you associate with integrity and honesty. You trust your mind to guide you forward. You have no time for secondhand opinions and conventional wisdom. You look up to people who have insight and can impart it to others. Your streak of skepticism keeps you from following anyone who hasn't earned your respect for telling the truth. In your mind, you distinguish between appearances and reality. There are moments when reality seems quite mysterious to you. The material world doesn't tell the whole story. You want to go beyond, or transcend. The way you do this is primarily by going deeper into your personal understanding and self-awareness. At your best, you feel secure enough to open new doors that take you into the unknown.

The Awakening Process: Finding Your Beauty in the Light

A beautiful transformation begins to take place when you see that you belong in the light. When people successfully find a way to live in the light, their experiences on the path turn out to be very similar, because there are certain stages that apply to almost everyone.

Stage 1: First Signs of Awakening

Stage 2: Opening the Door

Stage 3: Dedication to the Path

Stage 4: Resting into Existence

Stage 5: The True Self Becomes the Only Self

Radical Beauty is universal. These are stages of awakening experienced for thousands of years in every culture. Even though social roles have changed dramatically and society has become much more secular, you will discover that your personal journey will repeat the same soul journey that was undertaken at the time of the Buddha, Jesus, Saint Teresa, and anyone alive today who lives in the light. Let's look more closely at how the five stages unfold.

Being beautiful means seeing yourself that way, and for this, you must be wide awake. Because the light of awareness exists in everyone, it's hard to imagine a life that doesn't contain moments of awakening. But many other things happen during a typical day, and it's quite common not to notice the first signs. Let's say that you wake up one day and there's a sense of lightness and ease as you begin your day. The lightness stays with you and even increases instead of fading. You may think to yourself, "I'm having a good day." People smile at you more than usual; the things you need to accomplish are done more easily—it's as if all the gears are lubricated, with minimal friction. You go to bed feeling a sense of ease and fulfillment, yet when you wake up the next morning, everything has gone back to normal. You face a day of duties and demands that feels like every other day. The memory of your very good day quickly vanishes.

Yet what you actually experienced that day was a sign of awakening, giving you a clue to the inner beauty you could be radiating all the time. We said that when you are struck by something beautiful outside yourself, you are actually communicating with your own inner beauty. Likewise, when your existence feels lighter and easier, that's your inner beauty also being reflected. You are glimpsing the truth of who you really are, because beauty and truth cannot be separated. They are qualities of pure consciousness, pure being.

At this early stage, terms like *pure consciousness* and *pure being* hardly seem relevant, because they are too foreign to your daily experience. Even so, every-one's life contains glimpses of beauty, love, joy, and fulfillment that register on the emotional level. The problem is that we need to do more on the mental level.

We need to recognize that a sign of awakening has appeared.

We need to give significance to this experience.

We need to value and pursue it.

People get stuck in everyday existence and accept as normal a life where there's no expectation of waking up. Glimpses of the light, however striking, don't propel them into a new kind of normal, which is higher and better. But if you mentally notice what's happening to you and give it significance, instead of saying to yourself, "I'm having a good day," you'll say, "I'm being touched by the light." This simple shift is enough to reframe your whole experience, making it a clue to higher consciousness.

Please glance back at the list on page 258 that outlined the most common signs of awakening—each is a moment in the light. Keep noticing such moments and pause to let them sink in. Turn inward and relish what is happening instead of simply letting it pass. Let every image of beauty you see—from those you love, from children at play, from glorious nature—really sink in. Savor the moment as a precious gift. You are venturing into the experience of communing with your true self. The more you do this, the more you will naturally want to pursue these beautiful experiences. You are beginning to wake up to your spiritual beauty.

STAGE 2: OPENING THE DOOR

Once you taste beauty, you want more. At a certain point, once you notice and value the signs of awakening, you feel the desire to explore what's happening to you. There's a sense of curiosity about what your life might be like if it changed in unexpected ways. You might also feel restless and dissatisfied with how things are going presently. At this stage people make a conscious decision to let in the light. A major decision involves being kinder and more compassionate to yourself. Let's look into this shift, which brings in much more light the more you experience it.

When we are kind to other people, we let them know that they are good and lovable just as they are. Self-compassion is saying the same thing to yourself. Pause for a moment here. Do you love yourself just as you are? The way that people answer this question reveals a great deal about themselves, because quite often we are waiting for the day that someone else will treat us as good and lovable, without criticism or reservation.

If you are fortunate, this has already happened to you. But the world's wisdom traditions teach that the love you receive from outside is a reflection of the love you have inside. The most perfect love comes from your true self, which always sees you in the light. When you open the door to the light, you are asking to experience a new relationship inside yourself. Right at this moment, you are likely to be experiencing love and light only in bursts, as if the door was being opened and then quickly closed—passing moments when you can relate to yourself as worthy of love. At other times this isn't your experience. Negative reflections from the outside keep you from seeing your inner beauty.

It would be ideal if all of us were perfectly loved from the time we were small children. But the way you feel about yourself is almost always the result of mixed messages that you have heard all your life. When you needed love, kindness, and compassion, you learned that these would be given only under certain conditions. We've all received messages like the following:

> *I love you as long as you love me.*
>
> *I love you as long as you are being good.*
>
> *I love you only as much as you deserve.*
>
> *I love you, but don't ask for too much or you'll be spoiled.*

You may remember such messages as you were growing up or perhaps in your present relationships today. They place conditions on the love you experience, and these conditions come to feel normal. But if love is always limited, so is how beautiful you feel. The old game of comparison stays alive because we feel there is not enough love and beauty to go around, and somehow other people get more than their fair share compared with us.

Can you change your inner image of how much you are loved? You will never feel secure in your beauty until it is merged with love. The path to unconditional love only asks for you to open the door. No one else can open it for you; there is no source of unconditional love outside yourself. Right this minute you have the ability to find the place inside you where unconditional love exists. To show you how easy this is, try the following simple exercise:

Sit comfortably by yourself in a quiet place. Now say to yourself, "I am _____," using your name to fill in the blank, for example, "I am Sharon Thompson." Wait a few seconds and let this thought settle. Now shorten it: "I am Sharon." Sit for a moment to let this thought settle. Then shorten the thought to "I am," then to "I," and then sit in silence. Most people experience this sequence of thoughts as a natural way to find the inner silence inside themselves. It's a pleasant experience, which may last only briefly or several minutes—that part doesn't matter. What's important is to see that your identity can shift from "I am X" to simply "I am" and then silence.

You don't have to use your name in this exercise. Any X will work, because whenever you say to yourself "I am angry" or "I'm bored" or "I'm cooking dinner," you are placing a condition on who you are. These conditions come and go all the time. They rise and fall, while your true self remains constant. Sadly, we've developed the habit of living with labels and thinking they tell us who we are. "I am X, thirty-six years old of mixed race, religiously unaffiliated, a lawyer, with a husband and two children."

In the game of labeling, we'd all like to pin the label "beautiful" on ourselves. But once you do, insecurity sets in. The label could always wear out or fall off. All labels are temporary. Therefore, be very clear that beauty isn't a label—it's a state of being.

All of these labels that we identify with serve as distractions from who we really are: children of the light. When you stop being distracted by thinking "I am X," you easily find the path to simply being yourself. There's no huge spiritual secret beyond this. The spiritual path is all about clearing away labels, images, old memories, and outworn conditioning that prevent you from the simple experience of your true place in the light.

You can't turn conditional love into unconditional love any more than you can turn muddy water to pure, clean water. Instead, you must go to the place inside where you can simply be yourself and, without judgment or comparison, where you feel beautiful, loved, and lovable. Getting to this place isn't difficult. You just did it through a simple exercise. So why didn't you suddenly experience bliss, joy, and ecstasy, which are supposed to be there? Because it takes repeated experience to become accustomed to "I am" in place of "I am all the labels that apply to me." The quality of bliss, joy, and ecstasy is already part of you—in Indian the term for this state is *Ananda*. *Ananda* isn't held out as a faraway ideal that is only reached by a few gifted people after years of faith and devotion. *Ananda* is a quality of consciousness itself, meaning that you experience it when you experience the silence of your own mind.

This is where self-compassion comes in. Knowing that you can experience unconditional love, bliss, and joy by going to the place where these things are natural means you don't have to work on your limited, conditioned self. You don't have to criticize it to find it lacking in any way. Rather, you can treat your conditioned self as an ally on your inner journey. After all, this is the self that has given you glimpses of love, bliss, and joy all your life. You face a simple choice. You can look at your imperfect, conditioned self and say, "You caused all my problems. Thanks to you, I have been wounded and suffered. You don't live up to my ideals. I'm frustrated and exasperated by you."

This is a very common attitude. You may not accuse and reject your limited self directly, but every time you think you aren't good enough, beautiful enough, thin enough, and so on, you are in fact rejecting yourself.

The other side of the coin is to look at your limited self and say, "Thank you for always being here. Because of you I have experienced the light. I have known love and beauty. Join with me now, and trust in me. We are going to find our true home in the light." That's how self-compassion begins, by changing blame and judgment to acceptance and optimism.

Having adopted this new attitude toward yourself, you want to sustain it. There are various ways to practice self-compassion every day, as follows.

To be kind to yourself, DO

Smile at your reflection in the mirror.

Let others compliment you.

Bask in other people's approval when it comes your way.

Accept and be nonjudgmental with your personal appearance and body.

Value who you are and stand up for yourself.

Get to know yourself like a friend.

Be easy about your personal quirks.

Be as natural as possible, not worrying if you are pleasing or displeasing others.

Speak your truth when you know you should.

The Do list is centered on relating to yourself with a nonjudgmental attitude. There is also a Don't list, which is about removing self-judgments, because in the end, all lack of self-love is rooted in judging yourself.

To stop self-judgment, DON'T

Brush away compliments.

Reject other people's appreciation.

Belittle yourself, even with self-deprecating humor.

Dwell on your faults as a topic of conversation.

Rationalize away the times when someone else hurts you.

Accept indifference from people who supposedly love you.

Associate with others who have low self-esteem and expect you to be the same way.

Silently swallow bad treatment when you know you should speak up.

The reflections of how you feel about yourself exist all around you. Even negative reflections are incredibly useful if you take them as guides for change. Are there people in your life who take you for granted when they shouldn't?

Rather than trying to change them, see this as a reflection of how much you value yourself—in this case, not enough. You might want to write out the following checklist, and over the next week check off each time something on the list happens to you. The list contains typical reflections in everyone's life, both positive and negative.

Positive Reflections

____ Someone appreciated me.

____ I liked the person I saw in the mirror.

____ I received a sincere compliment.

____ I felt proud of something I did for myself.

____ I felt as if I belonged.

____ Someone expressed love for me in a meaningful way.

____ I felt lovable.

____ I felt well loved.

____ The beauty of the life I'm living really hit me.

____ I felt like a unique person; there's no one in the world quite like me.

Negative Reflections

____ Someone criticized me to my face.

____ I frowned at myself in the mirror.

____ I felt guilty or embarrassed by something I remembered from long ago.

____ I put myself down while talking to someone else.

____ I felt unwanted, an outsider.

____ I received what felt like an empty word or gesture of love.

____ I felt unlovable.

____ I sat through someone else's litany of complaints.

____ Something pointless about my life really hit me.

____ I felt bored by my existence and the people I keep seeing every day.

Some people might resist filling out these two lists because they're afraid of what they'll find. Or they might think that noticing negative reflections is a sign of low self-esteem. It's not. You are taking a major step toward self-compassion by looking around and being truthful with yourself. Being kind to yourself requires a decision to embrace change. Self-judgment keeps us from loving who we are right this moment. Every step you take to walk away from negative reflections is a step in the direction of unconditional love.

Radical Beauty asks you to summon your inner courage. For some people, opening the door is harder than it is for others. They keep feeling the tug of anxiety or threat, and their mind resists the prospect of change. The following thoughts are typical when you are in a resisting frame of mind:

> *I'm alright where I am. Why rock the boat?*
>
> *If I change, my friends and family won't accept me anymore.*
>
> *Perhaps my experiences aren't even real—I'm just fooling myself.*
>
> *I'm not the kind of person who ever changes—it's just wishful thinking.*
>
> *I don't want to stick out from the crowd. Society will look on me as abnormal.*

This kind of resistance crops up in everyone, because we all have a social self. Your social self is where judgments come from, and if you don't see yourself as beautiful, it's the reason why. This self has learned, often through painful trial and error, how to get along. Fitting in isn't easy, and in every life there are guardians of the rules who will be quick to notice anyone who dares to break them. We are referring to rules of behavior, which have been ingrained in everyone since early childhood. So how do you get past the warning voices in your head? You can't open the door to your true self until this happens.

Reassuring yourself that everything will be okay isn't an effective tactic. Your social self has deep roots; it is used to guiding you through every daily encounter, constantly monitoring whether your behavior is safe and acceptable. (For the moment we are leaving aside the small band of misfits, artists, rebels, sages, and saints whose behavior transgresses social norms. Such people often lead extraordinary lives, but they also tend to pay extraordinarily high prices, too.)

You need to recognize that you have been influenced by years of conditioning; therefore, to escape this conditioning, it's necessary to substitute new, positive beliefs for the warnings that try to keep you from opening the door. Here are some examples:

Warning: I'm alright where I am. Why rock the boat?
New thought: I can keep what's good in my life. The changes I want will only add to them.

Warning: If I change, my friends and family won't accept me anymore.
New thought: If I bring more light into my life, at the same time I will be bringing it to my family and friends. They will welcome the change.

Warning: Perhaps my experiences aren't even real—I'm just fooling myself.
New thought: I can't deny that my experiences make me feel good. That's real enough to make me trust them.

Warning: I'm not the kind of person who ever changes—it's just wishful thinking.
New thought: There's a part of me that can't wait to break out into a new way of life. I should give it a chance. The only reason I need is that this is what I want.

Warning: I don't want to stick out from the crowd. Society will look on me as abnormal.
New thought: No one else needs to know about what's going on inside me. This is something just for me, something I entirely own.

These new thoughts aren't just reassurances. They put you in contact with your true self, which is what opening the door actually means. Radical Beauty is about seeing yourself in the light, which is where all positive thoughts originate. Spirit has never forgotten how beautiful you are and always have been.

Now that you have opened the door, love and beauty call out. You find them in the most unexpected places. At this point, it's only natural to desire a complete shift in your life, nothing less than transformation. As Radical Beauty unfolds, we promise that transformation is possible, simply because the most natural way to live is from the level of the true self. It puts beauty, grace, and love together in one place as a normal way of life. The path lies before you. So what comes next? You dedicate yourself to reaching your goal. This is a dedication that you renew every day. Yet as we all know, it's easy for the day to run away with us, because our time is already dedicated to work, family, errands, and unexpected duties and demands that eat up the clock.

Fortunately, you don't have to set aside your daily life to be spiritually dedicated. We do recommend one important change, which is to meditate twice a day for 10 to 15 minutes (or longer). You probably have an opinion about meditation already. It's become so popular that few people still regard the practice as something exotic and alien. The image that now comes to mind is of a young, vibrant woman sitting in lotus position in yoga class, not a white-bearded Indian guru in a cave.

Society has promoted meditation as a healthy habit, and in fact there is a mountain of evidence telling us that meditation is good for the entire body, particularly by lowering the risk of heart disease and counteracting the damaging effects of stress. If you've had a hard day and want to unwind with a peaceful round of meditation, we encourage you to go for it. But when it comes to transformation and achieving your highest potential for spiritual beauty, meditation is more than any of these things.

Even though brief, your meditation time brings you into the silent core of yourself; this is where you will meet the truth of your own beauty and where the door to unconditional love opens.

How to Meditate: Technique 1

Here's a simple meditation based on the breath that you can do anywhere. It's best to pick a quiet, lowly lit spot where you can be alone. Sit for a moment with your eyes closed in order to become settled. Now place your attention on your nose; sense the gentle flow of air as it goes in and out.

Don't try to alter your breathing or to maintain a rhythm—simply be aware of your normal breathing. If your attention wanders, gently and easily bring it back to your breath. Don't mind if you feel drowsy or even doze off. These are signs that your body needs to rest and discharge stresses.

Continue for 10 to 15 minutes, then sit quietly for a moment before you open your eyes and return to your regular activity. Don't leap out of your chair or skip this moment to return to normal awareness. Letting your mind remain in the meditative state is desirable and very worth cultivating as you continue your practice over the coming weeks and months.

How to Meditate: Technique 2

A second type of meditation uses a mantra, a word selected for its vibrational quality in settling the mind. Mantras go back thousands of years, and there's some striking research to indicate that they lead to a deeper state of meditation. A simple mantra suitable for everyone is *So Hum*. You can meditate with it in the following way.

As with your breath meditation, try to pick a quiet, lowly lit spot where you can be alone. Sit for a moment with your eyes closed in order to become settled. Now quietly think the mantra: *So Hum*. Think these syllables as easily as any other thought. Repeat the mantra a second time, then a third: *So Hum, So Hum*.

Repeat the mantra for 10 to 15 minutes, but don't try to set up a regular rhythm. This style of meditation isn't about mentally chanting your mantra with a regular beat. Instead, you think *So Hum* when it's natural and easy to do so. If your attention wanders, easily come back to your mantra. Don't mind if you get drowsy or doze off. Don't mind if you forget to say the mantra for what seems like a long time.

The object is to allow the vibration of *So Hum* to settle your awareness as naturally as possible. You don't need to manipulate it or control it in any way. After 10 to 15 minutes, sit quietly for a moment before returning to your daily activity. Easing back into activity helps to maintain the meditative state.

Meditation clears the path and makes it much easier to greet renewal and change. Your awareness becomes brighter and more alert; mental and emotional obstacles are dissolved. Therefore, nothing is more effective than adopting a regular meditation program. At the same time, there's another dimension to consider. As you clear the path, certain potentials begin to wake up inside. You glimpse that there could be more love, beauty, creativity, and fulfillment in your life. Many people have gotten to this stage in their seeking. But then they run into a problem staying in that place where meditation has taken them.

Here's a good place to lay a common fear to rest. Some people fear that if they start to meditate, they will stir up hidden thoughts, feelings, and memories they'd rather not face. By going deeper into your mind, aren't you stirring up the demons that everyone has? In reality, meditation is value neutral. It doesn't conform to labels like "good" and "bad," "positive" and "negative." All that happens is that you reach a deeper level of awareness. Nothing will leap out of the dark. The main experience is the release of stress, accompanied by layers of fatigue falling away. Stress can bring up images of why you feel stressed in the first place. But all you have to do when this happens is to open your eyes and take a deep breath. Being mental images, negative thoughts and images pass away. If you seriously want to delve into the hidden compartments of your mind—some people do, being spiritually adventurous—that's a conscious choice. If you would rather have your meditations be easy and light, that is also a choice. The mind delivers what is asked of it.

Finding your inner beauty is meant to be lasting, and it will be. The main thing that causes the deep experience of meditation to fade away is stress. When you sit alone to meditate, the outside world has been left behind for a few minutes, yet once you go back into it, the demands of the outside world can't be escaped. Those demands can create a constant stream of stress, as we all well know. The destructive effects of stress have been well studied for almost fifty years. When someone is put into a stressful situation, the brain and body respond with stress hormones like cortisol and adrenaline. These are very effective natural tools that jump-start the body into fight-or-flight mode.

The Damaging Effects of Chronic Stress

Radical Beauty involves getting back into balance and restoring the natural state of mind and body. Beauty is a healed state. Stress is the enemy of healing; we weren't designed to be stressed out for any lengthy period. Fight-or-flight is meant to persist for only a matter of minutes, but low-level chronic stress activates these hormones too often, and their effect lasts too long. What should be a temporary reaction becomes routine. The result is a biochemical imbalance that the brain and body have a hard time adjusting to. You can't be in a meditative state and a stressful state at the same time; the two don't mesh. By "meditative state," we mean a state of restful alertness, in which you feel calm and centered but very awake at the same time. Low-level chronic stress imposes a very different mind-body state. The following symptoms are quite common in modern life, even among people who think that they have adapted well to daily stresses (in fact, some high-performance types boast that they thrive on stress).

Is Chronic Stress Getting to You?
Some typical signs of low-level chronic stress

You feel irritable and on edge.

Your muscles feel tight, especially in the neck and back.

Your stomach is in knots.

You swing between feeling highly alert and very dull.

You lose energy quickly through the day.

You find it hard to focus and concentrate.

Your efficiency at work declines.

When you go to bed at night, your mind races with thoughts, making it hard to fall asleep.

Sleep is shortened or restless.

You wake up feeling tired.

Your sex drive decreases.

You feel slightly anxious without cause.

You become lethargic and depressed.

You find it hard to express enthusiasm and optimism.

You feel unexplained aches and pains.

You have digestive difficulties or intestinal pain.

You catch more colds and flus than normal.

As you can see, this is an extensive list. Millions of people ignore stress because they are willing to put up with less than ideal well-being, until they reach the point where lack of sleep, flagging energy, free-floating anxiety, and dull attention become normal. More damage is done to natural beauty by these over-looked factors than anything else. If someone sees wrinkles, pallor, sagging skin, dull eyes, and other signs of premature aging in the mirror, they are reading the story of how they managed stress in the past. Nothing caused by chronic stress is normal, however, and as long as your body is subjected to the chemical imbalances created by stress, you will be out of balance.

Why create such a valuable thing as the meditative state only to allow it to be disrupted by your daily experiences? Our focus here is on avoiding that. No one's life is perfectly stress-free. At the same time, everyone's life has areas where the stress can be reduced. To simplify the problem, at any given moment you are doing one of the following:

> Creating stress
>
> Reacting to stress caused by external forces
>
> Healing your stress and the stress around you

We'd like to help you get past the first two situations so that you can become something new: a healer of stress. In this way you will be able to maintain the restful alertness that is the true foundation of mind-body balance. Every cell in your body will respond positively when this happens.

The biggest step you can take is to reject the role of victim.

People make jokes like "Gray hair is inherited. You get it from your children." They complain about the stress and strain of modern life. It's as if stress is like air pollution, existing all around us with very little we can do about it. But there's a lot you can do about it, once you escape the role of victim. Earlier in this book we mentioned stress in passing, but not in terms of achieving real, lasting control over it. By understanding how stress is created, you can begin to lower the stress level anywhere you find yourself—at work, in family situations, in everyday crises and challenges.

It's true but often ignored that each of us is a creator of the stress we suffer from. Stress is viral. Once someone creates it, the stressful results spread to others. The most infamous example is shouting "Fire!" in a crowded theater. The spread of panic in a crowd seems like an extreme example, yet in smaller, less glaring ways, any of us can contribute to the virus of stress. Here are some examples of how this happens. Since one main area of stress for most people is at work, let's start there.

How Stress Goes Viral at Work
Common conditions that create needless stress:

Someone is demanding, critical, and a perfectionist.

The person in charge gives erratic orders prone to unpredictable changes.

Co-workers show disrespect for one another or their work.

An undignified work environment exists (e.g., a place where bad language, gossip, and sexual remarks are allowed).

Personal issues are brought to work and become everybody's business.

Workers are criticized in public.

The people in authority can't be trusted.

There is constant pressure to meet deadlines.

Worker loyalty isn't valued.

The threat of losing your job is present.

A worker's experience and knowledge are undervalued.

Work rules are rigid, leaving little room for creativity and personal suggestions.

Reading over the list, consider the three options that face you every day.

Are you creating the stress?

Are you reacting to stress from the outside?

Are you helping to reduce and heal the stress?

Some of the stressful behaviors on the list may seem very ordinary to you. But that's generally a sign of denial. Each of these behaviors puts pressure on you or someone else, and with pressure the mind-body system reacts stressfully. Stress experts often refer to how ancient the stress response is, because the chemical triggers for it are located at the base of the skull in the oldest section of the brain, known as the reptilian brain. The reptilian brain doesn't think about what is causing a sense of threat. The example is often given of someone stuck in a traffic jam on the way home from work. The frustration of the situation causes the secretion of the same fight-or-flight hormones as our ancestors experienced at the approach of a saber-toothed tiger. The lower brain doesn't register the difference, which means that our response is primitive and chemical, not intelligent and rational.

Therefore, even when you think you are doing something quite harmless and necessary, such as criticizing another person for poor performance, the lower brain doesn't register anything reasonable—it just feels threatened. The same holds true outside the workplace in how we behave with our family and friends. It's often said that modern life is stressful because we're exposed to so much noise, speed, and complex tasks compared with our grandparents' generation. Those are stressful factors, no doubt, but the worst stress is psychological. We fall into the careless habit of putting pressure on others without realizing it.

Psychological Stress—It's All in the Family
The stressful habits of everyday life include the following:

Constant teasing, putting others down, picking on the weak

Blaming someone else

Harping on someone else's faults and mistakes

Not listening

Not letting everyone have their say

Being disrespectful

Using verbal or emotional abuse

Resorting to physical violence

Refusing to take responsibility for your own actions

Putting pressure on children to perform

Making seniors feel old, useless, and unwanted

Creating an atmosphere of resentment and complaint

Filling the air with constant arguments

Repeatedly rehashing old grievances

Imposing rigid rules

Making someone feel inferior or unwanted

Being a harsh authority figure, or living under one

Creating an atmosphere of emotional repression, where genuine
feelings cannot be expressed

Unloving behavior in general

As before, when you read over this list, you need to ask the following questions:

Are you creating the stress?

Are you reacting to stress from the outside?

Are you helping to reduce and heal the stress?

Millions of people would say that they have a loving family while the reality is that stressful behavior is going on under their roof. It's easy to forget that the family is a place that should be as stress-free as possible. It's not the place where you go to dump your "stuff"—the complaints, negativity, anger, and frustration accumulated during the day.

We hate to say it, but many people who sincerely believe that they are on a spiritual path remain oblivious to the stressful behavior they exhibit or encourage in others. They lack self-awareness, which is what the spiritual path is really all about.

Once you understand how low-level stress is affecting you and those around you, you'll want to break the cycle. You don't have to adopt the role of victim. At the same time, you don't have to adopt the opposite role of abuser or aggressor. The cycle of stressful behavior affects everyone equally. Ultimately, your goal is to find your inner love, truth, and beauty, letting them shine all around you. Stress is incompatible with this goal, leaving aside all the other damage it creates.

How to Be a Healer of Stress

If stress can go viral, so can beauty. Radical Beauty is about radiating your beauty so that it uplifts those around you. This is a form of spiritual healing. *Stress* and *spiritual* aren't two words you see together very often—one seems very worldly while the other is very unworldly. But *healing, whole,* and *holiness* come from the same root word. When you are healed of the damage created by stress, you find your wholeness and your holiness.

To become a healer of stress, you stop pressuring others—and yourself—at the psychological level. Thinking psychologically doesn't come easily for most of us. Let's return to the workplace again. If you've been taught that a hard-boiled attitude, confrontational tactics, and constant pressure are good for productivity, studies in the workplace do not bear this out. The best workplaces give workers their personal space, encourage creativity, allow flexible work hours, assign tasks according to everyone's unique strengths, and create an atmosphere of general respect. This is basic psychology turned into practice.

If you don't put much stock in psychology, look around you. If you are the focus or cause of stress in other people, the following things, either a few or a lot, will be evident: People don't look happy around you or working for you. They avoid direct eye contact. They seem nervous in your presence. The atmosphere grows quiet and tense when you enter a room or give orders. There is silent resistance to giving you what you ask for—you have to ask a second time, and even then there are delays. People under you make excuses, or else they have lost their motivation to perform.

The real eye-opener, however, is to take the same look around the family setting. Instead of workplace, substitute the home. In place of workers, substitute children or spouse. You may be shocked at how viral the stress around you actually is. Society sends us messages about rebellious teenagers who won't do what they're told, who act uncomfortable around adults, slack off at school, and exhibit a sullen, resentful attitude. These behaviors fit a stereotype, but that doesn't make them normal. They are signs of stress. We aren't saying that adolescence doesn't have its special challenges, because it certainly does. The point is that adding to those challenges with stressful pressures at home is just as damaging as if the pressure was applied at work.

It is generally futile to approach someone else and say, "I'm sorry, but your behavior is stressing me out." All you'll get is a defensive response that pushes you away. The focus must be on you instead.

By reversing your own stressful behavior, you become a healer of stress, breaking the circle once and for all. This is actually a powerful approach that can cause other people who have caused you stress to change before your eyes. We've seen it work with all kinds of difficult people, both at home and in the office.

TWELVE WAYS YOU CAN HEAL STRESS

Behaviors that reduce pressure on yourself and others:

1. Back away from being demanding, critical, and a perfectionist.

2. Be more consistent and less changeable in what you ask of others.

3. Never show disrespect for other people.

4. Maintain a dignified environment (e.g., a place where bad language, gossip, and sexual remarks are not condoned).

5. Give other people their own space.

6. Deal with your own stress instead of passing it down the line.

7. Don't create pets and favorites at the expense of someone who gets excluded or demeaned.

8. Never offer criticism in public or at the dinner table.

9. Take a personal interest in others, offering appreciation and praise generously.

10. Be loyal; show that you can be trusted.

11. When someone else is talking, pay attention and then follow through if they need something.

12. Ask for more input from others, showing that you value their experience and knowledge.

Think of these things in terms of letting inner beauty go viral. With small changes of behavior, along with self-awareness, you will be surprised to find that you are becoming a beacon of light. This is testimony to your new reality: you have truly dedicated yourself to the path. The gap between your social self and your true self is closing more and more, and the beauty of your true self is becoming a reality.

Every woman knows the feeling of not being enough. So much is asked of today's woman—and she asks even more of herself—that insecurity is just the beginning. There is a constant struggle against feeling anxious or depressed. There is doubt about how one set of values—being successful and highly competent—can really be compatible with another set of values—being loved, cherished, and honored. The nagging question "Can I have it all?" hangs over the minds of millions of women every day.

The answer to "Can I have it all?" isn't easy to find in our society, but we feel that there is an answer that gets overlooked. You can have it all when you realize that *you are all*. There's nothing you can buy in any store that will fill any empty feeling of lack. But when you find inner fulfillment, having it all is replaced by inner contentment with yourself, here and now, lacking nothing.

Let's say this is the right answer. How do you arrive at this state of total inner fulfillment? By realizing your spiritual beauty. And how do you do that? By following the most powerful instructions on the spiritual path:

Surrender

Let go

Accept

Be

These instructions aren't easy to follow. We all feel a powerful desire *to do something*. We hate putting up with the bad things in our lives. Society promotes the image of the go-getting, competitive person who is constantly on the move. It's no surprise, then, that we've lost the skill—and the wisdom—of just letting go. We equate hanging loose with doing nothing. Yet at a deeper level, each of those words implies a hidden action that goes on beneath the surface:

Surrendering means you aren't struggling anymore.

Letting go means that you aren't so attached and frustrated.

Accepting means that you can appreciate and be grateful for your life.

Being means that you trust a power beyond your own ego and
limited understanding.

When you grasp what the words mean in spiritual terms, it dawns on you that a much better life can be yours once you surrender, let go, accept, and simply be. We've put this in a single phrase: *Resting into existence.* In every spiritual tradition, importance is placed on surrendering to God, but it's an idea that doesn't seem applicable in modern times. In the past, when our distant ancestors were preoccupied every day with getting enough to eat, disaster struck if crops failed or game was scarce. Trusting in God to provide was the only way anyone had of connecting with nature's external forces. But today the vast majority of work is done in offices and corporations; these are settings where people feel they have much more control over what happens. There is little or no need to trust in a higher power except in unforeseen emergencies and crises. Even then, many people place their trust only on human agencies like law enforcement.

So asking you to place your trust in your own existence is asking a lot. As a strategy for living, this might sound quite strange, in fact. But consider the following possibilities:

> What if life is meant to flow, bringing fulfillment as a natural unfoldment?
>
> What if you are connected to a deep source of intelligence that knows how to take care of you and your needs?
>
> What if there's a higher plan that is guiding your life?

None of these ideas is completely foreign. We've all been exposed to sayings like "Everything happens for a reason" and "God has a plan." The problem is that the divine plan, if it exists, is invisible and unpredictable. Not to mention that putting the argument in religious terms runs against the grain of modern life, where the secular world is based on real-life events and things we can see, hear, and touch.

In other words, there's a gap between a beautiful idea—that every life has a meaning that unfolds in the best possible way—and our daily experience. You may have read of a life strategy that consists of always saying yes and never saying no. This is a form of complete surrender, because saying yes to literally everything implies enormous trust that something won't go terribly wrong. (Would you say yes to every stranger who offers you a ride, every unsolicited phone caller who asks for money, every request made by your five-year-old child?) On the other hand, saying no puts you in opposition to other people, creating clashes and disagreements along with missed opportunities. (Would you have said no twenty years ago if you were offered shares in Apple at its lowest price in the stock market?)

Deciding when to say yes and when to say no is, in fact, one of the hardest challenges in everyone's life. Who you marry and what kind of work you do depend on giving the right answer, as do thousands of smaller choices. But if saying yes all the time doesn't work, and neither does saying no all the time, what's the alternative? Must we muddle through trying to figure out the right answer on a case-by-case basis?

Most people are already doing that. If there's a better way, perhaps the world's wisdom traditions offer it. From their perspective, the soul knows best. So what would the soul do? That's an intimate matter. Your soul sees every situation through fresh eyes, and they aren't the eyes of anyone else. Even so, there's a pattern of trust that needs to develop inside each of us, in which we rely on the true self to bring the right solutions to everyday challenges.

You can't trust and be in total control at the same time; the two aren't compatible. Letting go is how trust develops. You stop worrying that everything depends on you. There's a parable from India that begins to shed light on why a person can rest easy and trust in their own existence. The parable isn't couched in religious terms at all. It's about a coachman driving a team of six horses. The horses are spirited, and the coachman whips them to go faster and faster.

Suddenly from inside the coach a quiet voice says, "Stop the coach." At first the driver can't believe his ears, and he cracks his whip even harder. But soon the same voice inside the coach whispers, "Stop the coach." Now the driver feels nervous, and he says aloud, "Why should I stop? I know how to drive, and I want to go faster." To which the voice replies, "But I own this coach, and I say stop." At this point the driver has no choice, and the coach comes to a halt.

The meaning of the parable is only revealed when you know that the coachman is the ego, the six horses are the five senses and the mind, and the owner of the coach is the higher self. We spend our lives with the ego acting as if it is in charge, and it takes control over the five senses and the mind, which obey the ego's commands willingly. Like horses in harness, our five senses and the mind can be directed this way and that. We see what the ego wants us to see; we hear what it wants us to hear. As for the mind, it can be conditioned to believe whatever story the ego tells it.

We've all been told a similar story, as it turns out, which keeps being repeated generation after generation. It's the story of life as a constant struggle where humans are puny things confronted by the inexorable powers of nature. No one is immune from danger and looming catastrophe. Because life isn't fair and nature is blind, we have no choice but to struggle if we want to survive.

The parable of the coachman contradicts this story by saying that despite all appearances, the ego isn't actually in charge of how life unfolds. The owner of the coach is *Atman,* the higher self, which we have been calling the true self. We've been describing the true self as the source of beauty, intelligence, truth, and creativity inside everyone. It has been in control of our lives from the moment of birth, but the ego, with its convincing story about life as a constant struggle, has taken over. As long as the ego dominates our awareness, we lose sight of how reality actually works, the same way the coachman lost sight of the fact that he didn't own the coach.

At some point in your personal growth, you will want to test the possibility that you could be living a new story. You don't have to test this new story by fighting against the ego and its constant demands, fears, old memories, and outworn conditioning. All you have to do is rest into existence. This is really the process of accepting your own spiritual beauty. On a daily basis you do the following things.

The Practical Side of Surrender
How to let your spiritual beauty shine through:

When there's a problem, look inside for the solution, knowing that it will be there.

Even when the details aren't perfect, accept that the larger picture will turn out alright in the end.

Don't act when you feel upset, angry, afraid, or uncertain.

Stay centered, and when you realize you aren't centered, take a few moments to restore your sense of balance and calm.

As much as possible, don't put up resistance to other people. Be open-minded and tolerant toward their point of view.

Maintain a seamless flow in your activity.

Don't exert yourself to the point of exhaustion but don't slack off.

Look for hints from your higher self about which way to turn.
Learn to trust your instincts.

Don't do what you already know to be wrong.

Look upon outward situations as a reflection of your inner situation.

Take responsibility for what you say, think, and do, without projecting blame or depending on someone else to take care of things.

Each of these items can be tested at your own pace. For most people, changing their story only begins when they see hope that it can be changed. Inertia is a powerful force. If you have landed in a bad relationship or a job you hate, if you feel lonely all the time or struggle with depression, it's unrealistic to say, "I'll just trust that everything's okay and go with the flow." We aren't advising you to do that. Instead, you need to be reasonably centered to begin with, which comes about through meditation. You need to feel reasonably free of damaging stress and have enough room to make some new choices. If these preconditions aren't met, this doesn't mean you are in a hopeless predicament; it only means that you should look to earlier stages of growth as your starting point.

Many people, however, are ready to change the story of life as a struggle, and therefore they can begin to experience a more open, relaxed, and trusting way of life. One drawback of religious and spiritual traditions, however beautiful their message, is a lack of practicality. Too often the hard world is regarded as the enemy of spirit, which also implies that you must choose one or the other. Either it's worldly success or living in the light, with no middle ground. On this basis, or something similar, millions of people yearn for spirituality but keep postponing it, for fear of what they might lose in worldly satisfactions.

But if your outer situation is good, your inner situation is probably good, too. Most of us experience a mixture of good and bad in both realms, which is why we can't see a clear path forward. We are more likely to deal with worldly things—work, family, politics, relationships, community activities—on their own terms, sealing our inner lives off as something private and isolated. But the message that needs to come through is that inner and outer are never separate, and when you begin to trust that you are safe and cared for from a deep level within yourself, the two halves of your life can be united. In wholeness lies the beauty of the soul—the essence of Radical Beauty—which is yours to claim as your own and to celebrate forever.

We've painted a picture of spiritual beauty that can entirely change your life—it's the most radical kind of beauty there is. Beginning with experiences that everyone has had—being loved, or observing the innocence of children and seeing a glorious sunset—a new way of life opens. The choice is yours. You can walk the path to inner beauty or hold back instead. Because there is so much potential inside you for love, truth, and beauty, you have the support of those things simply by being here on this planet. The choice to walk the path is an option that is never canceled, because the world's wisdom traditions declare that love, truth, and beauty are eternal.

Today your true self awaits you, as it has patiently waited every day. If you choose to, you can journey to where your true self lives, deep inside your awareness. What happens then? You will be transformed in the image of your true self. You will experience as your daily reality something beautifully expressed by the great Indian poet Rabindranath Tagore: "Love is the only reality and it is not a mere sentiment. It is the ultimate truth that lies at the heart of creation." To find the heart of creation, you must explore your own heart. Inside it are stored many experiences of love and non-love.

The Promise of Transformation

Radical Beauty is a journey of transformation. This hardly seems possible in our time, when so many people struggle to maintain meaning and purpose in their lives. There is no model for accepting unconditional love as the ultimate reality. In a celebrity culture, outer beauty is accepted as a sign of inner beauty—perhaps—but the connection could be imaginary. The real connection between inner and outer beauty begins inside, as we have emphasized in this book. When that connection is unbreakable, you will find yourself transformed completely.

The Signs of Transformation
The qualities of the true self dawning in your life:

Complete self-acceptance: "I am here, and I am enough."

Self-love as a natural state that never changes: "My purpose has always been about love."

A life filled with meaning and purpose: "I find joy pursuing my vision."

Inner peace: "I find fulfillment in stillness."

Reverence for life: "I take tender care of everything in creation."

A sense of common humanity with all other people: "The world is my family."

Empathy without judgment: "Let me embrace you, whoever you are."

A sense of unbounded possibilities: "My creativity finds a new way to express itself every day."

The expansion of personal identity as "I" becomes connected to cosmic consciousness: "I see myself in all I behold."

The expression of love, truth, and beauty appears in daily activity: "There is no difference between the truth I live, the beauty I behold, and the love I feel."

You may think that these are fairy-tale qualities never achieved in the rough-and-tumble of daily existence. Perhaps only a few exceptional individuals, born with unshakable faith, are fated to get anywhere near the true self. But faith isn't by any means what you need the most if you want to journey to the true self. Far more important are knowledge and experience. At this moment, you have your share of both. You have experienced how beautiful life can be, even if this has happened only in scattered glimpses. You have the knowledge of how inner beauty unfolds after reading this book. Therefore, the keys to transformation are already in your hands—there is no ancient, hidden secret that must be mysteriously imported.

Only one thing is left for you to do: activate your evolution. How? By putting your attention on the good things you want to increase in your life. In a word, *become the change you want to see.*

The qualities of the true self never go away, but people don't activate them. When we find ourselves pulled back into the demands of our busy lives, the desire to grow and evolve becomes blurred and overlooked. At that point, there's a disconnect. On a clear night you can walk outside and gaze at thousands of stars and galaxies; on any clear morning you can watch the sunrise in all its delicate beauty. Choosing to see external beauty is a possibility for everyone. What takes dedication is to turn inward and discover the same awe and wonder when you behold yourself.

Mirabai was a princess in medieval India who also happened to be a great mystical poet. She speaks poignantly of the life that is possible only through transformation:

> *Take me to that place no one can travel to*
> *Where death is afraid*
> *And swans alight to play*
> *On the overflowing lake of love.*
> *There the faithful gather*
> *Ever true to their Lord.*

Mirabai lived in religious times, during an age of faith, but "that place no one can travel to" is the same true self we have been discussing. You can't travel to it because there's nowhere to go "out there" in the world. Once you dedicate yourself to the path, you are making a personal promise to participate in a completely transformed reality. That's what personal evolution can achieve, and only personal evolution. It allows transformation to take place on the inside, and when this happens, transformation on the outside follows effortlessly. You can't force it. Of course you can work toward separate changes in your life—we all do that. You can lose weight, treat depression, find a new partner, quit smoking, and so on. Such efforts can be difficult, because they require you to break old habits or to make drastic changes that bother the people around you.

But transformation is different, because it involves the whole person, not individual changes that occur one at a time. Spiritual traditions around the world often use the same term—a *second birth*—to describe what inner transformation is like. A second birth erases all the mistakes of the past and returns the person to a state of innocence, a completely fresh start.

It's a beautiful ideal, but in practical terms, there's a problem. No one needs to change everything about themselves. In everyone's life there are good and bad parts. Looking at yourself today, you could list many aspects of your current situation that you value and love, along with achievements you're proud of and years of maturation that turned you into a worthy person.

Would you really want to give up all of this for the promise of a fresh start? No, of course not—and you don't have to. As a process, transformation mirrors what happens every day to an infant as it develops, stage by stage, from the moment of birth. An infant does nothing except be itself. On Tuesday the things it experiences aren't very different from the experiences on Monday.

Yet at a deeper level—in this case the unfolding of the potential inside human DNA—each day isn't the same as the day before. The infant is growing and developing, without actually making any special effort. One day a small child may be fascinated with paper dolls and playing in a sandbox. Turn around, and six months later these are playthings of the past, and something new, like alphabet blocks and learning a song, are fascinating instead. What's happening, and what continues to happen throughout a lifetime, is inner growth—evolution.

This tells us that evolution is natural; there's almost nothing about you as a two-year-old that is the same as the self you are today. What was hidden inside you back then were seeds and potentials. Why does it feel, as so many people report, that they aren't achieving their full potential? Because as adults we must consciously *choose* to evolve.

We've shown you many facets of Radical Beauty, and we've saved the most important for last: renewal. Whatever path you take, please, please renew yourself, forever and without end. Life is a process of endless renewal, and you stand at the switch, doing what it takes to move your evolution forward or the opposite, causing it to slow down or come to a halt.

From this moment forward, you can become as beautiful as anything in creation, surpassing even the most perfect rose by virtue of this rare gift called self-awareness. We'll leave you with the words of Rumi, the Persian poet who testifies to the hidden beauty behind all things.

The Open Door
People are constantly crossing
The threshold of eternity.
The door is open
If you can stay awake.

Radical Beauty Recipes

Note: As with all Radical Beauty recipes throughout the book and this section, we encourage you to use organic ingredients as much as possible.

Radical Beauty Salads

ANTIOXIDANT VEGGIE AND CHICKPEA SALAD

SERVES 3 TO 4

> 7^1/$_2$ oz (225 g) cooked and drained chickpeas
> 1^1/$_2$ oz (40 g) roughly chopped rocket
> 5 oz (150 g) chopped red pepper
> 4 oz (125 g) chopped seeded cucumber
> 1 small yellow tomato, diced
> 1^1/$_2$ oz (40 g) chopped celery
> 1^1/$_2$ tablespoons lime juice
> 2 fl oz (50 ml) extra-virgin olive oil or avocado oil
> 1 tablespoon chopped fresh basil
> ^{1}/$_4$ teaspoon sea salt, or to taste
> Freshly ground black pepper to taste
> ^{1}/$_4$ teaspoon dried oregano

In a medium bowl, mix the chickpeas and all the vegetables together. In a separate bowl, whisk together the lime juice, oil, basil, sea salt, pepper, and oregano. Pour the dressing over the salad and toss gently.

KALE QUINOA SALAD WITH BASIL DRESSING

8 fl oz (250 ml) coconut milk (low-fat is always an option)
8 fl oz (250 ml) vegetable broth or water
6 oz (175 g) red quinoa, soaked overnight and rinsed
Pinch of sea salt
1 small bunch of kale, stems removed, leaves chopped fine

BASIL DRESSING

$^1/_2$ oz (15 g) fresh whole basil leaves (no stems), rinsed and dried
$^1/_2$ oz (15 g) rocket leaves, rinsed and dried
$7^1/_2$ oz (225 g) spinach leaves, rinsed and dried
1 small garlic clove
1 tablespoon fresh lemon juice
Sea salt to taste
Freshly ground black pepper to taste
2 fl oz (50 ml) olive oil

Diced peppers, for topping
Diced tomatoes, for topping
Sliced avocado, for topping

In a medium saucepan, combine the coconut milk and the vegetable broth and bring to a boil. Add the quinoa and a pinch of sea salt, cover, and simmer on medium heat for about 15 minutes, until cooked. Remove from the heat and set aside to cool.

Meanwhile, make the dressing: Place the basil, rocket, spinach, garlic, lemon juice, sea salt, and pepper in a food processor. Start processing the mixture, and slowly drizzle in the olive oil. Process until well blended.

In a medium serving bowl, combine the cooked quinoa, chopped kale, and dressing. Mix well with a big spoon and season to taste with salt and pepper, as desired. Top with diced peppers, tomatoes, and avocado slices.

SKIN SMOOTHING GREEN BOUNTY SALAD

SERVES 1

4 leaves cos or round lettuce, torn
3/4 oz (20 g) torn rocket
7 1/2 oz (225 g) baby spinach leaves
1/2 oz (15 g) watercress, leaves and some stems
1 tablespoon roughly chopped walnuts
2 oz (50 g) diced red or yellow pepper
3 1/2 oz (100 g) quartered roasted or steamed beetroot
Drizzle of extra-virgin olive oil or avocado oil
1 tablespoon fresh lemon juice
Pinch of sea salt

Place all the ingredients in a bowl and toss well (and with love!). Enjoy immediately.

Radical Beauty Soups

INDIAN SPICED BUTTERNUT SQUASH SOUP

SERVES 2

2 teaspoons coconut oil
Pinch of red chili flakes
3 oz (75 g) chopped onions or leeks
2 teaspoons minced peeled fresh ginger
1 clove fresh garlic, peeled and minced (optional)
2–3 lbs (1–1.5 kg) cubed peeled butternut squash
1 sweet potato, peeled and cut into cubes
1 1/2 teaspoons garam masala
1/2 teaspoon ground cumin
1/4 teaspoon white pepper

2½ pints (1.4 litres) vegetable broth
4 fl oz (125 ml) cup coconut milk (low-fat is always an option)
2 teaspoons lemon juice
Sea salt to taste
Fresh coriander, for garnish
Gluten-free bread or brown rice, for serving (optional)

In a large soup pot over medium-high heat, combine the oil, red chili flakes, onions, ginger, garlic (if using), butternut squash, sweet potato, garam masala, cumin, and white pepper. Sauté for 5 minutes. Add the vegetable broth, lower the heat to low, cover the pot with a lid, and let the soup cook for about 30 minutes, or until the squash and sweet potato have cooked down. Set aside to cool. When cooled add the coconut milk and lemon juice. Blend the cooled soup to a smooth, creamy consistency with a hand blender, food processor, or blender. Reheat the soup before serving, add sea salt as desired, and garnish with fresh chopped coriander or whole coriander leaves. Serve with your favorite gluten-free bread or some brown rice, if desired.

LENTIL AND KALE SOUP

SERVES 4

1 teaspoon olive or coconut oil
5 oz (150 g) chopped leeks
3½ oz (100 g) sliced celery, ¼ inch thick
2 cloves garlic, crushed, or ½ teaspoon garlic granules
1 teaspoon minced peeled fresh ginger
1 pinch red chili flakes
1 teaspoon chopped fresh rosemary
5 oz (150 g) diced carrots
1 teaspoon ground cumin
½ teaspoon allspice
7 oz (200 g) brown lentils, sorted, rinsed, drained, and ideally soaked overnight
2–2½ pints (1.2–1.4 litres) vegetable broth, plus more as needed
2 bay leaves

(recipe continues)

2 tablespoons tomato paste or $^1/_2$ cup diced fresh tomatoes
5 oz (150 g) chopped kale
Sea salt to taste
Freshly ground black pepper to taste
2 tablespoons chopped fresh parsley or coriander, for garnish
Cooked quinoa or brown rice, for serving

In a soup pot over medium heat, heat the oil. Add the leeks, celery, garlic, ginger, red chili flakes, and rosemary. Sauté for 2 minutes. Add the carrots, cumin, allspice, lentils, vegetable broth, and bay leaves. Bring the soup to a boil, then reduce the heat to low simmer until the lentils are tender, 30 to 45 minutes. Add more broth as necessary. Add the tomato paste and kale and simmer another 5 minutes. Season with sea salt and black pepper, as desired. Remove bay leaves before serving. Ladle the soup into bowls and garnish with fresh parsley or coriander. Serve with cooked quinoa or brown rice.

NUTTY BROCCOLI SOUP

SERVES 4

1 large head broccoli
1 teaspoon olive oil
5 oz (150 g) chopped leeks or onions
2 teaspoons tamari
1 teaspoon dried or 1 tablespoon fresh minced thyme
1 teaspoon dried or 1 tablespoon fresh minced marjoram
1 teaspoon dried or 1 tablespoon fresh minced dill
1 teaspoon ground nutmeg
$^1/_2$ teaspoon black pepper
1.5 pints (850 ml) vegetable broth
2 oz (50 g) almonds, finely chopped, or 2 tablespoons almond butter for richer taste
2 teaspoons lemon juice
2 tablespoons chopped fresh parsley, for garnish

Cut the broccoli head into florets. Peel and chop the stalk.

In a soup pot over medium heat, heat the oil. Add the leeks, tamari, herbs, spices, and pepper. Cook for 2 or 3 minutes, then add the broccoli and stir frequently for several minutes.

Add the vegetable broth and bring to a boil. Simmer the soup until the broccoli is almost soft, but not overcooked. Let the soup cool for about 10 minutes, then add the almonds or almond butter and puree with a hand blender or in the food processor. Reheat gently, then add the lemon juice. Ladle into bowls and garnish with chopped parsley.

Radical Beauty Entrées

BUDDHA'S DELIGHT VEGETABLE STIR-FRY

SERVES 2

1 teaspoon plus $1/2$ tablespoon coconut oil or 2 tablespoons vegetable broth
1 clove garlic, minced
$1/2$ teaspoon grated fresh ginger
$1/8$ teaspoon red chili flakes
2 tablespoons tamari
$1^1/2$ tablespoons rice vinegar
$1/2$ tablespoon lemon juice
$1/2$ tablespoon maple syrup or coconut nectar
$1/2$ teaspoon dry mustard
6 fl oz (175 ml) vegetable broth
1 tablespoon arrowroot dissolved in 2 tablespoons water
3 oz (75 g) thinly sliced carrots, cut on the diagonal
2 oz (50 g) cauliflower florets
3 oz (75 g) bite-sized broccoli pieces, including peeled and sliced stalk
$1^1/2$ oz (40 g) thinly sliced bok choy, cur diagonally
$1^1/2$ oz (40 g) shredded white cabbage or Chinese leaf
$3^1/2$ oz (100 g) thinly sliced red or green peppers
7 oz (200 g) mung bean sprouts
$7^1/2$ oz (225 g) shredded spinach
$3^1/2$ oz (100 g) whole mangetout

(recipe continues)

2 teaspoons sesame oil, preferably untoasted
Steamed rice or udon noodles, for serving
Sliced spring onions, for garnish

In a small saucepan over medium heat, heat 1 teaspoon of the coconut oil or 1 tablespoonof the broth. Add the garlic, ginger, and red chili flakes and sauté briefly. Add the tamari, vinegar, lemon juice, maple syrup, and dry mustard. Whisk together, adding the vegetable broth slowly, and bring the mixture to a rolling boil.

Just as the sauce begins to boil, add the dissolved arrowroot, stirring constantly with a whisk until sauce is thickened. Remove from the heat and set aside.

In a large wok or sauté pan over high heat, heat the remaining $1/2$ tablespoon of coconut oil 1 tablespoon of vegetable broth. Begin adding the vegetables, one at a time and in the order listed, until all the vegetables are cooking in the wok or pan.

Allow the vegetables to cook until they are al dente—still a little crunchy—no more than 5 to 7 minutes.

Pour the sauce over the vegetables after they are cooked. Remove from the heat and add the sesame oil for flavor. Serve over steamed rice or udon noodles and garnish with sliced spring onions.

CREAMY MASALA VEGETABLE STEW

SERVES 2

$1/2$ teaspoon garlic powder (optional)
$1^1/2$ teaspoons ground cumin
$1^1/2$ teaspoons ground coriander
$1/4$ teaspoon ground turmeric
$1/4$ teaspoon ground cardamom
$1/4$ teaspoon ground allspice
2 teaspoons coconut oil
$1/2$ teaspoon brown mustard seeds
1 teaspoon fenugreek seeds
$1/4$ teaspoon red chili flakes

3 oz (75 g) chopped leeks or onions
1 tablespoon minced peeled fresh ginger
10 oz (300 g) diced tomatoes
3^1/$_2$ oz (100 g) diced celery
3^1/$_2$ oz (100 g) diced peppers
5 oz (150 g) green beans, ends trimmed
6 oz (175 g) diced courgette
1 pint (600 ml) vegetable broth
Sea salt to taste
10 oz (300 g) cubed yams or sweet potatoes
3^1/$_2$ oz (100 g) small cauliflower florets
8 fl oz (250 ml) coconut milk (low-fat is always an option)
2 tablespoons brown rice flour or chickpea flour
2 tablespoons chopped fresh coriander
2 tablespoons chopped fresh basil

In a small bowl, combine the garlic powder, cumin, coriander, turmeric, cardamom, and allspice. Set aside.

In a large saucepan or soup pot over medium-high heat, heat the coconut oil. Add the mustard seeds, fenugreek seeds, and red chili flakes. Let the seeds pop for a minute and add the leeks and ginger. Sauté for 2 minutes. Add the tomatoes and the previously prepared spice blend. Simmer on medium heat for 5 minutes. Add the celery, peppers, green beans, courgette, vegetable broth, and sea salt. Cover and let cook for 5 minutes.

Bring a pot of water to a boil and blanch the yams or sweet potatoes and the cauliflower for 3 minutes. Drain and add to the soup pot.

In a separate bowl, whisk the coconut milk and brown rice flour together until smooth, and add to the soup pot. Bring to a boil; reduce the heat to a low simmer until the vegetables are tender. Season with sea salt as desired. Add the fresh coriander and basil and serve.

AUBERGINE CAULIFLOWER CURRY

SERVES 3 TO 4

1^1/$_2$ lbs (750 g) peeled aubergine cut into 1-inch (2.5 cm) cubes

2 teaspoons coconut oil

1 tablespoon curry powder

1 tablespoon dried dill

1 teaspoon sea salt, plus more to taste

10 oz (300 g) cauliflower florets

5 oz (150 g) chopped leeks

2 teaspoons minced peeled fresh ginger

4 fl oz (125 ml) vegetable broth, plus more as needed

2 teaspoons ground cumin

2 teaspoons ground coriander

2 teaspoons garam masala

Pinch of red chili flakes

2 teaspoons lemon juice

6 fl oz (175 ml) coconut milk (low-fat is always an option), plus more as needed

8 fl oz (250 ml) unsweetened almond milk

1^1/$_2$ oz (15 g) chopped fresh coriander, plus more for garnish

Freshly ground black pepper to taste

Cooked quinoa, teff, or brown rice, for serving

Preheat the oven to 350°F/180°C.

In a large bowl, place the aubergine, 1 teaspoon of the coconut oil, the curry powder, dill, and sea salt, and mix well to coat the aubergine. Lay the aubergine cubes out on a sheet pan and roast for 20 minutes. Remove from the oven and cool. Meanwhile, bring 6^1/$_2$ pints (3.5 litres) of water to a boil, add the cauliflower, and blanch for 3 minutes. Drain and set aside.

In a 6^1/$_2$ pints (3.5-litre) soup pot over medium-high heat, heat the remaining 1 teaspoon of coconut oil. Add the leeks, ginger, vegetable broth, cumin, ground coriander, garam masala, and chili flakes. Reduce the heat to medium to low and simmer for 5 minutes, then add the lemon juice, coconut milk, almond milk, and fresh coriander. Add the roasted auberging and cauliflower and continue to simmer for another 4 or 5 minutes. If the mixture gets dry, add some additional vegetable broth and coconut milk. season with sea salt and black pepper, as desired. Serve with quinoa, teff, or brown roce. top with more fresh coriander.

MARINATED TOFU NORI WRAPS WITH NUTTY DIPPING SAUCE

SERVES 2

NUTTY DIPPING SAUCE

¼ teaspoon olive oil or sesame oil

1 clove garlic, minced

Pinch of red chili flakes

4 fl oz (125 ml) vegetable broth, plus more as needed

$1/2$ tablespoon tamari

$1/4$ tablespoon coconut nectar or maple syrup

2 tablespoons almond butter (preferably raw)

$1/4$ tablespoon sesame seeds

$1/4$ tablespoon chopped mint or fresh coriander

WRAPS

4 oz (125 g) thinly sliced organic firm tofu

2 nori wrappers (untoasted if you can find them)

2–3 tablespoons Nutty Dipping Sauce

2 tablespoons grated carrot

2 tablespoons grated courgettes

2 tablespoons thinly sliced red cabbage

2 tablespoons chopped fresh coriander

$3/4$ oz (20 g) sunflower sprouts

2 red-leaf or cos lettuce leaves

FOR THE SAUCE

In a saucepan over medium heat, heat the oil. Briefly sauté the garlic and red chili flakes. Add the vegetable broth, tamari, and coconut nectar. Simmer until heated through. Remove from heat. Add the mixture to a blender and puree along with the almond butter, sesame seeds, and mint. Add more vegetable broth if necessary to thin the sauce.

FOR THE WRAPS

Place half the tofu strips in the middle of each nori wrapper, and spread about 1 table-spoon Nutty Dipping Sauce over each.

Top each with half the carrots, courgette, cabbage, coriander, sprouts, and lettuce leaves. Drizzle some additional Nutty Dipping Sauce over the vegetables, then roll up or fold in half and enjoy.

GLUTEN-FREE MEDITERRANEAN PASTA

SERVES 4

> 5 oz (150 g) chopped leeks
> 2 tablespoons olive oil
> 5 oz (150 g) artichoke halves (marinated or nonmarinated)
> 4 oz (125 g) 1-inch (2.5-cm) asparagus pieces
> 5 oz (150 g) green beans, trimmed, cut in half, and split lengthwise
> 8 fl oz (250 ml) vegetable broth, plus more as needed
> 3½ oz (100 g) chopped watercress or red Swiss chard
> 2 tablespoons fresh lemon juice
> Sea salt to taste
> Freshly ground black pepper to taste
> 2 tablespoons chopped fresh basil
> 1 tablespoon chopped fresh oregano or 1 teaspoon dried oregano
> Cooked gluten-free pasta (pick your favorite shape!) or cooked quinoa

In a pan over low-medium heat, sauté the leeks with the olive oil. Simmer for 1 minute, and then add the artichokes, asparagus, and green beans. Simmer 2 to 3 minutes.

Add the broth, adding more if you like a thinner sauce. Add the watercress and simmer until the greens are wilted. Add the lemon juice, salt, pepper, basil, and oregano.

Pour the vegetable mixture over the cooked gluten-free pasta or the quinoa and stir gently. Serve immediately.

RAINBOW RISOTTO

SERVES 2

> 2 teaspoons coconut oil
> 3 oz (75 g) chopped leeks or shallots
> 1 tablespoon tamari
> 1½ teaspoons fresh or ½ teaspoon dried basil
> 1½ teaspoons fresh or ½ teaspoon dried rosemary
> 3½ oz (100 g) Arborio rice, rinsed and drained

1 pint (600 ml) hot vegetable broth, plus more as needed

1¹/₂ oz (40 g) thinly sliced carrots

1 oz (25 g) thinly sliced celery

3¹/₂ oz (100 g) sliced courgette (*Note:* cut the courgette in half lengthwise first, then into ¹/₄-inch (5-mm) slices)

3¹/₂ oz (100 g) coarsely torn spinach

1 tablespoon chopped fresh mint

2 teaspoons raw apple cider vinegar

Sea salt to taste

Freshly ground black pepper to taste

Chopped fresh parsley or coriander, for garnish

In a 4-pint (2.5-litre) soup pot over medium heat, heat 1 teaspoon of the coconut oil.

Sauté the leeks with the tamari, basil, and rosemary until the leeks are translucent.

Add the rice and sauté, stirring constantly until golden brown or caramelized. Lower the heat.

As the rice dries out, begin to add the hot broth, 8 fl oz (250 ml) at a time, stirring constantly and allowing the rice to absorb the broth before adding more. Keep stirring.

Risotto should have a soft (not mushy) texture with a creamy consistency. Be careful not to overcook or let the rice dry out. The cooking process will take about 20 to 30 minutes total. Taste the rice for creaminess, adding more broth if necessary.

Heat the remaining 1 teaspoon of the oil in a sauté pan over medium-high heat and add the carrots, celery, and courgette. Add some broth, if necessary, to keep the vegetables moist. Sauté until the carrots are al dente or almost soft.

Add the spinach and continue to sauté until just wilted. Pour all the ingredients from the sauté pan into the rice, add the mint and the raw apple cider vinegar and gently combine. Season with sea salt and black pepper, as desired.

Place the rice in a serving dish and garnish with freshly chopped parsley or coriander.

Radical Beauty Desserts

ALMOND BLISSFUL BEAUTY SHAKE

SERVES 1

8 fl oz (250 ml) unsweetened almond milk
1 tablespoon almond butter
2 teaspoons coconut nectar or raw, organic honey
Pinch of grated nutmeg
Pinch of ground cardamom
1/2 teaspoon chia seeds
1 teaspoon cacao nibs (optional)

Place all the ingredients in a blender and blend until smooth.

SILKY CHOCOLATE MOUSSE

SERVES 4

5 oz (150 g) organic dark chocolate chips or cacao nibs
1 tablespoon coconut oil
12 oz (375 g) organic low-fat, firm, silken tofu
2 fl oz (50 ml) maple syrup or coconut nectar
1 teaspoon pure vanilla extract
Shredded unsweetened coconut, for topping (optional)
Sliced or crushed raw almonds (optional)

In a small saucepan over low heat, melt the chocolate chips and heat the coconut oil. Stir frequently to avoid burning the chocolate. When the chips are melted, remove from the heat and stir to a creamy consistency. Set aside to cool.

In a blender or food processor place the tofu, maple syrup, and vanilla. Process or blend for about 1 minute. Scrape the sides down with a spatula; continue to blend to a smooth consistency. Add the cooled melted chocolate. Process and blend again until smooth. Serve the mousse in dessert bowls and top with shredded coconut and almonds, if desired.

CRANBERRY GODDESS SNACKS

MAKES 6 BALLS

2 oz (50 g) pine nuts

$1^1/2$ oz (40 g) sunflower seeds

2 oz (50 g) almonds

$3^1/2$ oz (100 g) dried cranberries

2 tablespoons maple syrup, plus more as needed

$1^1/2$ tablespoons coconut oil

$1/2$ teaspoon vanilla extract

$1/2$ teaspoon nutmeg

Pinch of sea salt

$1^1/2$ oz (40 g) finely shredded unsweetened coconut flakes

Note: Ideally soak seeds and nuts overnight and rinse well.

Place the pine nuts, sunflower seeds, and almonds in a food processor and pulse until coarsely ground. Add the dried cranberries and pulse again. Add the maple syrup, coconut oil, vanilla, nutmeg and sea salt. Continue to pulse until the mixture begins to stick together. Taste for sweetness, adding more maple syrup if necessary. Place the shredded coconut flakes in a flat bowl. Shape the nut and cranberry mixture into 1-inch balls (2.5-cm) and roll them in the coconut flakes to coat. Place them in the fridge for at least 1 hour before serving to harden. Store in the fridge in an airtight container.

Acknowledgments

From Deepak Chopra:

Every book calls upon a publishing team, and *Radical Beauty* was fortunate to have such a superb one, beginning with our astute and encouraging editor, Gary Jansen. Also many thanks to others at Harmony Books who constituted and managed the working team: Aaron Wehner, Publisher; Diana Baroni, Vice-President and Editorial Director; Tammy Blake, Vice President and Director of Publicity; Julie Cepler, Director of Marketing; Lauren Cook, Senior Publicist; Christina Foxley, Senior Marketing Manager; Jenny Carrow and Christopher Brand, our jacket design team; Elizabeth Rendfleisch, Director of Interior Design; Heather Williamson, Production Manager; and Patricia Shaw, Senior Production Editor.

We all know the pressures that book publishing is under today, and so a special thanks goes to the executives who must make tough decisions about which books to publish, including ours. Generous thanks to Maya Mavjee, President and Publisher of the Crown Publishing Group, and Aaron Wehner, Senior Vice President and Publisher of Harmony Books.

I want to take a moment to thank the people around me who are so selfless in their dedication. From the Chopra Center for Wellbeing: Sheila Patel, Valencia Porter, Lizabeth Weiss, Wendi Cohen, and Sara Harvey.

Deepak offers thanks to a fantastic team whose tireless efforts make everything possible from day to day and year to year: Carolyn Rangel, Felicia Rangel, Gabriela Rangel, and Tori Bruce. All of you have a special place in my heart. Thanks also goes to Poonacha Machaiah, cofounder of Jiyo, for helping to bring an online presence for a lot of my work. As always, my family remains at the center of my world and is cherished all the more as it expands: Rita, Mallika, Sumant, Gotham, Candice, Krishan, Tara, Leela, and Geeta.

From Kimberly Snyder:

I have so much deep appreciation for all those who contributed to the creation of *Radical Beauty*. First of all, I want to thank our fantastic editor, Gary Jansen, who made the collaboration process such a joy. We could not have asked for a more outstanding partner! Thank you also to the entire team at the Crown Publishing Group and Harmony books, including Aaron Wehner, Diana Baroni, Julie Cepler, Tammy Blake, Christina Foxley, Lauren Cook, and everyone who worked so hard to produce this book. Thank you to the Chopra Center for providing the base of the recipes used in the Radical Beauty Recipes section. And a big heartbeat thanks to my inspiring coauthor, Deepak. Thank you for the gifts of your collaboration and friendship.

I have immeasurable gratitude for the talented and brilliant John Pisani, who is my co-creator in everything and has been a rock of support and love along my journey from day one. I also want to express my deep gratitude for my Beauty Detox superstars, Katelyn Hughes and Cheri Alberts, who so passionately and tirelessly work to make the world a better place, as well as Dorothy Lysek and all the Beauties who are part of the Beauty Detox tribe/community. A special thanks to my literary agent Hannah Brown Gordon, as well as Jodi Lipper, and Tony Flores for helping me organize the research material. Through everything is the influence of my beloved Guruji Paramahansa Yogananda.

Sending out a big thank-you to my family and friends, especially Forrest and Lisa Masters, who gifted me the use of the beautiful apartment at Tres Sirenas in Rincon, Puerto Rico, where I secluded myself for a few weeks to start writing this book. I am so thankful for my son, Emerson, whom I was pregnant with during the writing of *Radical Beauty* and who helped spark creativity and inspiration in me in new and unexpected ways. And, for my love, Mick, who brings infinite sunshine and bliss into my life. I love you all.

Notes

Shift 1: Let Go of Your Preconceived Notions About Food

1. Benoit Chassaing, Omry Koren, Julia K. Goodrich, et al., "Dietary Emulsifiers Impact the Mouse Gut Microbiota Promoting Colitis and Metabolic Syndrome," *Nature* 519 (March 5, 2015): 92–96, doi:10.1038/nature14232.

2. Dora Anne Mills, "Chronic Disease: The Epidemic of the Twentieth Century," *Maine Policy Review* 9.1 (2000): 50–65, http://digitalcommons.library.umaine.edu/mpr/vol9/iss1/8.

3. "The Top 10 Causes of Death," World Health Organization, accessed February 7, 2016, http://www.who.int/mediacentre/factsheets/fs310/en/index2.html.

4. Stephanie Watson, "Healthy Aging: What Can You Control?" WebMD, last reviewed July 12, 2013, http://www.webmd.com/healthy-aging/features/healthy-aging.

Shift 2: Regain Control over Your Body's Natural Processes

1. Nicholas Wade, "Your Body Is Younger Than You Think," *New York Times,* August 2, 2005, http://www.nytimes.com/2005/08/02/science/02cell.html.

2. Ibid.

3. Angela Epstein, "Believe It or Not, Your Lungs Are Six Weeks Old—and Your Taste Buds Just Ten Days! So How Old Is the Rest of Your Body?" *Daily Mail,* updated October 13, 2009, http://www.dailymail.co.uk/health/article-1219995/Believe-lungs-weeks-old—taste-buds-just-days-So-old-rest-body.html#ixzz3bS9ZL4Ij.

4. Wade, "Your Body Is Younger Than You Think."

5. E. B. Lohman, K. S. B. Sackiriyas, G. S. Bains, et al., "A Comparison of Whole Body Vibration and Moist Heat on Lower Extremity Skin Temperature and Skin Blood Flow in Healthy Older Individuals," *Medical Science Monitor: International Medical Journal of Experimental and Clinical Research* 18, no. 7 (2012): CR415–CR424, doi:10.12659/MSM.883209.

6. "Is There a Connection Between Heavy Metals and Aging?" Buck Institute for Research on Aging, January 15, 2015, http://www.thebuck.org/buck-news/there-connection-between-heavy-metals-and-aging.

7. N. Anim-Nyame, S. R. Sooranna, M. R. Johnson, et al., "Garlic Supplementation Increases Peripheral Blood Flow: A Role for Interleukin-6?" *Journal of Nutritional Biochemistry* 15, no. 1, 30–36.

8. Mohammad El-Sayed Yassin El-Sayed Haggag, Rafaat Mohamed Elsanhoty, and Mohamed Fawzy Ramadan, "Impact of Dietary Oils and Fats on Lipid Peroxidation in Liver and Blood of Albino Rats," *Asian Pacific Journal of Tropical Biomedicine* 4, no. 1 (2014): 52–58, doi:10.1016/S2221-1691(14)60208-2.

9. See www.fda.gov/ForConsumers/ConsumerUpdates/ucm094550.htm.

10. Harvard T. H. Chan School of Public Health, *The Nutrition Source,* "Calcium and Milk: What's Best for Your Bones and Health?" www.hsph.harvard.edu/nutritionsource/calcium-full-story/.

11. A. J. Lanou, S. E. Berkow, and N. D. Barnard, "Calcium, Dairy Products, and Bone Health in Children and Young Adults: A Reevaluation of the Evidence," *Pediatrics* no. 115 (2005); 736–43.

12. D. Feskanich, W. C. Willett, and G. A. Colditz, "Calcium, Vitamin D, Milk Consumption, and Hip Fractures: A Prospective Study Among Postmenopausal Women," *American Journal of Clinical Nutrition* no. 77 (2003); 504–11.

13. L. H. Kushi, P. J. Mink, A. R. Folsom, et al., "Prospective Study of Diet and Ovarian Cancer," *American Journal of Epidemiology* no. 149 (1999); 21–31.

14. M. Zwolińska-Wcisło, D. Galicka-Latała, L. Rudnicka-Sosin, et al., "Coeliac Disease and Other Autoimmunological Disorders Coexistence" [in Polish], *Przegląd lekarski* 66, no. 7 (2009): 370–72.

15. Keeve E. Nachman, Patrick A. Baron, Georg Raber, et al., "Roxarsone, Inorganic Arsenic, and Other Arsenic Species in Chicken: A U.S.-Based Market Basket Sample," *Environmental Health Perspectives* 121, no. 7 (July 2013): 818–24, doi:10.1289/ehp.1206245.

16. James E. McWilliams, "Beware the Myth of Grass-Fed Beef: Cows Raised at Pasture Are Not Immune to Deadly E. Coli Bacteria." *Slate,* January 22, 2010, accessed February 11, 2016, http://www.slate.com/articles/health_and_science/green_room/2010/01/beware_the_myth_of_grassfed_beef.html.

17. "Growth Hormones Fed to Beef Cattle Damage Human Health," Organic Consumers Association, May 1, 2007, https://www.organicconsumers.org/scientific/growth-hormones-fed-beef-cattle-damage-human-health.

18. G. Paolella, C. Mandato, L. Pierri, et al., "Gut-Liver Axis and Probiotics: Their Role in Non-Alcoholic Fatty Liver Disease," *World Journal of Gastroenterology* 20, no. 42 (2014): 15518–31, doi:10.3748/wjg.v20.i42.15518.

19. Ibid.

20. A. Parodi, S. Paolino, A. Greco, et al., "Small Intestinal Bacterial Overgrowth in Rosacea: Clinical Effectiveness of Its Eradication," *Clinical Gastroenterology and Hepatology* 6, no. 7 (July 2008): 759–64, doi:10.1016/j.cgh.2008.02.054.

21. R. H. Siver, "Lactobacillus for the Control of Acne," *Journal of the Medical Society of New Jersey* 59 (1961): 52–53.

22. F. Marchetti, R. Capizzi, and A. Tulli, "Efficacy of Regulators of the Intestinal Bacterial Flora in the Therapy of Acne Vulgaris," *La Clinica Terapeutica* 122, no. 5 (September 15, 1987): 339–43.

23. T. F. Teixeira, M. C. Collado, C. L. Ferreira, et al., "Potential Mechanisms for the Emerging Link Between Obesity and Increased Intestinal Permeability," *Nutrition Research* 32, no. 9 (September 2012): 637–47, doi:10.1016/j.nutres.2012.07.003.

24. Ibid.

25. D. J. Jenkins, C. W. Kendall, D. G. Popovich, et al., "Effect of a Very-High-Fiber Vegetable, Fruit, and Nut Diet on Serum Lipids and Colonic Function," *Metabolism* 50, no. 4 (April 2001): 494–503. http://www.ncbi.nih.gov/pubmed/11288049.

26. Nick Ng, "B Vitamins and the Liver," Livestrong.com, last updated October 22, 2015, http://www.livestrong.com/article/280046-b-vitamins-the-liver/.

27. "Managing Women's Issues with Chinese Medicine," Pacific College of Oriental Medicine, accessed February 18, 2016, http://www.pacificcollege.edu/acupuncture-massage-news/articles/587 -managing-womens-issues-with-chinese-medicine.html.

28. Morgan E. Levine, Jorge A. Suarez, Sebastian Brandhorst, et al., "Low Protein Intake Is Associated with a Major Reduction in IGF-1, Cancer, and Overall Mortality in the 65 and Younger but Not Older Population," *Cell Metabolism* 19, no. 3 (March 4, 2014): 407–17.

29. Alice G. Walton, "Why High-Protein Diets May Be Linked to Cancer Risk," *Forbes*, http://www .forbes.com/sites/alicegwalton/2014/03/04/the-protein-puzzle-meat-and-dairy-may-significantly -increase-cancer-risk/.

30. Ioannis Delimaris, "Adverse Effects Associated with Protein Intake Above the Recommended Dietary Allowance for Adults," *ISRN Nutrition* 2013, article ID 126929 (2013), doi:10.5402/2013/126929.

31. "Metabolic Functions of the Liver," About.com, accessed February 18, 2016, http://biology.about .com/library/organs/bldigestliver5.htm.

32. Carolyn Robbins, "High-Protein Diet and the Liver," Livestrong.com, last updated October 8, 2015, http://www.livestrong.com/article/280961-high-protein-diet-and-the-liver/.

33. Salynn Boyles, "Study: Tylenol Liver Effect Stronger," WebMD, July 5, 2006, http://www.webmd .com/news/20060705/study-tylenol-liver-effect-stronger.

34. Paul Fassa, "Ten Reasons Why You Should Drink Warm Lemon or Lime Water Daily," *Natural News,* August 21, 2011, http://www.naturalnews.com/033383_lemon_juice_digestion.html.

35. K. E. Mayer, R. P. Myers, and S. S. Lee, "Silymarin Treatment of Viral Hepatitis: A Systematic Review," *Journal of Viral Hepatitis* 12, no. 6 (November 2005): 559–67.

36. Maurizio Battino, José L. Quiles, Jesús R. Huertas, et al., "Feeding Fried Oil Changes Antioxidant and Fatty Acid Pattern of Rat and Affects Rat Liver Mitochondrial Respiratory Chain Components," *Journal of Bioenergetics and Biomembranes* 34, no. 2 (April 2002): 127–34.

37. Jose L. Quiles, Jesus R. Huertas, Maurizio Battino, et al., "The Intake of Fried Virgin Olive or Sunflower Oils Differentially Induces Oxidative Stress in Rat Liver Microsomes," *British Journal of Nutrition* 88 (2002): 57–65, doi:10.1079/BJN2002588.

38. Will MacLean and Jane Lyttleton, *Clinical Handbook of Internal Medicine: The Treatment of Disease with Traditional Chinese Medicine,* vol. 2, *Spleen and Stomach* (Sydney, Australia: University of Western Sydney, 2002).

39. I. Alvarez-Gonzalez, E. Madrigal-Bujaidar, and V. Y. Sanchez-Garcia, "Inhibitory Effect of Grapefruit Juice on the Genotoxic Damage Induced by Ifosfamide in Mouse," *Plant Foods Human Nutrition* 65, no. 4 (December 2010): 369–73.

40. John L. Ingraham, "Understanding Congeners in Wine: How Does Fusel Oil Form, and How Important Is It?" *Wines & Vines,* May 2010, accessed February 19, 2016, http://www.winesandvines .com/template.cfm?section=features&content=74439&ftitle=Understanding%20Congeners %20in%20Wine.

41. "Whisky Hangover 'Worse Than Vodka,' Study Suggests," BBC News, last updated December 19, 2009, http://news.bbc.co.uk/2/hi/health/8416431.stm.

42. "Find a Vitamin or Supplement: Hops," WebMD, accessed February 19, 2016, http://www.webmd .com/vitamins-supplements/ingredientmono-856-HOPS.aspx?activeIngredientId=856&active IngredientName=HOPS.

Shift 3: Radical Beauty Ratios and Macronutrient Balance

1. Apostolos Pappas, "The Relationship of Diet and Acne: A Review," *Dermato-Endocrinology* 1, no. 5 (2009): 262–67.

2. C. C. Zouboulis, "Is Acne Vulgaris a Genuine Inflammatory Disease?" *Dermatology* 203, no. 4 (2001): 277–79.

3. A. P. Simopoulos, "The Importance of the Ratio of Omega-6/Omega-3 Essential Fatty Acids," *Biomedicine and Pharmacotherapy* 56, no. 8 (October 2002): 365–79.

4. E. M. Conner and M. B. Grisham, "Inflammation, Free Radicals, and Antioxidants," *Nutrition* 12, no. 4 (April 1996): 274–77.

5. Ying Chen and John Lyga, "Brain-Skin Connection: Stress, Inflammation and Skin Aging," *Inflammation and Allergy Drug Targets* 13, no. 3 (2014): 177–90, doi:10.2174/1871528113666140522104422.

6. J. G. Robinson, N. Ijioma, and W. Harris, "Omega-3 Fatty Acids and Cognitive Function in Women," *Women's Health* 6, no. 1 (2010): 119–34, doi:10.2217/whe.09.75.

7. Marianne Klokk, Karl Gunnar Gotestam, and Arnstein Mykletun, "Factors Accounting for the Association Between Anxiety and Depression, and Eczema: The Hordaland Health Study (HUSK)," *BMC Dermatology* 10 (2010): 3, doi:10.1186/1471-5945-10-3.

8. C. Y. Chang, D. S. Ke, and J. Y. Chen, "Essential Fatty Acids and Human Brain," *Acta Neurologica Taiwanica* 18, no. 4 (December 2009): 231–41.

9. Brian Hallahan and Malcolm R. Garland, "Essential Fatty Acids and Mental Health," *British Journal of Psychiatry* 186, no. 4 (March 2005): 275–77, doi:10.1192/bjp.186.4.275.

10. Simopoulos, "The Importance of the Ratio of Omega-6/Omega-3 Essential Fatty Acids."

11. Dr. Joseph Mercola, "Major Trouble Ahead if You Don't Fix Omega-3 Fat Deficiency," Mercola.com, January 12, 2012, http://articles.mercola.com/sites/articles/archive/2012/01/12/aha-position-on-omega-6-fats.aspx.

12. Dr. Susan E. Brown and Larry Trivieri Jr., *The Acid Alkaline Food Guide: A Quick Reference to Foods and Their Effect on pH Levels* (Garden City Park, NY: Square One Publishers, 2006), 2.

13. G. K. Schwalfenberg, "The Alkaline Diet: Is There Evidence That an Alkaline pH Diet Benefits Health?" *Journal of Environmental and Public Health* 2012 (2012): 727630, doi:10.1155/2012/727630.

14. Ibid., 33.

15. Ibid., 3.

16. Russell Blaylock, MD, *Excitotoxins: The Taste That Kills* (Santa Fe, NM: Health Press, 2006).

17. D. C. Willcox, B. J. Willcox, W.-C. Hsueh, et al., "Genetic Determinants of Exceptional Human Longevity: Insights from the Okinawa Centenarian Study," *Age* 28, no. 4 (2006): 313–32, doi:10.1007/s11357-006-9020-x.

18. X. Ouyang, P. Cirillo, Y. Sautin, et al., "Fructose Consumption as a Risk Factor for Nonalcoholic Fatty Liver Disease," *Journal of Hepatology* 48, no. 6 (2008): 993–99, doi:10.1016/j.jhep.2008.02.011.

19. "Nutrition Recommendations and Interventions for Diabetes: A Position Statement of the American Diabetes Association," supplement, *Diabetes Care* 31, suppl. 1 (January 2008): S61–S78, http://care.diabetesjournals.org/content/31/Supplement_1/S61.full.pdf.

20. Elena Conis, "Is Crystalline Fructose a Better Choice of Sweetener?" *Los Angeles Times,* February 2, 2009, http://articles.latimes.com/2009/feb/02/health/he-nutrition2.

21. R. J. Wurtman and J. J. Wurtman, "Brain Serotonin, Carbohydrate-Craving, Obesity and Depression," supplement, *Obesity Research* 3, no. S4 (November 1995): 477S–480S, http://www.ncbi.nlm.nih.gov/pubmed/8697046.

22. R. E. Strecker, M. M. Thakkar, T. Porkka-Heiskanen, et al., "Behavioral State-Related Changes of Extracellular Serotonin Concentration in the Pedunculopontine Tegmental Nucleus: A Microdialysis Study in Freely Moving Animals," *Sleep Research Online* 2, no. 2 (1999): 21–27.

23. Linda Ray, "Ketosis and Acidosis," Livestrong.com, last updated August 11, 2015, http://www.livestrong.com/article/449496-ketosis-acidosis/.

24. Mardia López-Alarcón, Otilia Perichart-Perera, Samuel Flores-Huerta, et al., "Excessive Refined Carbohydrates and Scarce Micronutrients Intakes Increase Inflammatory Mediators and Insulin Resistance in Prepubertal and Pubertal Obese Children Independently of Obesity," *Mediators of Inflammation* 2014, article ID 849031 (2014), doi:10.1155/2014/849031.

25. Rebecca Adams, "Why Sugar Is Just as Bad for Your Skin as It Is for Your Waistline," *Huffington Post,* October 10, 2013, http://www.huffingtonpost.com/2013/10/10/sugar-bad-for-skin_n_4071548.html.

26. Patrick J. Skerrett, "Is Fructose Bad for You?," Harvard Health Publications, Harvard Medical School, April 26, 2011, http://www.health.harvard.edu/blog/is-fructose-bad-for-you-201104262425.

27. T. Colin Campbell, *The Low-Carb Fraud* (Dallas, TX: Benbella Books, 2013), 54.

28. L. Cordain, J. B. Miller, S. B. Eaton, et al., "Plant-Animal Subsistence Ratios and Macronutrient Energy Estimations in Worldwide Hunter-Gatherer Diets," *American Journal of Clinical Nutrition* 71, no 3 (March 2000): 682–92; L. Cordain, S. B. Eaten, J. B. Miller, et al., "The Paradoxical Natural of Hunter-Gatherer Diets: Meat-Based, Yet Non-atherogenic," supplement, *European Journal of Clinical Nutrition* 56 (2002): S42–S52.

29. Quoted in Campbell, *The Low-Carb Fraud,* 54.

30. Ibid.

31. Quoted in Campbell, *The Low-Carb Fraud,* 54. R. B. Lee, *What Humans Do for a Living, or How to Make Out on Scarce Resources* (Chicago: Aldine Publishing House, 1968).

32. Quoted in Campbell, *The Low-Carb Fraud,* 54. L. Cordain, J. Brand Miller, S. B. Eaten, et al., "Plant-Animal Subsistence Ratios and Macronutrient Energy Estimations in Worldwide Hunter-Gatherer Diets," *American Journal of Clinical Nutrition* 71 (2000): 682–92.

33. Quoted in Campbell, *The Low-Carb Fraud,* 54. K. Milton, "Hunter-Gatherer Diets: A Different Perspective," *American Journal of Clinical Nutrition* 71 (2000): 665–67.

34. K. Milton, "Nutritional Characteristics of Wild Primate Foods: Do the Diets of Our Closest Living Relatives Have Lessons for Us?" *Nutrition* 15, no. 6 (1999): 488–98.

35. K. K. Carroll, "Experimental Evidence of Dietary Factors and Hormone-Dependent Cancers," *Cancer Research* 35 (November 1975): 3374–83; World Cancer Research Fund / American Insti-

tute for Cancer Research, *Food, Nutrition, Physical Activity, and Prevention of Cancer: A Global Perspective* (Washington, DC: American Institute for Cancer Research, 2007).

36. L. D. Youngman and T. C. Campbell, "Inhibition of Aflatoxin B1-induced Gamma-Glutamyl Transpeptidase Positive (GGT+) Hepatic Preneoplastic Foci and Tumors by Low Protein Diets: Evidence That Altered GGT+ Foci Indicate Neoplastic Potential," *Carcinogenesis* 13, no. 9 (1992): 1607–13.

37. G. L. G. Hildenbrand, L. C. Hildenbrand, K. Bradford, et al., "Five-Year Survival Rates of Melanoma Patients Treated by Diet Therapy After the Manner of Gerson: A Retrospective Review," *Alternative Therapies in Health and Medicine* 1, no. 4 (September 1995): 29–37.

38. Caldwell B. Esselstyn, MD, "Updating a 12-Year Experience with Arrest and Reversal Therapy for Coronary Heart Disease (An Overdue Requiem for Palliative Cardiology)," *American Journal of Cardiology* 84, no. 3 (August 1, 1999): 339–41; L. M. Morrison, "Diet in Coronary Atherosclerosis," *Journal of the American Medical Association* 173, no. 8 (June 25, 1960): 884–88; D. Ornish, S. E. Brown, L. W. Scherwitz, et al., "Can Lifestyle Changes Reverse Coronary Heart Disease?" *Lancet* 336, no. 8708 (July 21, 1990): 129–33.

39. R. J. Barnard, L. Lattimore, R. G. Holly, et al., "Response of Non-insulin-dependent Diabetic Patients to an Intensive Program of Diet and Exercise," *Diabetes Care* 5, no. 4 (July–August 1982): 370–74.

40. Dr. T. Colin Campbell and Thomas M. Campbell II, *The China Study: The Most Comprehensive Study of Nutrition Ever Conducted and the Startling Implications for Diet, Weight Loss, and Long-Term Health* (Dallas, TX: Benbella Books, 2006).

41. Olfa Saidi, Nadia Ben Mansour, Martin O'Flaherty, et al., "Analyzing Recent Coronary Heart Disease Mortality Trends in Tunisia between 1997 and 2009," *PLoS One* 8, no. 5 (May 3, 2013), doi:10.1371/journal.pone.0063202.

42. Julia Critchley, Jing Liu, Dong Zhao, et al., "Explaining the Increase in Coronary Heart Disease Mortality in Beijing Between 1984 and 1999," *Circulation* 110 (2004): 1236–44, doi:10.1161/01.CIR.0000140668.91896.AE.

43. Taina Backstrom and Sarah Wamala, "Folkhälsan i Sverige" [in Swedish], March 26, 2013, www.socialstyrelsen.se.

44. Morgan E. Levine, Jorge A. Suarez, Sebastian Brandhorst, et al., "Low Protein Intake Is Associated with a Major Reduction in IGF-1, Cancer, and Overall Mortality in the 65 and Younger but Not Older Population," *Cell Metabolism* 19, no. 3 (March 4, 2014): 407–17.

45. "Your Body Recycling Itself—Captured on Film," McGill University Department of Biochemistry, September 13, 2010, https://www.mcgill.ca/channels/news/your-body-recycling-itself-%E2%80%93-captured-film-167428.

46. Linda Ray, "Ketosis and Acidosis," Livestrong.com, May 23, 2011, http://www.livestrong.com/article/449496-ketosis-acidosis/.

47. N. Kazerouni, R. Sinha, C.-H. Hsu, et al., "Analysis of 200 Food Items for Benzo[a]pyrene and Estimation of Its Intake in an Epidemiologic Study," *Food Chemistry and Toxicology* 39, no. 5 (May 2001): 423–36.

48. M. J. Kaiserman and W. S. Rickert, "Carcinogens in Tobacco Smoke: Benzo[a]pyrene from Canadian Cigarettes and Cigarette Tobacco," *American Journal of Public Health* 82, no. 7 (July 1992): 1023–26.

49. Cai Weijing, Jaimie Uribarri, Li Zhu, et al., "Oral Glycotoxins Are a Modifiable Cause of Dementia and the Metabolic Syndrome in Mice and Humans," *Proceedings of the National Academy of Sciences* 111, no. 13 (April 1, 2014): 4940–45, doi:10.1073/pnas.1316013111.

50. Ibid.

51. Morgan E. Levine, Jorge A. Suarez, Sebastian Brandhorst, et al., "Low Protein Intake Is Associated with a Major Reduction in IGF-1, Cancer, and Overall Mortality in the 65 and Younger but Not Older Population," *Cell Metabolism* 19, no. 3 (March 4, 2014): 407–17.

52. Ibid.

53. T. Sugimura, K. Wakabayashi, H. Nakagama, et al., "Heterocyclic Amines: Mutagens/Carcinogens Produced During Cooking of Meat and Fish," *Cancer Science* 95, no. 4 (April 2004): 290–99.

54. S. C. Larsson, L. Bergkvist, and A. Wolk, "Processed Meat Consumption, Dietary Nitrosamines and Stomach Cancer Risk in a Cohort of Swedish Women," *International Journal of Cancer* 119, no. 4 (August 2006): 915–19.

55. L. Li, P. Wang, X. Xu, et al., "Influence of Various Cooking Methods on the Concentrations of Volatile N-nitrosamines and Biogenic Amines in Dry-Cured Sausages," *Journal of Food Science* 77, no. 5 (May 2012): C560–655, doi:10.1111/j.1750-3841.2012.02667.x.

Shift 4: Feel a Connection to Your Food

1. "National Organic Program," US Department of Agriculture, accessed February 20, 2016, http://www.ams.usda.gov/AMSv1.0/nop.

2. Polly Walker, Pamela Rhubart-Berg, Shawn McKenzie, et al., "Public Health Implications of Meat Production and Consumption," *Public Health Nutrition* 8, no. 4 (2005): 348–56, doi:10.1079/PHN2005727.

3. "Food Program: Animal Feed," Grace Communications Foundation, accessed February 20, 2016, http://www.sustainabletable.org/260/animal-feed.

4. Dr. A. Velimirov, Dr. C. Binter, and Dr. J. Zentek, *Biological Effects of Transgenic Maize NK603x-MON810 Fed in Long Term Reproduction Studies in Mice* (Vienna: Department/Universitätsklinik für Nutztiere und öffentliches Gesundheitswesen in der Veterinärmedizin, 2008).

5. Joël Spiroux de Vendômois, François Roullier, Dominique Cellier, et al., "A Comparison of the Effects of Three GM Corn Varieties on Mammalian Health," *International Journal of Biological Sciences* 5, no. 7 (2009): 706–26, doi:10.7150/ijbs.5.706.

6. B. Markaverich, S. Mani, M. A. Alejandro, et al., "A Novel Endocrine-Disrupting Agent in Corn with Mitogenic Activity in Human Breast and Prostatic Cancer Cells," *Environmental Health Perspectives* 110, no. 2 (February 2002): 169–77.

7. B. M. Markaverich, J. R. Crowley, M. A. Alejandro, et al., "Leukotoxin Diols from Ground Corncob Bedding Disrupt Estrous Cyclicity in Rats and Stimulate MCF-7 Breast Cancer Cell Proliferation," *Environmental Health Perspectives* 113, no. 12 (December 2005): 1698–1704, doi:10.1289/ehp.8231.

8. Walker, Berg, McKenzie, et al., "Public Health Implications of Meat Production and Consumption."

9. Ibid.

10. J. P. F. D'Mello, "Contaminants and Toxins in Animal Feeds," accessed February 20, 2016, http://www.fao.org/docrep/article/agrippa/x9500e04.htm.

11. "Dioxins and Their Effects on Human Health," World Health Organization, last updated June 2014, http://www.who.int/mediacentre/factsheets/fs225/en/.

12. Ibid.

13. D'Mello, "Contaminants and Toxins in Animals Feeds."

14. T. V. Lynn, D. D. Hancock, T. E. Besser, et al., "The Occurrence and Replication of *Escherichia Coli* in Cattle Feeds," *Journal of Dairy Science* 81, no. 4 (April 1998): 1102–8.

15. D. S. Krytenburg, D. D. Hancock, D. H. Rice, et al., "A Pilot Survey of *Salmonella enterica* Contamination of Cattle Feeds in the Pacific Northwestern USA," *Animal Feed Science and Technology* 75, no. 1 (September 30, 1998): 75–79.

16. "Beef Recall: 50,000 Pounds of Meat Recalled Due to Possible E. Coli Contamination," Huffington Post Healthy Living, August 5, 2013, http://www.huffingtonpost.com/2013/07/31/beef-recall_n_3685744.html.

17. N. K. Dhand, D. V. Joshi, and S. K. Jand, "Fungal Contaminants of Dairy Feed and Their Toxigenicity," *Indian Journal of Animal Sciences* 68, no. 10 (1998): 1095–96.

18. J. P. F. D'Mello, A. M. C. Macdonald, and M. P. Cochrane, "A Preliminary Study of the Potential for Mycotoxin Production in Barley Grain," *Aspects of Applied Biology* 36 (1993): 375–82.

19. J. P. F. D'Mello and A. M. C. Macdonald, "Fungal Toxins as Disease Elicitors," in *Environmental Toxicology: Current Developments,* ed. J. Rose (Amsterdam: Gordon and Breach Science Publishers, 1998), 253–89.

20. C. M. Placinta, J. P. F. D'Mello, and A. M. C. Macdonald, "A Review of Worldwide Contamination of Cereal Grains and Animal Feed with *Fusarium* Mycotoxins," *Animal Feed Science and Technology* 78, nos. 1–2 (March 31, 1999): 21–37.

21. D'Mello, "Contaminants and Toxins in Animal Feeds."

22. F. G. Peers and C. A. Linsell, "Dietary Aflatoxins and Liver Cancer—a Population Based Study in Kenya," *British Journal of Cancer* 27, no. 6 (June 1973): 473–84.

23. D'Mello, "Contaminants Toxins in Animal Feeds."

24. L. Lynas, D. Currie, W. J. McCaughey, et al., "Contamination of Animal Feedingstuffs with Undeclared Antimicrobial Additives," *Food Additives and Contaminants* 15, no. 2 (February–March 1998): 162–70.

25. Walker, Berg, McKenzie, et al., "Public Health Implications of Meat Production and Consumption."

26. Ibid.

27. "Arsenic Toxicity: What Are the Physiologic Effects of Arsenic Exposure?" Agency for Toxic Substances and Disease Registry, October 1, 2009, http://www.atsdr.cdc.gov/csem/csem.asp?csem=1&po=11.

28. Dr. Joseph Mercola, "Environmental Toxins Linked to Rise in Autism," Mercola.com, April 2, 2014, http://articles.mercola.com/sites/articles/archive/2014/04/02/environmental-toxin-exposure .aspx.

29. Please see the documentary *Cowspiracy* and visit cowspiracy.com.

Shift 5: Incorporate Top Radical Beauty Foods and Routines

1. "Routine Periodic Fasting Can Reduce Risk of Coronary Heart Disease," News-Medical, April 4, 2011, http://www.news-medical.net/news/20110404/Routine-periodic-fasting-can-reduce-risk -of-coronary-heart-disease.aspx.

2. Dr. Mee Lain Ling, "8 Reasons to Drink Warm Water," February 17, 2013, http://drmeelainling .com/8-reasons-to-drink-warm-water/.

3. Ibid.

4. Doris Chung, "Mythbusters: Will Drinking Water Help With . . . ?" The Whole U, The University of Washington, September 17, 2014, http://www.washington.edu/wholeu/2014/09/17/water/.

5. Xiaoshuang Dai, Joy M. Stanilka, Cheryl A. Rowe, et al., "Consumption of *Lentinula edodes* Modulates Human Immune Function by Altering Cytokine Secretion of PBMC *ex Vivo*," *FASEB Journal* 27 (2013): 643.15.

6. Dr. Joseph Mercola, "The Health Benefits of Mushroom Consumption," Mercola.com, May 13, 2013, http://articles.mercola.com/sites/articles/archive/2013/05/13/mushroom-benefits.aspx #_edn6.

7. Dr. Zhimin Xu, "Black Rice Rivals Pricey Blueberries as Source of Healthful Antioxidants," August 26, 2010. Presented at the 240th National Meeting of the American Chemical Society. http://www.acs.org/content/acs/en/pressroom/newsreleases/2010/august/black-rice-rivals-pricey-blueberries-as-source-of-healthful-antioxidants.html.

8. "Aloe Vera," Memorial Sloan Kettering Cancer Center, last updated August 28, 2015, https:// www.mskcc.org/cancer-care/integrative-medicine/herbs/aloe-vera.

9. Jörn Söhle, Anja Knott, Ursula Holtzmann, et al., "White Tea Extract Induces Lipolytic Activity and Inhibits Adipogenesis in Human Subcutaneous (Pre)-Adipocytes," *Nutrition and Metabolism* 6 (May 1, 2009): 20, doi:10.1186/1743-7075-6-20.

10. Goran Bjelakovic, Dimitrinka Nikolova, Lise Lotte Gluud, et al., "Mortality in Randomized Trials of Antioxidant Supplements for Primary and Secondary Prevention: Systematic Review and Meta-analysis," *Journal of the American Medical Association* 297, no. 8 (2007): 842–57, doi:10.1001 /jama.297.8.842.

11. Adam M. Bernstein, Eric Ding, Walter Willett, et al., "A Meta-analysis Shows That Docosa-hexaenoic Acid from Algal Oil Reduces Serum Triglycerides and Increases HDL-Cholesterol and LDL-Cholesterol in Persons Without Coronary Heart Disease," *Journal of Nutrition* 142, no. 1 (January 2012): 99–104, doi:10.3945/jn.111.148973.

Shift 6: Incorporate Natural Skin-Care Ingredients

1. Elissa S. Epel , Elizabeth H. Blackburn, Jue Lin, et al., "Accelerated Telomere Shortening in Response to Life Stress," *Proceedings of the National Academy of Sciences* 101, no. 49 (December 2004): 17312–15, doi:10.1073/pnas.0407162101.

2. Rob Stein, "Study Is First to Confirm That Stress Speeds Aging, *Washington Post,* November 30, 2004, A01.

3. Suzanna Wright, "Beyond First Blush: An Up-Close Look at Natural Skin Care Products," WebMD, reviewed on March 17, 2009, http://www.webmd.com/beauty/skin/beyond-first-blush -an-upclose-look-at-natural-skin-care-products.

4. R. E. Black, F. J. Hurley, and D. C. Havery, "Occurrence of 1,4-Dioxane in Cosmetic Raw Materials and Finished Cosmetic Products," *Journal of AOAC International* 84, no. 3 (May–June 2001): 666–70.

5. P. D. Darbre and P. W. Harvey, "Paraben Esters: Review of Recent Studies of Endocrine Toxicity, Absorption, Esterase and Human Exposure, and Discussion of Potential Human Health Risks," *Journal of Applied Toxicology* 28, no. 5 (July 2008): 561–78, doi:10.1002/jat.1358.

6. Pumori Saokar Telang, "Vitamin C in Dermatology," *Indian Dermatology Online Journal* 4, no. 2 (April–June 2013): 143–46, doi:10.4103/2229-5178.110593.

7. R. E. Fitzpatrick and E. F. Rostan, "Double-Blind, Half-Face Study Comparing Topical Vitamin C and Vehicle for Rejuvenation of Photodamage," *Dermatologic Surgery* 28, no. 3 (March 2002): 231–36.

8. "Retinyl Palmitate (Vitamin A Palmitate)," EWG's Skin Deep Cosmetics Database, accessed February 20, 2016, http://www.ewg.org/skindeep/ingredient/705545/RETINYL_PALMITATE _%28VITAMIN_A_PALMITATE%29/#.

9. S. K. Katiyar, "Skin Photoprotection by Green Tea: Antioxidant and Immunomodulatory Effects," *Current Drug Targets: Immune, Endocrine and Metabolic Disorders* 3, no. 3 (September 2003): 234–42.

10. Mark H. J. Sturme, Michiel Kleerebezem, Jiro Nakayama, et al., "Cell to Cell Communication by Autoinducing Peptides in Gram-Positive Bacteria," *Antonie van Leeuwenhoek* 81, no. 1 (December 2002): 233–43.

11. T. D. Phillips, "Dietary Clay in the Chemoprevention of Aflatoxin-Induced Disease," supplement, *Toxicological Sciences* 52, S2 (1999): 118–26.

12. "FDA Authority over Cosmetics," US Food and Drug Administration, last updated August 3, 2013, http://www.fda.gov/Cosmetics/GuidanceRegulation/LawsRegulations/ucm074162.htm.

13. "Regulation of Nonprescription Products," US Food and Drug Administration, last updated February 24, 2015, http://www.fda.gov/AboutFDA/CentersOffices/OfficeofMedicalProductsand Tobacco/CDER/ucm093452.htm.

14. "FDA Authority over Cosmetics."

15. "Ingredients Prohibited and Restricted by FDA Regulations," US Food and Drug Administration, updated May 30, 2000, http://www.fda.gov/Cosmetics/ProductandIngredientSafety /SelectedCosmeticIngredients/ucm127406.htm.

16. "Considering Whether an FDA-Regulated Product Involves the Application of Nanotechnology: Guidance for Industry," US Food and Drug Administration, last updated January 25, 2016, http:// www.fda.gov/RegulatoryInformation/Guidances/ucm257698.htm.

17. "Ingredients Found Unsafe for Use in Cosmetics (11 Total, Through February, 2012), Cosmetic Ingredient Review," accessed November 2013, http://www.cir-safety.org/sites/default/files /U-unsafe%202-02-2012%20final.pdf.

18. "How FDA Evaluates Regulated Products: Cosmetics," US Food and Drug Administration, last updated February 18, 2016, http://www.fda.gov/AboutFDA/Transparency/Basics/ucm262353 .htm.

19. Samin Özen and Darcan Şükran, "Effects of Environmental Endocrine Disruptors on Pubertal Development," *Journal of Clinical Research in Pediatric Endocrinology* 3, no.1 (March 2011): 1–6, doi:10.4274/jcrpe.v3i1.01.

20. Åke Bergman, Jerrold J. Heindel, Susan Jobling, et al., eds., *The State-of-the-Science of Endocrine Disrupting Chemicals—2012* (Geneva: World Health Organization / United Nations Environment Programme, 2013), http://www.who.int/ceh/publications/endocrine/en/index.html.

21. "Hypoallergenic Cosmetics," US Food and Drug Administration, http://www.fda.gov/cosmetics/ cosmeticlabelinglabelclaims/labelclaimsandexpirationdating/ucm2005203.htm.

22. Julia R. Barrett, "Chemical Exposures: The Ugly Side of Beauty Products," *Environmental Health Perspectives* 113, no. 1 (January 2005): A24.

23. Danielle Dellorto, "Avoid Sunscreens with Potentially Harmful Ingredients, Group Warns," CNN.com, May 16, 2012, http://www.cnn.com/2012/05/16/health/sunscreen-report/index .html.

24. M. S. Wolff, S. M. Engel, G. S. Berkowitz, et al., "Prenatal Phenol and Phthalate Exposures and Birth Outcomes," *Environmental Health Perspectives* 116, no. 8 (2008): 1092–97.

25. A. Ziolkowska, A. S. Belloni, G. G. Nussdorfer, et al., "Endocrine Disruptors and Rat Adrenocortical Function: Studies on Freshly Dispersed and Cultured Cells," *International Journal of Molecular Medicine* 18, no. 6 (2006): 1165–68.

26. N. R. Janjua, B. Mogensen, A. M. Andersson, et al., "Systemic Absorption of the Sunscreens Benzophenone-3, Octyl-Methoxycinnamate, and 3-(4-Methyl-Benzylidene) Camphor After Whole-Body Topical Application and Reproductive Hormone Levels in Humans," *Journal of Investigative Dermatology* 123, no. 1 (2004): 57–61.

27. H. S. Sharma, S. Hussain, J. Schlager, et al., "Influence of Nanoparticles on Blood-Brain Barrier Permeability and Brain Edema Formation in Rats," supplement, *Acta Neurochirurgica* 106 (2010): 359–64, doi:10.1007/978-3-211-98811-4_65.

28. B. Kiss, T. Bíró, G. Czifra, et al., "Investigation of Micronized Titanium Dioxide Penetration in Human Skin Xenografts and Its Effect on Cellular Functions of Human Skin-Derived Cells," *Experimental Dermatology* 17, no. 8 (August 2008): 659–67, doi:10.1111/j.1600-0625.2007.00683.x.

29. "EWG Asks FDA, NTP to Wind Up Study of Vitamin A in Sunscreen," Environmental Working Group, May 28, 2010, http://www.ewg.org/news/news-releases/2010/05/28/ewg-asks-fda-ntp -wind-study-vitamin-sunscreen.

30. L. R. Gaspar, J. Tharmann, P. M. Maia Campos, et al., "Skin Phototoxicity of Cosmetic Formulations Containing Photounstable and Photostable UV-Filters and Vitamin A Palmitate." *Toxicology In Vitro* 27, no. 1 (February 2013): 418–25, doi:10.1016/j.tiv.2012.08.006.

31. "PABA," EWG's Skin Deep Cosmetics Database, accessed February 21, 2016, http://www.ewg .org/skindeep/ingredient/704390/PABA/#.

32. "Antiperspirant Safety: Should You Sweat It?" WebMD, reviewed June 1, 2011, http://www .webmd.com/skin-problems-and-treatments/features/antiperspirant-facts-safety?page=3.

Shift 7: Practices to Nourish Your Skin from the Outside In

1. Anatoliy A. Gashev and Victor Chatterjee, "Aged Lymphatic Contractility: Recent Answers and New Questions," *Lymphatic Research and Biology* 11, no. 1 (2013): 2–13.

2. M. Y. Cho, E. S. Min, M. H. Hur, et al., "Effects of Aromatherapy on the Anxiety, Vital Signs, and Sleep Quality of Percutaneous Coronary Intervention Patients in Intensive Care Units," *Evidence-Based Complementary and Alternative Medicine* 2013 (2013): 381381, doi:10.1155/2013/381381.

Shift 8: Address Specific Skin Issues

1. C. A. Adebamowo, D. Spiegelman, F. W. Danby, et al., "High School Dietary Dairy Intake and Teenage Acne," *Journal of the American Academy of Dermatology* 52, no. 2 (February 2005): 207–14.

2. Yvonne B. D'Souza and Colin D. Short, "The Eye—a Window on the Kidney," *Nephrology Dialysis Transplantation* 24, no. 12 (2009): 3582–84, doi:10.1093/ndt/gfp406.

3. "10 Anti-inflammatory Foods to Know: Reduce Inflammation and Fight Disease with These Grocery List Staples," Cleveland Clinic Health Essentials, April 11, 2012, http://health.cleveland clinic.org/2012/04/10-anti-inflammatory-foods-to-know/.

4. "Varicose Veins," Mayo Clinic, last updated January 22, 2016, http://www.mayoclinic.org/diseases -conditions/varicose-veins/basics/causes/con-20043474.

Shift 9: Nourish Strong, Healthy Hair and Nails

1. "Final Report on the Safety Assessment of Sodium Lauryl Sulfate," *International Journal of Toxicology* 2, no. 7 (December 1983): 127–81, doi:10.3109/10915818309142005.

2. Ibid.

3. US Department of Health and Human Services, Public Health Service, and National Institute of Environmental Health Sciences, *Sixth Annual Report on Carcinogens: Summary 1991* (Washington, DC: US Department of Health and Human Services, 1991), 192–95.

4. "Sodium Lauryl Sulfate Ammonium Lauryl Sulfate," in *1996 CIR Compendium* (Washington, DC: Cosmetic Ingredient Review, 1996), 134–35.

5. S. C. DaSilva, R. P. Sahu, R. L. Konger, et al., "Increased Skin Barrier Disruption by Sodium Lauryl Sulfate in Mice Expressing a Constitutively Active STAT6 in T Cells," *Archives of Dermatological Research* 304, no. 1 (January 2012): 65–71.

6. Matthew J. Zirwas and Sarah A. Stechschulte, "Moisturizer Allergy: Diagnosis and Management," *Journal of Clinical and Aesthetic Dermatology* 1, no. 4 (November 2008): 38–44.

7. "Propylene Glycol," EWG's Skin Deep Cosmetics Database, accessed February 21, 2016, http://www.ewg.org/skindeep/ingredient/705315/PROPYLENE_GLYCOL/.

8. Ibid.

9. H. Lessmann, W. Uter, A. Schnuch, et al., "Skin Sensitizing Properties of the Ethanolamines Mono-, Di-, and Triethanolamine. Data Analysis of a Multicentre Surveillance Network (IVDK) and Review of the Literature," *Contact Dermatitis* 60, no. 5 (May 2009): 243–55, doi:10.1111/j.1600 -0536.2009.01506.x.

10. "Ingredients, IFRA Survey: Transparency List," International Fragrance Association, accessed February 21, 2016, http://www.ifraorg.org/public/index_ps/parentid/1/childid/15/leafid/111.

11. Environmental Working Group and Campaign for Safe Cosmetics, "Not So Sexy: Hidden Chemicals in Perfume and Cologne," May 12, 2010, http://www.safecosmetics.org/article.php?id=644.

12. Dr. Daniel Zagst, "The Vagus Nerve: Your Friend in Weight Loss and a Better Mood," Natural News, December 27, 2012, http://www.naturalnews.com/038473_Vagus_nerve_weight_loss_moods.html.

13. California Environmental Protection Agency, Department of Toxic Substances Control, "Summary of Data and Findings from Testing a Limited Number of Nail Products," April 2012, http://www.dtsc.ca.gov/PollutionPrevention/upload/NailSalon_Final.pdf.

Shift 10: Understand the Sleep-Beauty-Wellness Connection

1. Max Hirshkowitz, PhD; Kaitlyn Whiton; Steven M. Albert,et al.,"National Sleep Foundation's Sleep Time Duration Recommendations Methodology and Results Summary," *Sleep Health* 1, no. 1 (March 2015); 40–43, https://sleepfoundation.org/how-sleep-works/how-much-sleep-do-we-really-need/page/0/1.

2. "Unhealthy Sleep-Related Behaviors—12 States, 2009," Centers for Disease Control and Prevention, *Morbidity and Mortality Weekly Report* 60, no. 8 (March 4, 2011): 1, http://www.cdc.gov/mmwr/PDF/wk/mm6008.pdf.

3. Shawn D. Youngstedt and Daniel F. Kripke, "Long Sleep and Mortality: Rationale for Sleep Restriction," *Sleep Medicine Reviews* 8, no. 3 (June 2004): 159–74.

4. Cheri D. Mah, MS; Kenneth E. Mah, MD, MS; Eric J. Kezirian, MD, MPH; et al., "The Effects of Sleep Extension on the Athletic Performance," *Sleep* 34, no. 7 (July 2011): 943–50, http://dx.doi.org/10.5665/sleep.1132.

5. "Healthy Sleep: Why Do We Sleep Anyway?" Division of Sleep Medicine, Harvard Medical School, last reviewed December 18, 2007, http://healthysleep.med.harvard.edu/healthy/matters/benefits-of-sleep/why-do-we-sleep.

6. P. Oyetakin-White, A. Suggs, B. Koo, et al., "Does Poor Sleep Quality Affect Skin Ageing?" *Clinical and Experimental Dermatology* 40, no. 1 (January 2015): 17–22, doi:10.1111/ced.12455.

7. "Sleep Deprivation Linked to Aging Skin, Study Suggests," *Science Daily*, July 23, 2013, http://www.sciencedaily.com/releases/2013/07/130723155002.htm.

8. Ibid.

9. Ibid.

10. Ibid.

11. "Study Reveals the Face of Sleep Deprivation," *Science Daily*, August 30, 2013, http://www.sciencedaily.com/releases/2013/08/130830161323.htm.

12. S. R. Patel and F. B. Hu, "Short Sleep Duration and Weight Gain: A Systematic Review," *Obesity* 16, no. 3 (March 2008): 643–53.

13. "Sleep Deprivation Linked to Aging Skin, Study Suggests."

14. Patricia Prinze, "Sleep, Appetite, and Obesity—What Is the Link?" *PLoS Medicine* 1, no. 3 (December 2004): e61, http://www.ncbi.nlm.nih.gov/pmc/articles/PMC535424/.

15. S. R. Patel, A. Malhotra, D. P. White, et al., "Association Between Reduced Sleep and Weight Gain in Women," *American Journal of Epidemiology* 164, no. 10 (November 2006): 947–54.

16. "The Nutrition Source: Sleep Deprivation and Obesity," Harvard T. H. Chan School of Public Health, accessed February 21, 2016, http://www.hsph.harvard.edu/nutritionsource/sleep/.

17. Ibid.

18. S. Taheri, L. Lin, D. Austin, et al., "Short Sleep Duration Is Associated with Reduced Leptin, Elevated Ghrelin, and Increased Body Mass Index," *PLoS Medicine* 1, no. 3 (December 2004): e62, doi:10.1371/journal.pmed.0010062.

19. Stephanie M. Greer, Andrea N. Goldstein, and Matthew P. Walker, "The Impact of Sleep Deprivation on Food Desire in the Human Brain," *Nature Communications* 4 (August 6, 2013), http://www.nature.com/ncomms/2013/130806/ncomms3259/full/ncomms3259.html.

20. J. F. Bell and F. J. Zimmerman, "Shortened Nighttime Sleep Duration in Early Life and Subsequent Childhood Obesity," *Archives of Pediatrics and Adolescent Medicine* 164, no. 9 (September 2010): 840–45, doi:10.1001/archpediatrics.2010.143.

21. Ibid.

22. "Health and Aging: Can We Prevent Aging?" National Institute on Aging, last updated October 23, 2015, https://www.nia.nih.gov/health/publication/can-we-prevent-aging.

23. E. Barrett-Connor, T.-T. Dam, K. Stone, et al., "The Association of Testosterone Levels with Overall Sleep Quality, Sleep Architecture, and Sleep-Disordered Breathing," *Journal of Clinical Endocrinology and Metabolism* 93, no. 7 (July 2008): 2602–9, doi:10.1210/jc.2007-2622.

24. R. Leproult and F. Van Cauter, "Effect of 1 Week of Sleep Restriction on Testosterone Levels in Young Healthy Men," *Journal of the American Medical Association* 305, no. 21 (June 2011): 2173–74, doi:10.1001/jama.2011.710.

25. A. W. Evers, E. W. Verhoeven, F. W. Kraaimaat, et al., "How Stress Gets Under the Skin: Cortisol and Stress Reactivity in Psoriasis," *British Journal of Dermatology* 163, no. 5 (November 2010): 986–91, doi:10.1111/j.1365-2133.2010.09984.x.

26. Alex Groberman, "Cortisol Levels and Weight Gain," PsyWeb.com, May 4, 2012, http://www.psyweb.com/articles/mental-health/cortisol-levels-and-weight-gain.

27. Camille Peri, "10 Things to Hate About Sleep Loss," WebMD, February 13, 2014, http://www.webmd.com/sleep-disorders/excessive-sleepiness-10/10-results-sleep-loss.

28. L. Besedovsky, T. Lange, and J. Born, "Sleep and Immune Function," *Pflugers Archive* 463, no. 1 (January 2012): 121–37, doi:10.1007/s00424-011-1044-0.

29. Penelope A. Bryant, John Trinder, and Nigel Curtis, "Sick and Tired: Does Sleep Have a Vital Role in the Immune System?" *Nature Reviews Immunology* 4, no. 6 (June 2004): 457–67, doi:10.1038/nri1369.

30. Besedovsky, Lange, and Born, "Sleep and Immune Function."

31. Glen Gordon, MD, "Beating Free Radicals: The Basis for Injury, Illness and Death," Natural News, May 22, 2008, http://www.naturalnews.com/023285_free_radicals_injury_antioxidant.html.

32. Lulu Xie, Hongyi Kang, Qiwu Xu, et al., "Sleep Drives Metabolite Clearance from the Adult Brain," *Science* 342, no. 6156 (October 18, 2013): 373–77, doi:10.1126/science.1241224.

33. D. Dinges, F. Pack, K. Williams, et al., "Cumulative Sleepiness, Mood Disturbance, and Psycho-motor Vigilance Decrements During a Week of Sleep Restricted to 4–5 Hours Per Night," *Sleep* 20, no. 4 (April 1997): 267–77.

34. "Sleep Deprivation and Memory Loss," WebMD, accessed February 21, 2016, http://www.webmd.com/sleep-disorders/sleep-deprivation-effects-on-memory.

35. D. Neckelmann, A. Mykletun, and A. A. Dahl, "Chronic Insomnia as a Risk Factor for Developing Anxiety and Depression," *Sleep* 30, no. 7 (July 2007): 873–80.

36. M. M. Weissman, S. Greenwald, G. Nuño-Murcia, et al., "The Morbidity of Insomnia Uncompli-cated by Psychiatric Disorders," *General Hospital Psychiatry* 19, no. 4 (July1997): 245–50.

37. June C. Lo, Kep Kee Loh, Hui Zheng, et al., "Sleep Duration and Age-Related Changes in Brain Structure and Cognitive Performance," *Sleep* 37, no. 7 (2014): 1171–78, doi:10.5665/sleep.3832.

38. J. Zhang, Y. Zhu, G. Zhan, et al., "Extended Wakefulness: Compromised Metabolics in and Degenera-tion of Locus Ceruleus Neurons," *Journal of Neuroscience* 34, no. 12 (March 2014): 4418–31.

39. "Penn Medicine Researchers Show How Lost Sleep Leads to Lost Neurons: First Report in Pre-clinical Study Showing Extended Wakefulness Can Result in Neuronal Injury," Penn Medicine, March 18, 2014, http://www.uphs.upenn.edu/news/News_Releases/2014/03/veasey.

40. Ibid.

41. A. Di Meco, Y. B. Joshi, and D. Practicò, "Sleep Deprivation Impairs Memory, Tau Metabolism, and Synaptic Integrity of a Mouse Model of Alzheimer's Disease with Plaques and Tangles," *Neu-robiology of Aging* 35, no. 8 (August 2014): 1813–20.

Shift 11: Tune In to Your Body's Natural Rhythms

1. "Circadian Rhythms Fact Sheet," National Institute of General Medical Sciences, last reviewed October 1, 2015, http://www.nigms.nih.gov/Education/Pages/Factsheet_CircadianRhythms.aspx.

2. Tina L. Huang and Christine Charyton, "A Comprehensive Review of the Psychological Effects of Brainwave Entrainment," *Alternative Therapies in Health and Medicine* 14, no. 5 (September–October 2008): 38–50.

3. Paul Israel, *Edison: A Life of Invention* (New York: John Wiley and Sons, 2000).

4. "Brain's SCN Is the Master Clock That Synchronizes Other Biological Clocks in the Body," News-Medical, September 10, 2009, http://www.news-medical.net/news/20090910/Brains-SCN-is-the-master-clock-that-synchronizes-other-biological-clocks-in-the-body.aspx.

5. M. Gradisar, A. R. Wolfson, A. G. Harvey, L. Hale, R. Rosenberg, and C. A. Czeisler, "The Sleep and Technology Use of Americans: Findings from the National Sleep Foundation's 2011 Sleep in America Poll," *Journal of Clinical Sleep Medicine* 9, no. 12 (2013): 1291–99 http://doi.org/10.5664/jcsm.3272.

6. H. Noguchi and T. Sakaguchi, "Effect of Illuminance and Color Temperature on Lowering of Physiological Activity," *Applied Human Science* 18, no. 4 (July 1999): 117–23.

7. J. Bellingham, S. S. Chaurasia, Z. Melyan, et al., "Evolution of Melanopsin Photoreceptors: Discov-ery and Characterization of a New Melanopsin in Nonmammalian Vertebrates," *PLoS Biology* 4, no. 8 (July 2006): e254, doi:10.1371/journal.pbio.0040254.

8. "Untangling the Biological Effects of Blue Light," *Science Daily,* October 20, 2014, https://www.sciencedaily.com/releases/2014/10/141020212752.htm.

9. M. Spitschan, S. Jain, D. H. Brainard, et al., "Opponent Melanopsin and S-cone Signals in the Human Pupillary Light Response," *Proceedings of the National Academy of Sciences* 111, no. 43 (2014): 15568–72, doi:10.1073/pnas.1400942111.

10. Daniel A. Cohen, Wei Wang, James K. Wyatt, et al., "Uncovering Residual Effects of Chronic Sleep Loss on Human Performance," *Science Translational Medicine* 2, no. 14 (January 13, 2010): 14ra3, doi:10.1126/scitranslmed.3000458.

11. National Sleep Foundation, *2011 Sleep in America Poll: Communications Technology in the Bedroom; Summary of Findings* (Crofton, MD: WBA Market Research, 2011), http://sleepfoundation.org/sites/default/files/sleepinamericapoll/SIAP_2011_Summary_of_Findings.pdf.

12. Ibid.

13. Jeanne F. Duffy and Charles A. Czeisler, "Effect of Light on Human Circadian Physiology," *Sleep Medicine Clinics* 4, no. 2 (June 2009): 165–77.

14. "Annual Sleep in America Poll Exploring Connections with Communications Technology Use and Sleep," National Sleep Foundation, March 7, 2011, http://sleepfoundation.org/media-center/press-release/annual-sleep-america-poll-exploring-connections-communications-technology-use-.

15. Anne-Marie Chang, Daniel Aeschbach, Jeanne F. Duffy, et al., "Evening Use of Light-Emitting eReaders Negatively Affects Sleep, Circadian Timing, and Next-Morning Alertness," *Proceedings of the National Academy of Sciences* 112, no. 4 (January 27, 2015): 1232–37, www.pnas.org/cgi/doi/10.1073/pnas.1418490112.

16. J. Dyche, A. M. Anch, K. A. Fogler, et al., "Effects of Power Frequency Electromagnetic Fields on Melatonin and Sleep in the Rat," *Emerging Health Threats Journal* 5 (2012), doi:10.3402/ehtj.v5i0.10904.

Shift 12: Establish Healthy Sleep Routines
1. Kathryn J. Reid, Kelly Glazer Baron, Brandon Lu, et al., "Aerobic Exercise Improves Self-Reported Sleep and Quality of Life in Older Adults with Insomnia," *Sleep Medicine* 11, no. 9 (October 2010): 934–40.

2. Ibid.

3. P. Oyetakin-White, A. Suggs, B. Koo, et al., "Does Poor Sleep Quality Affect Skin Ageing?" *Clinical and Experimental Dermatology* 40, no. 1 (January 2015): 17–22, doi:10.1111/ced.12455.

4. L. C. Lack, M. Gradisar, E. J. Van Someren, et al., "The Relationship Between Insomnia and Body Temperatures," *Sleep Medicine Reviews* 12, no. 4 (August 2008): 307–17, doi:10.1016/j.smrv.2008.02.003.

5. "Touch: A Great Night's Sleep Can Depend on the Comfort You Feel in Your Bedroom Environment," National Sleep Foundation, accessed February 21, 2016, http://sleepfoundation.org/bedroom/touch.php.

6. Joshua J. Gooley, Kyle Chamberlain, Kurt A. Smith, et al., "Exposure to Room Light Before Bedtime Suppresses Melatonin Onset and Shortens Melatonin Duration in Humans," *Journal of Clinical Endocrinology and Metabolism* 96, no. 3 (March 2011): E463–E472, doi:10.1210/jc.2010–2098.

7. Stephanie Watson, "The Best Mattress for a Better Night's Sleep: Buying a New Mattress? Here Are Some Tips for Finding the Right Mattress for You," WebMD, last reviewed March 3, 2014, http://www.webmd.com/sleep-disorders/excessive-sleepiness-10/best-mattress-good-nights-sleep.

8. Ibid.

9. "Choosing the Best Mattress: Simple Guide for Mattress Shopping," Better Sleep Council, accessed February 21, 2016, http://www.bettersleep.org/mattresses-and-more/choosing-the-best-mattress/.

10. "Dog Tired? It Could Be Your Pooch," *Science Daily,* February 15, 2002, https://www.sciencedaily.com/releases/2002/02/020215070932.htm.

11. Wilfred R. Pigeon, Michelle Carr, Colin Gorman, et al., "Effects of a Tart Cherry Juice Beverage on the Sleep of Older Adults with Insomnia: A Pilot Study," *Journal of Medicinal Food* 13, no. 3 (June 2010): 579–83, doi:10.1089/jmf.2009.0096.

12. S. J. Edwards, I. M. Montgomery, E. Q. Colquhoun, et al., "Spicy Meal Disturbs Sleep: An Effect of Thermoregulation?" *International Journal of Psychophysiology* 13, no. 2 (September 1992): 97–100.

13. Ibid.

14. C. Drake, T. Roehrs, J. Shambroom, et al., "Caffeine Effects on Sleep Taken 0, 3, or 6 Hours Before Going to Bed," *Journal of Clinical Sleep Medicine* 9, no. 11 (2013): 1195–1200.

15. "Alcohol Interferes with the Restorative Functions of Sleep," *Science Daily,* August 16, 2011, https://www.sciencedaily.com/releases/2011/08/110815162220.htm.

Shift 13: Harness the Beauty of the Seasons

1. "Health Benefits of Sea Salt," Organic Facts, accessed February 22, 2016, https://www.organicfacts.net/health-benefits/other/health-benefits-of-sea-salt.html.

Shift 14: Balance Solar and Lunar Energy and All the Earth's Elements

1. Robyn M. Lucas, Anthony J. McMichael, Bruce K. Armstrong, et al., "Estimating the Global Disease Burden Due to Ultraviolet Radiation Exposure," *International Journal of Epidemiology* 37, no. 3 (July 2008): 654–67, doi:10.1093/ije/dyn017.

2. "Melatonin—Overview," WebMD, Sleep Disorders Health Center, accessed February 22, 2016, http://www.webmd.com/sleep-disorders/tc/melatonin-overview.

3. Ibid.

4. Dr. Michael Holick, *The Vitamin D Solution: A 3-Step Strategy to Cure Our Most Common Health Problems* (New York: Hudson Street Press, 2010).

5. S. Pilz, S. Frisch, H. Koertke, et al., "Effect of Vitamin D Supplementation on Testosterone Levels in Men," *Hormone and Metabolic Research* 43, no. 3 (March 2011): 223–25.

6. J. A. Knight, J. Wong, K. M. Blackmore, et al., "Vitamin D Association with Estradiol and Progesterone in Young Women," *Cancer Causes and Control* 21, no. 3 (March 2010): 479–83.

7. Sian Geldenhuys, Prue H. Hart, Raelene Endersby, et al., "Ultraviolet Radiation Suppresses Obesity and Symptoms of Metabolic Syndrome Independently of Vitamin D in Mice Fed a High-Fat Diet." *Diabetes* 63, no. 11 (November 2014): 3759–69, doi:10.2337/db13-1675.

8. Donald Liu, Bernadette O. Fernandez, Alistair Hamilton, et al., "UVA Irradiation of Human Skin Vasodilates Arterial Vasculature and Lowers Blood Pressure Independently of Nitric Oxide Synthase," *Journal of Investigative Dermatology* 134, no. 7 (2014): 1839–46, doi:10.1038/jid .2014.27.

9. L. Yang, M. Lof, M. B. Veierød, et al., "Ultraviolet Exposure and Mortality Among Women in Sweden," *Cancer Epidemiology Biomarkers and Prevention* 20, no. 4 (April 2011): 683–90.

10. P. Brøndum-Jacobsen, B. G. Nordestgaard, S. F. Nielsen, et al., "Skin Cancer as a Marker of Sun Exposure Associates with Myocardial Infarction, Hip Fracture and Death from Any Cause," *International Journal of Epidemiology* (2013): 1–11, doi:10.1093/ije/dyt168.

11. Liu, Fernandez, Hamilton, et al., "UVA Irradiation of Human Skin . . ."

12. W. B. Grant, "An Estimate of Premature Cancer Mortality in the U.S. Due to Inadequate Doses of Solar Ultraviolet-B Radiation," *Cancer* 94, no. 6 (March 2002): 1867–75, doi:10.1002/cncr.10427.

13. H. J. van der Rhee, E. de Vries, and J. W. Coebergh, "Does Sunlight Prevent Cancer? A Systematic Review," *European Journal of Cancer* 42, no. 14 (September 2006): 2222–32.

14. Hekla Sigmundsdottir, Junliang Pan, Gudrun F. Debes, et al., "DCs Metabolize Sunlight-Induced Vitamin D3 to 'Program' T Cell Attraction to the Epidermal Chemokine CCL27," *Nature Immunology* 8, no. 3 (March 2007): 285–93, doi:10.1038/ni1433.

15. Salynn Boyles, "Early Research Suggests That Sunlight in Small Doses May Protect Skin from Damage," WebMD, January 29, 2007, http://www.webmd.com/beauty/sun/20070130/could -some-sun-be-good-your-skin.

16. Ibid.

17. Stephanie Watson, "Skin Care Vitamins and Antioxidants," WebMD, last reviewed April 24, 2012, http://www.webmd.com/vitamins-and-supplements/lifestyle-guide-11/beauty-skin-care-vitamins -antioxidants?page=1.

18. C. Xu, J. Zhang, D. M. Mihai, et al., "Light-Harvesting Chlorophyll Pigments Enable Mammalian Mitochondria to Capture Photonic Energy and Produce ATP," *Journal of Cell Science* 127, pt. 2 (January 2014): 388–99, doi:10.1242/jcs.134262.

19. Ibid.

20. Sayer Ji, "Amazing Discovery: Plant Blood Enables Your Cells to Capture Sunlight Energy," GreenMedInfo.com, May 12, 2015, http://www.greenmedinfo.com/blog/chlorophyll-enables- your-cells-captureuse-sunlight-energy-copernican-revolution.

21. Defeng Wu, PhD, and Arthur I. Cederbaum, PhD, "Alcohol, Oxidative Stress, and Free Radical Damage," National Institute on Alcohol Abuse and Alcoholism, October 2004, http://pubs.niaaa .nih.gov/publications/arh27-4/277-284.htm.

22. Paul Kristiansen and Charles Mansfield, "Overview of Organic Agriculture," in *Organic Agriculture: A Global Perspective*, eds. Paul Kristiansen, Acram Taji, and John Reganold (Collingwood, Australia: CSIRO Publishing, 2006), 1–24.

23. "The Planting Calendar Rhythms," Bio-Dynamic Association of India (BDAI), accessed February 22, 2016, http://biodynamics.in/Rhythm.htm.

24. M. Zimecki, "The Lunar Cycle: Effects on Human and Animal Behavior and Physiology," *Postepy Higieny i Medycyny Doswiadczalnej* 60 (January 2007): 1–7.

Shift 15: Get Closer to Nature Indoors and Out

1. G. Chevalier, "Grounding the Human Body Improves Facial Blood Flow Regulation: Results of a Randomized, Placebo Controlled Pilot Study," *Journal of Cosmetics, Dermatological Sciences and Applications* 4 (2014): 293–308, doi:10.4236/jcdsa.2014.45039.

2. David Holiday, Robert Resnick, and Jearl Walker, *Fundamentals of Physics*, 4th ed. (New York: Wiley, 1993).

3. James L. Oschman, "Can Electrons Act as Antioxidants? A Review and Commentary," *Journal of Alternative and Complementary Medicine* 13, no. 9 (2007): 955–67, doi:10.1089/acm.2007.7048.

4. P. Brondum-Jacobsen, B.G. Nordestgaard, S.F. Nielsen, et al. (2013), "Skin Cancer as a Marker of Sun Exposure Associates with Myocardial Infarction, Hip Fracture and Death from Any Cause," *International Journal of Epidemiology*.

5. G. Chevalier, S. T. Sinatra, J. L. Oschman, and R. M. Delany, "Earthing (Grounding) the Human Body Reduces Blood Viscosity—a Major Factor in Cardiovascular Disease," *Journal of Alternative and Complementary Medicine,* 19, no. 2 (2013): 102–10, doi:10.1089/acm.2011.0820.

6. Elissa S. Epel, Elizabeth H. Blackburn, Jue Lin, et al., "Accelerated Telomere Shortening in Response to Life Stress," *Proceedings of the National Academy of Sciences* 101, no. 49 (December 2004): 17312–15, doi:10.1073/pnas.0407162101.

7. R. Brown, G. Chevalier, and M. Hill, "Pilot Study on the Effect of Grounding on Delayed-Onset Muscle Soreness," *Journal of Alternative and Complementary Medicine* 16, no. 3 (2010): 265–73.

8. K. Sokal and P. Sokal, "Earthing the Human Body Influences Physiologic Processes," *Journal of Alternative and Complementary Medicine* 17, no. 4 (2011): 301–8.

9. "Questions About Your Community: Indoor Air," United States Environmental Protection Agency, http://www.epa.gov/region1/communities/indoorair.html.

10. "PBDES—Fire Retardants in Dust: Dust and Indoor Pollution," Environmental Working Group, May 12, 2004, http://www.ewg.org/research/pbdes-fire-retardants-dust/dust-and-indoor-pollution.

11. A. C. Steinemann, I. C. MacGregor, S. M. Gordon, et al., "Fragranced Consumer Products: Chemicals Emitted, Ingredients Unlisted," *Environmental Impact Assessment Review* 31, no. 3 (April 2010): 328–33, doi:10.1016/j.eiar.2010.08.002.

12. "PBDES—Fire Retardants in Dust . . ."

13. B. C. Wolverton, Anne Johnson, and Keith Bounds, *Indoor Landscape Plants for Indoor Air Pollution Abatement* (Stennis Space Center, MS: National Aeronautics and Space Administration, 1989), http://maison-orion.com/media/1837156-NASA-Indoor-Plants.pdf.

14. United States Environmental Protection Agency, "Dry Cleaning Emission Standards: Basic Information—About Perchloroethylene, or 'Perc,'" accessed February 22, 2016, http://www.epa.gov/drycleaningrule/basic.html.

15. US Environmental Protection Agency, *Integrated Risk Information System (IRIS) on Tetrachloro-ethylene* (Washington, DC: National Center for Environmental Assessment, Office of Research and Development, 2012).

16. L. Kheifets, A. Ahlbom, C. M. Crespi, et al., "Pooled Analysis of Recent Studies on Magnetic Fields and Childhood Leukaemia," *British Journal of Cancer* 103, no. 7 (September 28, 2010): 1128–35, doi:10.1038/sj.bjc.6605838.

17. International Agency for Research on Cancer / World Health Organization, "IARC Classifies Radiofrequency Electromagnetic Fields as Possibly Carcinogenic to Humans" (press release), May 31, 2011, http://www.iarc.fr/en/media-centre/pr/2011/pdfs/pr208_E.pdf.

18. *BioInitiative 2012: A Rationale for Biologically-Based Exposure Standards for Low-Intensity Electromagnetic Radiation* (2013), http://www.bioinitiative.org/table-of-contents/.

19. Richard Quan, MD; Christine Yang, MS; Steven Rubinstein, MD; et al., "Effects of Microwave Radiation on Anti-infective Factors in Human Milk," *Pediatrics* 89, no. 4 (1992): 667–69.

Pillar 5: Beautiful Movement

1. "Exercise and Immunity," Medline Plus, last updated May 11, 2014, http://www.nlm.nih.gov/medlineplus/ency/article/007165.htm.

Shift 16: Incorporate Fluid Movement Throughout Your Day

1. I. J. Kullo, M. Khaleghi, and D. D. Hensrud, "Markers of Inflammation Are Inversely Associated with VO2 Max in Asymptomatic Men," *Journal of Applied Physiology* 102, no. 4 (May 2007): 1374–79, doi:10.1152/japplphysiol.01028.2006.

2. "Exercise and Depression," WebMD, reviewed February 19, 2014, http://www.webmd.com/depression/guide/exercise-depression#1.

3. J. L. Etnier, P. M. Nowell, D. M. Landers, et al., "A Meta-regression to Examine the Relationship Between Aerobic Fitness and Cognitive Performance," *Brain Research Reviews* 52, no. 1 (August 2006): 119–30.

4. E. Puterman, J. Lin, E. Blackburn, et al., "The Power of Exercise: Buffering the Effect of Chronic Stress on Telomere Length," *PLoS One* 5, no. 5 (May 2010): e10837, doi:10.1371/journal.pone.0010837.

5. "2008 Physical Activity Guidelines for Americans: Summary," Health.gov, Office of Disease Prevention and Health Promotion, accessed February 22, 2016, http://health.gov/paguidelines/guidelines/summary.aspx.

6. Paul B. Laursen and David G. Jenkins, "The Scientific Basis for High-Intensity Interval Training," *Sports Medicine* 32, no. 1 (2002): 53–73, doi:10.2165/00007256-200232010-00003.

7. Patti Neighmond, "Sitting All Day: Worse for You Than You Might Think," NPR.org, updated April 25, 2011, http://www.npr.org/2011/04/25/135575490/sitting-all-day-worse-for-you-than-you-might-think.

8. Diana Gerstacker, "Sitting Is the New Smoking: Ways a Sedentary Lifestyle Is Killing You," Huffington Post Healthy Living, last updated November 26, 2014, http://www.huffingtonpost.com/the-active-times/sitting-is-the-new-smokin_b_5890006.html.

9. D. Schmid and M. Leitzmann, "Television Viewing and Time Spent Sedentary in Relation to Cancer Risk: A Meta-analysis," *Journal of the National Cancer Institute* 106, no. 7 (2013): 1–19.

10. E. G. Wilmot, C. L. Edwardson, F. A. Achana, et al., "Sedentary Time in Adults and the Association with Diabetes, Cardiovascular Disease and Death: Systematic Review and Meta-analysis,". *Diabetologia* 55, no. 11 (2012): 2895–905, doi:10.1007/s00125-012-2677-z.

11. "Depression and Anxiety: Exercise Eases Symptoms," Mayo Clinic, October 10, 2014, http://www.mayoclinic.org/diseases-conditions/depression/in-depth/depression-and-exercise/art-20046495?pg=1.

12. Jannique G. Z. van Uffelen, PhD; Yolanda R. van Gellecum; Nicola W. Burton, PhD, et al., "Sitting-Time, Physical Activity, and Depressive Symptoms in Mid-Aged Women," *American Journal of Preventive Medicine* 45, no. 3 (September 2013): 276–81, doi:10.1016/j.amepre.2013.04.009.

13. Nancy Klobassa Davidson and Peggy Moreland, "Diabetes: Is Sitting the New Smoking?" Mayo Clinic, February 1, 2013, http://www.mayoclinic.org/diseases-conditions/diabetes/expert-blog/sitting-and-health/BGP-20056537.

14. G. N. Healy, C. E. Matthews, D. W. Dunstan, et al., "Sedentary Time and Cardio-Metabolic Biomarkers in US Adults: NHANES 2003-06," *European Heart Journal* 32, no. 5 (March 2011): 590–97, doi:10.1093/eurheartj/ehq451.

15. D. W. Dunstan, B. A. Kingwell, R. Larsen, et al., "Breaking Up Prolonged Sitting Reduces Postprandial Glucose and Insulin Responses," *Diabetes Care* 35, no. 5 (May 2012): 976–83, doi:10.2337/dc11-1931.

16. L. Bey and M. T. Hamilton, "Suppression of Skeletal Muscle Lipoprotein Lipase Activity During Physical Inactivity: A Molecular Reason to Maintain Daily Low-Intensity Activity," *Journal of Physiology* 551 (2003): 673–82, doi:10.1113/jphysiol.2003.045591.

17. V. Lobo, A. Patil, A. Phatak, et al., "Free Radicals, Antioxidants and Functional Foods: Impact on Human Health," *Pharmacognosy Reviews* 4, no. 8 (2010): 118–26, doi:10.4103/0973-7847.70902.

18. D. J. Betteridge, "What Is Oxidative Stress?" *Metabolism* 49, no. 2, suppl. 1 (February 2000): 3–8.

19. U. Singh and I. Jialal, "Oxidative Stress and Atherosclerosis," *Pathophysiology* 13, no. 3 (August 2006): 129–42.

20. S. Reuter, S. C. Gupta, M. M. Chaturvedi, et al., "Oxidative Stress, Inflammation, and Cancer: How Are They Linked?" *Free Radical Biology and Medicine* 49, no. 11 (December 2010): 1603–16, doi:10.1016/j.freeradbiomed.2010.09.006.

21. D. Harman, "The Free Radical Theory of Aging," *Antioxidants and Redox Signaling* 5, no. 5 (October 2003): 557–61.

22. Mary F. Bennett, Michael K. Robinson, Elma D. Baron, et al., "Skin Immune Systems and Inflammation: Protector of the Skin or Promoter of Aging?" *Journal of Investigative Dermatology Symposium Proceedings* 13 (2008): 15–19, doi:10.1038/jidsymp.2008.3.

23. Ralph M. Trüeb, "Oxidative Stress in Ageing of Hair," *International Journal of Trichology* 1, no. 1 (2009): 6–14, doi:10.4103/0974-7753.51923.

24. R. J. Bloomer, "Effect of Exercise on Oxidative Stress Biomarkers," *Advances in Clinical Chemistry* 46 (2008): 1–50.

25. K. Fisher-Wellman and R. J. Bloomer, "Acute Exercise and Oxidative Stress: A 30 Year History," *Dynamic Medicine* 8 (2009): 1, doi:10.1186/1476-5918-8-1.

26. W. L. Knez, D. G. Jenkins, and J. S. Coombes, "Oxidative Stress in Half and Full Ironman Triathletes," *Medicine and Science in Sports and Exercise* 39, no. 2 (February 2007): 283–88.

27. Z. Radak, H. Y. Chung, E. Koltai, et al., "Exercise, Oxidative Stress and Hormesis," *Ageing Research Reviews* 7, no. 1 (January 2008): 34–42.

28. J. H. O'Keefe, H. R. Patil, C. J. Lavie, et al., "Potential Adverse Cardiovascular Effects from Excessive Endurance Exercise," *Mayo Clinic Proceedings* 87, no. 6 (June 2012): 587–95, doi:10.1016/j .mayocp.2012.04.005.

29. "Run for Your Life! At a Comfortable Pace, and Not Too Far: James O'Keefe at TEDxUMKC," TEDx Talks YouTube video, 7:51, November 27, 2012, accessed December 13, 2012, http://goo.gl /D521F.

30. J. Finaud, G. Lac, and E. Filaire, "Oxidative Stress: Relationship with Exercise and Training," *Sports Medicine* 36, no. 4 (2006): 327–58.

31. Margaret E. Sears, Kathleen J. Kerr, and Riina I. Bray, "Arsenic, Cadmium, Lead, and Mercury in Sweat: A Systematic Review," *Journal of Environmental and Public Health* 2012, article ID 184745 (2012): 1–10, doi:10.1155/2012/184745.

32. Eman M. Alissa and Gordon A. Ferns, "Heavy Metal Poisoning and Cardiovascular Disease," *Journal of Toxicology* 2011, article ID 870125 (2011): 1–21, doi:10.1155/2011/870125.

33. Emma E. A. Cohen, Robin Ejsmond-Frey, Nicola Knight, et al., "Rowers' High: Behavioural Synchrony Is Correlated with Elevated Pain Thresholds," *Biology Letters* 6, no. 1 (2009): 106–8, doi: 10.1098/rsbl.2009.0670.

34. D. D. Cosca and F. Navazio, "Common Problems in Endurance Athletes," *American Family Physician* 76, no. 2 (July 15, 2007): 237–44.

35. K. De Bock, W. Derave, B. O. Eijnde, et al., "Effect of Training in the Fasted State on Metabolic Responses During Exercise with Carbohydrate Intake," *Journal of Applied Physiology* 104, no. 4 (April 2008): 1045–55, doi:10.1152/japplphysiol.01195.2007.

36. K. D. Tipton, B. B. Rasmussen, S. L. Miller, et al., "Timing of Amino Acid–Carbohydrate Ingestion Alters Anabolic Response of Muscle to Resistance Exercise," *American Journal of Physiology–Endocrinology and Metabolism* 281, no. 2 (August 2001): E197–206.

37. S. M. Phillips and L. J. Van Loon, "Dietary Protein for Athletes: From Requirements to Optimum Adaptation," *Journal of Sports Sciences* 29, suppl. 1 (2011): S29–38, doi:10.1080 /02640414.2011.619204.

38. Blake B. Rasmussen, Kevin D. Tipton, Sharon L. Miller, et al., "An Oral Essential Amino Acid–Carbohydrate Supplement Enhances Muscle Protein Anabolism after Resistance Exercise," *Journal of Applied Physiology* 88, no. 2 (February 2000): 386–92.

39. Ikuma Murakami, Takayuki Sakuragi, Hiroshi Uemura, et al., "Significant Effect of a Pre-exercise High-Fat Meal After a 3-Day High-Carbohydrate Diet on Endurance Performance," *Nutrients* 4, no. 7 (2012): 625–37.

40. Y. Yang, L. Breen, N. A. Burd, et al., "Resistance Exercise Enhances Myofibrillar Protein Synthesis with Graded Intakes of Whey Protein in Older Men," *British Journal of Nutrition* 108, no. 10 (November 2012): 1780–88, doi:10.1017/S0007114511007422.

Shift 17: Practice Breathing and Yoga Exercises for Beauty
1. B. K. S. Iyengar, *Light on Yoga,* rev. ed. (New York: Schocken, 1977).

Index

About the Authors

DEEPAK CHOPRA, M.D., founder of the Chopra Foundation and cofounder of the Chopra Center for Well-Being, is a world-renowned pioneer in integrative medicine and personal transformation. He is the author of a great many books, translated into over 43 languages, including numerous *New York Times* bestsellers. *Time* magazine has described Dr. Chopra as "one of the top 100 heroes and icons of the century". The *WorldPost* and *Huffington Post* global Internet survey ranked Dr. Chopra #10 of the most influential thinkers in the world and "#1 in medicine." Visit him at DeepakChopra.com.

KIMBERLY SNYDER, C.N., is a nutritionist and the *New York Times* bestselling author of the Beauty Detox book series. Snyder has appeared as a nutrition and beauty expert on *Dr. Oz, Ellen*, and *Today*, and has been featured in the *New York Times*, the *Wall Street Journal, Vogue, Elle*, and *InStyle*. She is also the creator of Glow Bio, an organic juice and smoothie company, and she hosts the popular podcast Beauty Inside Out. For her wellness products and more great health and beauty information, visit KimberlySnyder.com.